GASTROINTESTINAL HEMORRHAGE

GRUNE & STRATTON RAPID MANUSCRIPT REPRODUCTION

GASTROINTESTINAL HEMORRHAGE

Edited by

Richard G. Fiddian-Green, M.A., M.D., F.R.C.S.
*Associate Professor of Surgery
Director of Gastrointestinal Endocrine Laboratory
University of Michigan Medical Center
Ann Arbor, Michigan*

Jeremiah G. Turcotte, M.D.
*Professor of Surgery
Chairman, Department of Surgery
University of Michigan Medical Center
Ann Arbor, Michigan*

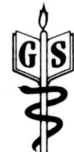

Grune & Stratton
A Subsidiary of Harcourt Brace Jovanovich, Publishers
New York   London   Toronto   Sydney   San Francisco

Library of Congress Cataloging in Publication Data

Symposium on Gastrointestinal Hemorrhage,
   University of Michigan, 1980.
      Gastrointestinal hemorrhage.

   Includes bibliographies and index.
   1. Gastrointestinal hemorrhage—Congresses.
I. Fiddian-Green, Richard G.   II. Turcotte,
Jeremiah G.   III. Title.
RC803.S95   1980   616.3   80-11318
ISBN 0-8089-1267-4

© 1980 by Grune & Stratton, Inc.
All rights reserved. No part of this publication
may be reproduced or transmitted in any form or
by any means, electronic or mechanical, including
photocopy, recording, or any information storage
and retrieval system, without permission in
writing from the publisher.

Grune & Stratton, Inc.
111 Fifth Avenue
New York, New York 10003

Distributed in the United Kingdom by
Academic Press, Inc. (London) Ltd.
24/28 Oval Road, London, NW 1

Library of Congress Catalog Number 80-11318
International Standard Book Number 0-8089-1267-4

Printed in the United States of America

Compiled from the manuscripts of papers presented at a multidisciplinary symposium on Gastrointestinal Hemorrhage held at the University of Michigan under the auspices of the Departments of General Surgery and Postgraduate Medicine and Health Professions Education.

PROGRAM COMMITTEE

    Richard G. Fiddian-Green, M.A., M.D., F.R.C.S., Chairman
        Jeremiah G. Turcotte, M.D.
        James C. Stanley, M.D.
        Gerald B. Zelenock, M.D.
        Frederic E. Eckhauser, M.D.

Contents

Preface JEREMIAH G. TURCOTTE	xi
Contributors	xiii

Evaluation of the Bleeding Patient

Clinical Evaluation of the Bleeding Adult TERENCE KENNEDY	3
Gastrointestinal Bleeding in Infants and Children ARNOLD G. CORAN	13
Evaluation of Chronic Gastrointestinal Blood Loss JEAN-PIERRE RAUFMANN AND WILLIAM O. DOBBINS, III	23
Diagnostic Endoscopy THOMAS L. DENT	39
Diagnostic Angiography in Gastrointestinal Hemorrhage KYUNG J. CHO AND DOUGLASS F. ADAMS	51

Peptic Ulcer Disease

The Natural History of Bleeding Peptic Ulcers TIMOTHY T. NOSTRANT AND JEAN-PIERRE RAUFMANN	81
Pathophysiological Considerations in the Management of Patients With Bleeding Ulcers AARON S. FINK AND RICHARD G. FIDDIAN-GREEN	95
Medical Treatment of Bleeding Ulcers GEORGE WILLEFORD AND CHARLES T. RICHARDSON	113
Surgery for Massive Upper Gastrointestinal Hemorrhage PHILIP E. DONAHUE AND LLOYD M. NYHUS	129
Rebleeding After Surgery for Bleeding Ulcers TERENCE KENNEDY	147
Pathophysiology of Erosive Gastritis and Stress Ulceration W. P. RITCHIE, JR.	155
Prevention and Treatment of Acute Gastric Erosions and Stress Ulcerations CHARLES E. LUCAS	167
Therapeutic Endoscopy: Photocoagulation and Electrocoagulation ROBERT L. PROTELL AND FRED E. SILVERSTEIN	189
Therapeutic Angiography in Gastrointestinal Hemorrhage KYUNG J. CHO AND DOUGLASS F. ADAMS	203

Variceal Bleeding

Prognosis in the Cirrhotic With Gastrointestinal Hemorrhage THOMAS C. CHALMERS AND HENRY SACKS	233
Hemodynamics in Portal Hypertension FREDERIC E. ECKHAUSER, WILLIAM E. STRODEL, AND JEREMIAH G. TURCOTTE	235

Gastrointestinal Hemorrhage, Portacaval Shunts,
and Hepatic Reserve ... 253
    KEITH S. HENLEY, H. CLIFFORD LANE,
    AND TIMOTHY T. NOSTRANT

Vasopressin in the Management of Variceal Hemorrhage ... 261
    MILTON G. MUTCHNICK

Control of Gastroesophageal Variceal Bleeding With
Balloon Tamponade ... 275
    STEPHEN R. RAMSBURGH AND JEREMIAH G. TURCOTTE

Esophageal Variceal Injection Using the Fiberoptic Endoscope ... 291
    JOHN G. ALLISON, JEFFREY W. LEWIS,
    AND RALPH S. CHUNG

Emergency Portacaval Shunt for Bleeding Esophageal Varices ... 295
    MARSHALL J. ORLOFF AND RICHARD H. BELL, JR.

Elective Portosystemic Shunts ... 311
    JEREMIAH G. TURCOTTE AND FREDERIC E. ECKHAUSER

Miscellaneous Causes of Gastrointestinal Bleeding

Gastrointestinal Hemorrhage in the Immunosuppressed Patient ... 329
    DUANE T. FREIER

Hemobilia ... 339
    S. MARTIN LINDENAUER

Splanchnic Artery Aneurysms and Gastrointestinal Hemorrhage ... 345
    JAMES C. STANLEY, WALTER M. WHITEHOUSE, JR.,
    AND LINDA M. GRAHAM

Morphologic Features of Right Colonic Vascular Ectasias
in Elderly Patients ... 359
    HENRY D. APPELMAN

Vascular Ectasias and Colonic Diverticula:
Common Causes of Lower Gastrointestinal
Hemorrhage in the Aged ... 375
    NORMAN W. THOMPSON

Intestinal Ischemia: A Paradoxical Cause of
 Gastrointestinal Hemorrhage   389
>GERALD B. ZELENOCK AND ERROL E. ERLANDSON

Drug-related and Hematological Disorders Associated
 With Gastrointestinal Bleeding   407
>WILLIAM W. COON

Index   419

Preface

The University of Michigan Section of General Surgery in conjunction with our Department of Postgraduate Medicine has sponsored a continuing education course in surgery for many years. Our goal has been to review and update a subject of current interest to practicing surgeons. We have selected subjects in which there is interest and expertise within our department, and then have supplemented our own faculty with distinguished scientists from throughout the world. An improved understanding of the etiology and pathogenesis of disease as well as a concise summary of new developments in diagnosis and treatment have been emphasized. Vascular surgery, surgical oncology, and socioeconomic problems confronting surgeons have been the subjects of courses in recent years.

This year the usual format of this program has been altered to appeal to a wider audience. A multidisciplinary "Symposium on Gastrointestinal Hemorrhage" has been organized. The faculty is composed of gastroenterologists, radiologists, and pathologists, as well as surgeons from the United States and England. Each faculty member has contributed a chapter to this text. The book will be distributed at the time of the course and be available for purchase later through outlets of our publisher, Grune & Stratton. We have attempted to provide a most current and authoritative summary of selected topics which will be useful to practitioners from the several disciplines concerned with the management of gastrointestinal hemorrhage. Emphasis has been given to those areas in which new information or techniques have become available in recent years. For those who attend the course, the text is intended as a handy reference to reinforce and record the subject matter presented.

Gastrointestinal hemorrhage is a subject that lends itself well to such a symposium. Our understanding of and the therapeutic strategy for the management of gastrointestinal hemorrhage have changed substantially in recent years. Routine fiberoptic endoscopy and mesenteric angiography have proved to be powerful diagnostic tools and have also been instrumental in defining the natural history of such lesions as stress gastritis and the Mallory-Weiss syndrome. Several therapeutic applications of these techniques are currently under investigation. Coagulation of gastric and duodenal lesions, sclerotherapy of varices, infusion of pharmacologic agents, and clotting of bleeding vascular lesions and ulcers using angiographic catheters are all topics of intense current interest and investigation. New operations such as highly selective vagotomy and the distal splenorenal shunt have been developed and are under clinical evaluation. Our understanding of the pathogenesis and treatment of bleeding diverticulitis and arteriovenous malformation of bowel has progressed, but remains imperfect. These and other subjects do provide a fertile ground for a two-day course and a monograph.

Special thanks should be given to our faculty and, most particularly, to our guests from other institutions. They have worked faithfully and have risen to the challenge of providing a written manuscript on very short notice, as well as preparing for participation in the course itself. Our program planning committee and the chairman and coeditor of this text, Dr. Richard Fiddian-Green, have spent many hours selecting, organizing, and editing the material. Without the help of our editorial associate, Jeanne Tashian, our publisher, Grune & Stratton, and our secretarial staff, the text and course could not have been assembled within the short time frame necessary to ensure that information is truly current. This book is planned as the first of many Michigan symposia designed to summarize the latest information on a variety of surgical topics in the years to come. We hope after studying this first effort you will share our enthusiasm for the project.

Jeremiah G. Turcotte, M.D.

Contributors

Douglass F. Adams, M.D.
Professor and Chairman
Department of Radiology
University of Michigan Medical Center
Ann Arbor, Michigan

John G. Allison, M.D., M.B.Ch.B., F.R.C.S. (Ed.), F.C.S. (S.A.)
Assistant Professor
Department of Surgery
University of Iowa College of Medicine
Iowa City, Iowa

Henry D. Appelman, M.D.
Professor of Pathology
Department of Pathology
University of Michigan Medical Center
Ann Arbor, Michigan

Richard H. Bell, Jr., M.D.
Assistant Professor of Surgery
Department of Surgery
University of California Medical Center
San Diego, California

Thomas C. Chalmers, M.D.
President and Dean
Mount Sinai School of Medicine
New York, New York

Kyung J. Cho, M.D.
Associate Professor
Department of Radiology
Director, Division of Cardiovascular Radiology
University of Michigan Medical Center
Ann Arbor, Michigan

Raphael S. Chung, M.D., F.A.C.S.
Associate Professor
Department of Surgery
University of Iowa College of Medicine
Iowa City, Iowa

William W. Coon, M.D.
Professor of Surgery
Department of Surgery
University of Michigan Medical Center
Ann Arbor, Michigan

Arnold G. Coran, M.D.
Professor of Surgery
Head, Section of Pediatric Surgery
Department of Surgery
University of Michigan Medical School
Ann Arbor, Michigan

Thomas L. Dent, M.D.
Professor of Surgery
Chief, Division of Gastrointestinal Surgery
Section of General Surgery
University of Michigan Medical Center
Ann Arbor, Michigan

William O. Dobbins, III, M.D.
Associate Chief of Staff for Research
Ann Arbor Veterans Administration Medical Center
Professor of Internal Medicine
University of Michigan Medical Center
Ann Arbor, Michigan

Philip E. Donahue, M.D.
Assistant Professor of Surgery
Department of Surgery
University of Illinois Hospital
Chief, General Surgery
West Side Veterans Administration Hospital
Chicago, Illinois

Frederic E. Eckhauser, M.D.
Assistant Professor of Surgery
Department of Surgery
University of Michigan Medical Center
Assistant Chief, Surgical Service
Ann Arbor Veterans Administration Medical Center
Ann Arbor, Michigan

Errol E. Erlandson, M.D.
Assistant Professor of Surgery
Division of Peripheral Vascular Surgery
Department of Surgery
University of Michigan Medical Center
Ann Arbor, Michigan

Aaron S. Fink, M.D.
Chief Resident
Department of Surgery
University of Michigan Medical Center
Ann Arbor, Michigan

Duane T. Freier, M.D.
Chief, Surgical Service
Veterans Administration Medical Center
Associate Professor of Surgery
University of Michigan Medical Center
Ann Arbor, Michigan

Linda M. Graham, M.D.
Research Fellow in Vascular Surgery
Resident in General Surgery
Department of Surgery
University of Michigan Medical Center
Ann Arbor, Michigan

Keith S. Henley, M.D.
Professor of Internal Medicine
Head, Section of Gastroenterology
Section of Gastroenterology
University of Michigan Medical Center
Ann Arbor, Michigan

CONTRIBUTORS

Terence Kennedy, M.S. (Lond.), F.R.C.S. (England), F.R.C.S.I.
Consultant Surgeon
Royal Victoria Hospital
Honorary Lecturer in Gastrointestinal Surgery
The Queens University
Belfast, Northern Ireland

H. Clifford Lane, M.D.
Clinical Associate
Division of Allergy and Infectious Diseases
National Institutes of Health
Washington, D.C.

Jeffrey W. Lewis, M.D.
Assistant Professor
Department of Surgery
University of Iowa College of Medicine
Iowa City, Iowa

S. Martin Lindenauer, M.D.
Professor of Surgery
Department of Surgery
University of Michigan Medical Center
Chief of Staff
Veterans Administration Medical Center
Ann Arbor, Michigan

Charles E. Lucas, M.D.
Professor of Surgery
Wayne State University
Chief, Emergency Surgical Service
Detroit General Hospital
Detroit, Michigan

Milton G. Mutchnick, M.D.
Assistant Professor of Internal Medicine
University of Michigan Medical Center
Chief, Liver Disease Section
Veterans Administration Medical Center
Ann Arbor, Michigan

Timothy T. Nostrant, M.D.
Instructor
Section of Gastroenterology
Department of Internal Medicine
University of Michigan Medical Center
Ann Arbor, Michigan

Lloyd M. Nyhus, M.D., F.A.C.S.
Warren H. Cole Professor
Head, Department of Surgery
University of Illinois at the Medical Center
Chicago, Illinois

Marshall J. Orloff, M.D.
Professor and Chairman
Department of Surgery
University of California Medical Center
San Diego, California

Robert L. Protell, M.D.
Assistant Professor of Internal Medicine
Department of Medicine
University of Washington
Director, Harborview Medical Center Endoscopy Clinic
Seattle, Washington

Stephen R. Ramsburgh, M.D.
Instructor
Department of Surgery
University of Michigan Medical Center
Ann Arbor, Michigan

Jean-Pierre Raufmann, M.D.
Fellow in Gastroenterology
Department of Internal Medicine
University of Michigan Medical Center
Ann Arbor, Michigan

Charles T. Richardson, M.D.
Chief, Gastroenterology
Veterans Administration Medical Center
Associate Professor of Internal Medicine
Department of Internal Medicine
University of Texas Health Sciences Center
Dallas, Texas

W. P. Ritchie, Jr., M.D., Ph.D.
Professor of Surgery
University of Virginia School of Medicine
Charlottesville, Virginia

Henry Sacks, Ph.D., M.D.
Instructor
Departments of Medicine and Biostatistics
Mount Sinai School of Medicine
New York, New York

Fred E. Silverstein, M.D.
Associate Professor of Medicine
Department of Medicine
University of Washington
Seattle, Washington

James C. Stanley, M.D.
Associate Professor of Surgery
Head, Division of Peripheral Vascular Surgery
Department of Surgery
University of Michigan Medical Center
Ann Arbor, Michigan

William E. Strodel, M.D.
Instructor in Surgery
Department of Surgery
University of Michigan Medical Center
Staff Surgeon
Veterans Administration Medical Center
Ann Arbor, Michigan

Norman W. Thompson, M.D., F.A.C.S.
Henry King Ransom Professor of Surgery
Department of Surgery
University of Michigan Medical Center
Ann Arbor, Michigan

George Willeford, M.D.
Fellow in Gastroenterology
Veterans Administration Medical Center
Department of Internal Medicine
University of Texas Health Science Center
Dallas, Texas

Walter M. Whitehouse, Jr., M.D.
Assistant Professor of Surgery
Division of Peripheral Vascular Surgery
Department of Surgery
University of Michigan Medical Center
Ann Arbor, Michigan

Gerald B. Zelenock, M.D.
Instructor in Surgery
Division of Peripheral Vascular Surgery
Department of Surgery
University of Michigan Medical Center
Ann Arbor, Michigan

Evaluation of the Bleeding Patient

Terence Kennedy, M.S. (Lond),
F.R.C.S. England, F.R.C.S.I.

Clinical Evaluation
of the Bleeding Adult

ABSTRACT

Priority in the physical examination of the bleeding adult is given to the hemodynamic assessment. The finding of stigmata of liver disease or an abdominal mass, suggestive of carcinoma, is also important. Laboratory investigation is directed towards a grouping and cross-matching of blood and towards assessment of the patient's coagulation status. In determining the source of the hemorrhage, barium meal is informative but will not identify the bleeding site with certainty. Endoscopy may be hazardous but will identify the bleeding site with certainty.

Monitoring is of paramount importance and is directed towards identifying those patients who will require emergency operation to stop their bleeding. The occurrence of perforation or catastrophic hemorrhage constitutes absolute indications for surgical intervention. Other factors of importance in making the decision to operate include age, rate of bleeding, presence of hypertension, firm diagnosis of a chronic ulcer, and recurrent bleeding after admission to hospital.

Emergency operation carries a mortality rate of around 6-8% compared with mortality of under 1% in elective surgery. It is important to select those patients who will require surgical intervention early and to avoid emergency surgery unless it is clearly indicated.

It is a curious fact that in most hospitals, patients with hematemesis or melena are routinely admitted to medical rather than surgical wards. Although in the great majority, bleeding will cease spontaneously, in a few, operation is essential if the patient is to survive. The proportion coming to emergency operation varies, in different series, between 5 and 30%. The kernel of the problem is to filter out this supremely important minority group.

Terence Kennedy, M.S. (Lond), F.R.C.S. England, F.R.C.S.I.: Consultant Surgeon, Royal Victoria Hospital, Belfast, and Honorary Lecturer in Gastrointestinal Surgery, The Queens University, Belfast, Northern Ireland.

Table 1
Causes of Hematemesis and Melena

	Walt (1978)	Avery-Jones and Gummer (1974)	Way (1977)
Gastric ulcer	17%	16%	15%
Duodenal ulcer	16%	35%	40%
Erosive gastritis	37%	24%	20%
Mallory-Weiss	11%	–	10%
Varices	9%	3%	10%
Tumor	3%	3%	–
Miscellaneous	7%	19%	5%

There are many causes of acute upper gastrointestinal bleeding and the more important are indicated in Table 1. These large series are not strictly comparable as all diagnoses were not confirmed endoscopically. Nevertheless there are important differences, notably the decreased incidence of varices in the British series. This experience is mirrored in other reports [8]. Mallory-Weiss ulcers appear to be recognized more often in the USA and acute erosive gastritis, perhaps the most difficult problem, is less common in Britain. Central to the problem of clinical evaluation is the need to arrive at an accurate diagnosis of the source of bleeding.

HISTORY

If the patient is very ill or in shock it may not be practicable to elicit a detailed history, but it will usually be possible to collect some useful clues. A history of heavy alcohol intake over a long period will suggest the possibility of cirrhosis and esophageal varices, but it must not be forgotten that alcoholics often have chronic gastric or duodenal ulcers which may bleed.

Drug ingestion is often a factor. If the patient has been taking aspirin or related drugs, the possibility of acute erosive gastritis becomes a probability and the same may be said for the ingestion of phenylbutazone. Where the patient has a preexisting chronic duodenal ulcer, any of these drugs may cause a flare-up, so it is not safe to assume that the bleeding is due to erosions. Some years ago, before we had emergency endoscopy, I encountered a 50 year old woman who had a massive hemorrhage. She had taken large amounts of aspirin for her "lumbago." I suspected erosive gastritis and refused to operate, but a day or two later she had a further massive, exsanguinating hemorrhage; I operated and was surprised to find a huge posterior duodenal ulcer which had eroded the gastroduodenal artery. Her "lumbago" was due to this penetrating duodenal ulcer.

The use of steroids must also be examined, although in my own experience steroid therapy has not been a common or particularly important cause of ulceration and hemorrhage. It is important to inquire whether the patient is on anticoagulant drugs following cardiac surgery or for other reasons.

The precise history of the onset of vomiting may be extremely important. Vomiting of food often associated with much retching, perhaps following overindulgence in food or alcohol, may precede the vomiting of blood. In such a case it is highly likely that the cause of the bleeding is a Mallory-Weiss mucosal tear.

It is a curious fact that patients admitted after an acute hemorrhage seldom experience pain once they are in the hospital. Usually there is a past history of ulcer type pain which tends to become more severe in the few days immediately before the hemorrhage. Pain persisting after admission generally indicates a deeply penetrating ulcer, one that is likely to erode a large artery such as the left gastric, splenic or gastroduodenal and require operation. Sometimes there is no history of pain at any time. This may suggest erosive gastritis but it is also characteristic of benign tumors.

PHYSICAL EXAMINATION

Priority is given to a rapid assessment of the patient's circulatory state — color, pulse rate and volume, blood pressure and peripheral perfusion. The rapid evaluation and proper management of shock must take precedence over everything else. The presence of liver palm or spider nevi may indicate hepatic cirrhosis. Occasionally the bleeding patient may have jaundice or ascites or splenomegaly any of which would point rather strongly towards portal hypertension.

A palpable mass in the epigastrium may be present if there is a carcinoma of the stomach, but this is not a common cause of massive bleeding.

Signs of bleeding at other sites should be sought including subcutaneous ecchymoses and petechiae, and when present they will lead to queries about the patient's bleeding tendency. Rarely there may be signs of Osler's hereditary telangiectasia.

LABORATORY INVESTIGATIONS

On admission blood should be taken for grouping and cross-matching. Screening of the patient's coagulation status, prothrombin and platelets is not important in the majority of patients, but in those with liver disease these investigations are mandatory. Routine biochemical screening tests may be helpful. Particular emphasis should be placed on bilirubin and transaminase levels in patients with liver disease. A low serum albumin level is of great importance in assessing the prognosis in a patient with bleeding esophageal varices.

RADIOLOGY AND ENDOSCOPY

There is no doubt that it is safe to perform an upper GI series within the first twenty four hours after a major hemorrhage, provided that the patient is not in a state of hypovolemic shock. Often information of the greatest value is obtained, particularly in patients with chronic gastric or duodenal ulcer. Carcinoma, though a relatively rare cause of severe bleeding, may be readily diagnosed and the appearance of a leiomyoma, an occasional cause of massive bleeding is absolutely characteristic. The radiologist will demonstrate a smooth rounded filling defect, often with a pit or crater in its center. The problem is to differentiate between filling defects due to tumor and those due to blood clots. Not too much should be read into the finding of evidence of a chronic duodenal ulcer, as this may be associated with a small relatively acute gastric ulcer which is the real source of the hemorrhage.

Radiology is very valuable in the demonstration of esophageal varices, but it does not indicate whether the varices are the source of active bleeding. It is probably easier to demonstrate varices by barium studies than by fiberoptic endoscopy, though bleeding is readily seen with the endoscope. Varices are more easily seen if the old fashioned rigid endoscope is used, but this requires a general anesthetic.

It is only the most skilled radiologists that are likely to demonstrate Mallory-Weiss ulcers and few will be able to diagnose erosive gastritis, both conditions that are readily diagnosed by endoscopy. The overall success rate of barium studies is little better than 60%.

With the advent of fiberoptic endoscopy many clinicians have now largely abandoned the use of barium studies as the first diagnostic tool. It is important to remember however that endoscopy has dangers in the patient who is actively bleeding at the time of examination when he may vomit and aspirate blood.

In most hospitals and clinics endoscopy is performed by an internist or full-time endoscopist, but in my hospital the examination is usually carried out by surgeons. I have found it to be most advantageous to see the actual bleeding point before embarking on operation. Sometimes the stomach is full of blood and clot and a clear view cannot be obtained; where there is much blood present it is usually advisable to operate without undue delay.

In some patients the source of bleeding cannot be determined by either endoscopy or barium studies. These may be very difficult clinical problems, though help can sometimes be obtained from selective angiography. The bleeding may be arising in the distal duodenum or upper jejunum, perhaps from an angiomatous lesion or perhaps from an intrahepatic lesion causing hemobilia. This technique can be remarkably sensitive and it is said that rates of bleeding as little as 1 ml per minute can be demonstrated. There are some risks and angiography should not be used routinely.

MONITORING

Every patient who has had an acute hematemesis or melena of any magnitude must be carefully observed in hospital. Blood will be cross matched and transfused as required and intravenous fluids, usually saline initially, should be given from the outset. Pulse rate and blood pressure must be carefully recorded and the hemoglobin should be measured. In cases of severe hemorrhage with shock it is helpful to set up a central venous pressure line; this will greatly assist both the assessment and the proper control of transfusion. We do not, however, use central venous pressure measurements in the routine management of slight to moderate bleeding. A catheter should be passed and urinary output carefully measured in all severe cases.

Nasogastric intubation is widely practiced, both to empty the stomach of blood and clots and to observe fresh bleeding at an early stage. The value of intubation has probably been exaggerated as clots can only be removed using a very large tube and then only with difficulty. Gastric lavage with iced saline has been recommended, though I am unable to find any objective evidence that it is of the slightest value. Where there is massive bleeding from the left gastric or gastroduodenal artery it is impossible to believe that iced saline can be effective.

RATE OF BLEEDING

It is important to make an estimate of the rate of blood loss. Anything over 1 liter in 24 hours can be considered a major hemorrhage. Often the rate is much greater and sometimes it is difficult with transfusion to keep up with the blood loss. This situation may be categorized as "catastrophic bleeding."

It is probably never possible to measure accurately all the blood lost, but an estimate can be arrived at indirectly by measuring the amount of blood transfusion required to restore circulatory equilibrium and a normal hemoglobin level. Whether the shed blood presents as hematemesis or melena may have some bearing. In general, rapid bleeding tends to cause hematemesis and less rapid bleeding causes melena. The site of the bleeding lesion also has an influence, esophageal varices or gastric ulcer tending to hematemesis and duodenal ulcer to melena.

Melena is not always dark and tarry; sometimes large amounts of dark red blood are passed per rectum, indicating very rapid bleeding. In these cases it may be difficult to decide whether the bleeding site is in the colon or duodenum. A useful diagnostic measure is to check the blood urea. If this is normal, the bleeding site is not in the stomach or duodenum because large amounts of blood passing through the whole small bowel will cause enough protein absorption to raise the BUN level appreciably. When BUN is normal the bleeding site is probably in the colon.

THE DECISION TO OPERATE

We know that around 90% of all patients will stop bleeding spontaneously, but a few will die if operation is withheld. We also know that operation in the acute phase carries a significant mortality — 6% [1], 8% [3], and 20% [8]. Mortality will vary with the proportion treated surgically and will be higher in older patients and those for whom emergency operation is unduly delayed. Mortality is virtually eliminated when it is possible to delay operation until it can be done as an elective procedure. Typical figures for elective operation are 0.7% for gastrectomy [6] and 0.23% for vagotomy [5]. The logical policy, therefore, is one of selective operation but the internist should not be encouraged to hang onto his patient until too late. It has been said that the ideal partnership is an enthusiastic, hawkish physician working with a reluctant surgeon.

Two factors constitute absolute indications for urgent operation:

1. Perforation, which may occur before, with or after the hematemesis. This situation is fortunately rare as it carries a high mortality. The diagnosis depends upon the finding of abdominal rigidity and or the demonstration of free gas in the abdomen.
2. Catastrophic hemorrhage, where the bleeding is so brisk that it is difficult or impossible to keep pace with transfusion. A very large vessel will be the source, perhaps the splenic artery in the base of a gastric ulcer, the gastroduodenal artery or perhaps an aortic aneurysm ruptured into the duodenum. An exception to the need for immediate operation applies in the case of esophageal varices which are probably best controlled by tamponade with a Sengstaken-Blakemore tube in the first instance.

In other cases the decision for or against emergency operation is made after considering various factors (Table 2):

1. Age. Younger patients are likely to stop bleeding spontaneously whereas older patients are more likely to continue and the effects of hemorrhage are more severe in the elderly. For practical purposes an age of 45-50 years can be taken as a watershed; over the age of 60-65 operation will more often be required. Much of the mortality from bleeding is in older patients. Avery-Jones and Gummer found a mortality rate of 2.4% under 60 years and 9.3% over this age in all cases whether treated medically or surgically.

Table 2
Factors Influencing Decision to Operate

	For	Against
Age	Over 50	Under 50
Hypertension	Yes	No
Diagnosis	Chronic duodenal or gastric ulcer	Uncertain erosions, Mallory-Weiss
Bleeding	> 1.5 liters/24 hours, recurrent after admission	< 1.5 liters/24 hours, stopped
Pain	Persistent	None
Drugs	None	Aspirin, steroids, anticoagulants
Transfusion problems	Rare blood group	None
Other chronic illness	Respiratory disease	Recent coronary occlusion, coagulopathies

2. Hypertension. In older patients there is an increased incidence of vascular disease and hypertension. These patients are more likely to bleed, less likely to stop bleeding spontaneously, and more likely to bleed again and again. They are in fact a group in whom relatively earlier operation is generally desirable.
3. Diagnosis. Where there is a clear cut diagnosis of chronic gastric or duodenal ulcer it is appropriate to take a hawkish attitude and recommend early operation. The decision to operate early is especially valid in those who have bled before. Where the diagnosis is uncertain and where erosive gastritis or Mallory-Weiss tears are proven or suspected the doves may well prevail.
4. Extent and rate of bleeding. Where there is only a small hemorrhage which stops spontaneously and is not associated with any signs of oligemic shock there is obviously no need for emergency surgery. Where there is massive continuing hemorrhage, the need for operation is obvious. Between these two extremes are many patients, some of whom should be treated surgically; when operation is indicated it should be done early rather than late because delayed emergency operation carries a very high mortality, around 25%. There is no precise total loss of blood or rate of bleeding that makes operation essential, but most clinicians would regard some 1.5-2 liters per 24 hours as an indication for serious consideration. Rates above this are a threat to life, especially in the older patient. Some internists like to wait until the patient has lost 5 or more liters of blood before alerting a surgical colleague. Such conservatism is rewarded only with a high mortality.

5. Continuing or recurrent bleeding. Where bleeding continues unabated the need for operation is obvious. In most patients bleeding ceases spontaneously at about the time of admission and usually it does not recur. When there is a second or subsequent episode of bleeding while the patient is in hospital, a hawkish attitude must be adopted. These patients often have a deep ulcer involving a large vessel and conservative management is dangerous. In patients aged 45-50 years and over with a proven chronic gastric or duodenal ulcer, recurrence of bleeding after admission to hospital is a very strong indication for operation.
6. Pain. It is usual for ulcer type pain to cease when the patient is admitted. Persistence or reappearance of pain may indicate perforation, an absolute indication for operation. More often it simply indicates a deeply penetrating ulcer of the kind that often has a large vessel such as the gastroduodenal artery or the left gastric artery in its base. This type of bleeding ulcer tends to do badly when treated conservatively.
7. Drugs. A history of ingestion of aspirin and antirheumatic drugs suggests the probability of erosive gastritis, a condition which is not easily treated surgically. If there is no evidence of chronic ulcer in these cases it is advisable, at least in the first instance, to avoid operation. Nevertheless it must be recognized that in some cases with erosive gastritis the bleeding does not cease spontaneously. In this situation operation must be undertaken though the results are generally poor with a mortality as high as 40% [2].
8. Tumors. Where there is radiological or endoscopic evidence of a carcinoma it is probably best to avoid emergency surgery. Hemorrhage from malignant tumors is seldom massive or life threatening. A delay of a few days may allow a calculated and more radical approach to remove the tumor. With leiomyoma bleeding is likely to be very much more massive and severe and operation need not be radical. In these patients a more aggressive policy with early operation is generally appropriate.
9. Esophageal varices constitute a special problem which will not be discussed here in detail. Emergency shunt has a mortality of around 50% [7]. Esophageal tamponade and injection sclerotherapy are perhaps more promising emergency measures with a much lower mortality [4].
10. Transfusion difficulties. Some patients with hematemesis and melena belong to rare or obscure blood groups or are difficult to transfuse for other reasons. Paradoxically this constitutes an important reason for early operation. If such a patient is treated medically and has a subsequent severe bleed it might be impossible to resuscitate him.
11. Associated medical conditions. We have already accepted hypertension as an indication for operation, but if the patient has had a coronary occlusion within two or three weeks of the hemorrhage most would agree that operation is contraindicated. If the patient is on anticoagulant therapy this must of course be stopped.

Other chronic unrelated diseases, such as chronic bronchitis are paradoxically often an incentive towards operation. It is better to operate early in these cases, since a competent anesthetist can handle obstructive airway disease. If such a patient rebleeds two or three times and then comes to operation, the risks are hideous.

It is important to appreciate that none of these factors constitutes an absolute indication for or against operation. It is a combination of them all that should guide the clinician. For example a hypertensive man aged 70 with a chronic duodenal ulcer will not require urgent operation if blood loss is only 0.5 liter. He will however need to be watched very closely and if there is any repetition of bleeding then it will be wise to operate without delay. Conversely a 20 year old woman with a history of taking aspirin may require operation for erosive gastritis if the blood loss continues over a period of days, ultimately constituting a threat to life.

Many authors advocate a more aggressive policy: Hunt, et al [3] in a prospective study in Australia lowered the overall mortality from bleeding duodenal ulcers from 12% to 5% by employing emergency operation in 43% of their admissions. My own view is that operation *in the acute phase* is required in perhaps 10% of duodenal ulcers, but that many others should be treated surgically (and safely) only when they have recovered from the acute hemorrhage.

Chronic Bleeding

The problem here is altogether less urgent and demanding. Blood loss is indicated by the finding of coffee ground vomiting, chronic melena or fecal occult bleeding. Once loss of blood is established it is important to record serial hemoglobin levels as an indication of the rate of loss. Diagnosis is made by endoscopy, barium series or angiography or a combination of these, though often it is extremely difficult to define the precise source of bleeding.

CONCLUSION

There are many causes of acute hematemesis and melena and in the great majority bleeding will cease spontaneously. Between 5 and 20% of patients, however, require emergency operation, even though it does carry a mortality of 6-10%. The purpose of assessment is to determine which patients should be treated surgically. The most important points in favor of operation are the patient's age, the rate of bleeding, the presence of hypertension, a firm diagnosis of chronic ulcer and recurrent bleeding after admission to hospital.

Emergency operation carries a mortality of around 6-8% compared with a mortality of under 1% in elective surgery. It is therefore important to avoid emergency operation unless it is clearly indicated. An operation rate of around 10% is probably appropriate in most series.

REFERENCES

1. Avery-Jones FA, Gummer JWP: Acute hematemesis and melaena from peptic ulceration. In Maingot R: Abdominal Operations, 6th Ed. New York, Appleton-Century-Crofts, 1974
2. Donahue PE, Nyhus LM: Massive upper gastrointestinal hemorrhage. In Nyhus LM, Wastell C (eds): Surgery of the Stomach and Duodenum, 3rd Ed. Boston, Little, Brown, 1977, p 405
3. Hunt PS, Korman MG, Hansky J, et al: Bleeding duodenal ulcer: reduction in mortality with a planned approach. Br J Surg 66:636, 1979
4. Johnston GW, Rodgers HW: A review of 15 years experience of sclerotherapy in hemorrhage from oesophageal varices. Br J Surg 60:797, 1973
5. Kennedy T: A critical appraisal of surgical treatment. In Truelove SC: Topics in Gastroenterology. Oxford, Blackwell, 1979, p 131
6. McKeown KC: A prospective study of the immediate and long term results of Polya gastrectomy for duodenal ulcer. Br J Surg 58:847, 1972
7. Orloff MJ, Charters AC, Chandler JG, et al: Portacaval shunt as emergency procedure in unselected patients with alcoholic cirrhosis. Surg Gynecol Obstet 141:58, 1975
8. Schiller KFR, Truelove SC, Williams DG: Haematemesis and melaena, with special reference to factors influencing the outcome. Br Med J 2:7, 1970
9. Walt AJ: Personal experiences with upper gastrointestinal bleeding. In Nyhus LM, Wastell C (eds): Surgery of Stomach and Duodenum, 3rd Ed. Boston, Little, Brown, 1977, p 435
10. Way LW: Upper gastrointestinal hemorrhage. In Dunphy JE, Way LW. Current Surgical Diagnosis and Treatment. Los Altos, Lange, 1977, p 482

Arnold G. Coran, M.D.

Gastrointestinal Bleeding in Infants and Children

ABSTRACT

Rectal bleeding in infants and children in most cases is minimal and the causes are usually easily detected and just as easily treated. Because the risk of malignancy in children with gastrointestinal bleeding is minimal, the type of diagnostic work-up employed is far less extensive than that used in an adult with a similar clinical presentation. The causes of rectal bleeding in infants and children are closely correlated with the age of the patient; therefore, if one evaluates the degree of rectal bleeding, the color of the blood in the stool, and the age of the patient, a definitive diagnosis of the etiology of the bleeding can be made 90% of the time.

GENERAL CONSIDERATIONS

Gastrointestinal bleeding in infants and children is quite different than in adults. Such conditions as diverticulosis and hemorrhoids are common in adults, but quite rare in children. In addition, the incidence of carcinoma associated with gastrointestinal bleeding in adults is sufficiently high to justify a thorough investigation even in the presence of a benign lesion capable of producing the complaint. This is not true in children. Therefore, in a child, if a cause is found, no further investigation is warranted [2, 3].

The first step in the evaluation of a child with gastrointestinal bleeding is a complete history and physical examination. Always check the anus for the presence of a fissure before doing a digital examination, since a fissure may result from the examination itself. All infants and children with bleeding abnormalities should have a "coagulation screen" which includes a platelet

---

Arnold G. Coran, M.D.: Professor of Surgery, Head, Section of Pediatric Surgery, Department of Surgery, University of Michigan Medical School, Ann Arbor, Michigan.

count, prothrombin time and thromboplastin time. The differential diagnosis of rectal bleeding is based on the volume and character of the blood loss, the age of the patient, and the general health of the child prior to bleeding. The color of the blood in instances of rectal bleeding varies considerably according to both the level of bleeding or the rate of blood loss. Large amounts of red blood per rectum may originate from brisk bleeding above the ligament of Treitz, but a small volume from the upper gastrointestinal tract will become so thoroughly mixed with the intestinal content that it will be invisible in the stool. In general, however, the character of the bleeding can help to define whether the blood is coming from the proximal or distal gastrointestinal tract. Bright red blood, especially when it coats, but is not mixed with the stool, most likely comes from the anorectal region. The higher in the intestinal tract the source of bleeding and the more intimately mixed with the feces, the darker in color is the blood likely to be. Upper gastrointestinal bleeding gives tarry, black, sticky stools (melena), the result of conversion of hemoglobin to acid hematin. If there is hematemesis associated with rectal bleeding, this almost always implies hemorrhage proximal to the ligament of Treitz. Profuse upper gastrointestinal bleeding can result in bright red blood per rectum because of the significant irritant effect of the blood itself. Currant-jelly stool, a result of blood mixed with mucous, is produced by inflammation or irritation in the lower gastrointestinal tract.

The degree of rectal bleeding will often suggest the origin of the hemorrhage. For example, anal fissures and juvenile colonic polyps usually result in a minimal amount of bleeding, whereas peptic ulcers, Meckel's diverticula and esophageal varices are often associated with major gastrointestinal bleeding, which can even result in shock and death.

Associated conditions and other symptoms and signs often suggest the underlying etiology of the rectal bleeding. For example, mucocutaneous pigmentation, diffuse lymphadenopathy, cutaneous hemangiomas, and hepatosplenomegaly are all conditions which give the physician a clue to the underlying diagnosis of bleeding. By correlating the age of the patient with the various above-mentioned signs and symptoms, one can come to a definitive diagnosis in most cases.

The common causes of rectal bleeding in various age groups are listed in Table 1.

SPECIFIC CONDITIONS

Anal Fissure

Anal fissure is a superficial mucosal tear of the anal mucosa usually located posteriorly and associated with small amounts of bright red blood coating the feces. It is the commonest cause of rectal bleeding in infants and is usually due to the passage of hard fecal material secondary to chronic constipation.

Table 1
Causes of Rectal Bleeding

	Neonates	Infants up to Age 2	Children Ages 2-12	Adolescents
Common causes	Hemorrhagic disease of the newborn (due to vitamin K deficiency)	Infectious diarrhea	Infectious diarrhea	Peptic ulcer
	Swallowed blood (diagnosed by the Apt test [1])	Anal fissure	Juvenile polyp	Inflammatory bowel disease
		Intussusception	Peptic ulcer	
	Anorectal trauma	Meckel's diverticulum	Esophageal varices	Esophageal varices
	Infectious diarrhea	Milk allergy	Inflammatory bowel disease	
	Necrotizing enterocolitis			
Less common causes	Volvulus	Peptic ulcer	Meckel's diverticulum	Polyps
	Vascular malformations	Intestinal duplication	Intestinal duplication	Infectious diarrhea
	Stress ulcer	Volvulus	Intussusception	Hemorrhoids
			Vascular malformation	Clotting abnormalities
			Anal fissure	
			Adenomatous intestinal polyps	
			Clotting abnormalities	

Occasionally anal trauma resulting from too vigorous a rectal examination or inappropriate placement of a rectal thermometer can cause an anal fissure. The condition is almost always well treated by the use of stool softeners and high fiber diets along with sitz baths. It is rare to have to perform a fissurectomy in an infant with this condition [7, 8, 9].

Intussusception

Intussusception occurs most frequently between the ages of 6 months and 2 years and about 20% of the cases follow an upper respiratory tract infection or gastroenteritis. In 80% of the patients, no lead point is found. This condition is usually accompanied by pain, bilious vomiting, the passage of "currant-jelly" stool and the presence of a palpable abdominal mass. The diagnosis is made with a barium enema examination showing a typical coiled-spring appearance in the transverse or ascending colon or both. In 80-90% of the patients, the barium enema will also effectively reduce the intussusception, thereby eliminating the need for operative therapy. In those cases in which the intussusception is not reduced hydrostatically, an operative manual reduction of the intussusception must be carried out.

Meckel's Diverticulum

Meckel's diverticulum is a vitelline duct anomaly which usually contains ectopic gastric and pancreatic mucosa. Bleeding is usually due to peptic ulceration of the adjacent ileal mucosa. The volume of bleeding can be quite significant, often leading to a major fall in the patient's hemoglobin. The bleeding may be painless and is usually associated with maroon-colored stool. Contrast studies of the small and large intestine are generally useless in making a diagnosis. The most effective diagnostic study is the radionuclide scan which will often show take-up of isotope in the region of a Meckel's diverticulum [5]. Angiography is useful only if the rate of bleeding is greater than 0.5 to 1.0 cc per minute. If a Meckel's diverticulum is strongly suspected clinically or is demonstrated with the radionuclide scan, then excision of the diverticulum is indicated.

Duplications

Duplications of the intestine can occur anywhere along the alimentary tract. They are either cystic or tubular, and in 20% of the cases, communicate with the normal intestine. The tubular forms of duplication share a common serosal wall with the normal adjacent bowel. They usually contain ectopic gastric mucosa and bleeding is due to peptic ulceration of the mucosa adjacent to ectopic mucosa.

Polyps [4]

Juvenile polyps. These are inflammatory or retention polyps which occur quite commonly in children under 15 years of age. The peak incidence of occurrence is between the ages of 4 and 8 years with 2% to 3% of children involved. Boys are affected more commonly than girls, and the polyps are usually solitary in over 70% of the cases. The majority of polyps occur in the rectum and sigmoid, usually within reach of the sigmoidoscope. These polyps are usually associated with small amounts of bright red rectal bleeding coating the feces. Occasionally, the polyp will prolapse outside the anus or cause an intussusception. Seventy-five percent of the polyps can be detected by proctosigmoidoscopy and the remainder can be easily diagnosed with an air-contrast barium enema, or, occasionally, with flexible colonoscopy. Since these polyps tend to autoamputate and slough, non-operative therapy is indicated. It is certainly inappropriate to do a colotomy to remove a juvenile polyp. Polyps that are seen during sigmoidoscopy should be removed at the time of the diagnostic procedure. If a polyp beyond the reach of a sigmoidoscope causes significant rectal bleeding, which is unusual, then removal with a flexible colonoscope is indicated.

Hereditary and generalized juvenile polyposis. Hereditary juvenile polyposis is an inherited disorder in which multiple juvenile polyps are seen throughout the colon and occasionally in the small bowel. The polyps tend to recur, and there is an increased incidence of gastrointestinal cancer in family members. The children often present with a clinical picture of mucous diarrhea, rectal bleeding, anemia, hypoproteinemia, hypocalcemia, clubbing, intussusception and prolapse. If the symptoms are severe, surgical therapy may be indicated.

Cronkhite-Canada syndrome. Cronkhite-Canada syndrome is a nonhereditary form of multiple juvenile polyposis. It is associated with alopecia, cutaneous hyperpigmentation, and atrophic nails.

Peutz-Jeghers syndrome. The Peutz-Jeghers syndrome is associated with hamartomatous polyps principally found in the small bowel, but with a substantial incidence of polyps in the colon also. Occasionally polyps are found in the stomach and duodenum. The syndrome is inherited as an autosomal dominant with both sexes equally affected. Pigmentation of the lips and buccal mucosa is characteristic. Rectal bleeding is common and is associated, in many cases, with significant anemia. Occasionally the polyps act as a lead point for an intussusception. Since there is no increased risk of gastrointestinal cancer, therapy should be conservative, with resectional surgery avoided whenever possible. Occasionally a polypectomy can be performed if clinically indicated. Ovarian tumors occur in about 5% of affected girls.

Adenomatous polyps. There are three syndromes associated with adenomatous colonic polyps: familial polyposis, Gardner's syndrome, and Turcot's syndrome. Familial polyposis is inherited as a Mendelian autosomal dominant with both sexes equally affected. Fifty percent of the offspring of an affected individual will develop these polyps. The symptoms usually start in adolescence and consist of diarrhea, often associated with mucous, together with rectal bleeding and anemia. The diagnosis is confirmed by the family history and diagnostic sigmoidoscopy and colonoscopy with biopsy of the polyps. These polyps are all premalignant with a sharp increase in the risk of carcinoma in late adolescence. Six percent of these patients will develop carcinoma before 15 years of age. Because of the premalignant nature of these polyps, a colectomy should be performed in all children between the ages of 10 and 15 years. The various procedures recommended at present are a total proctocolectomy with an ileostomy, a subtotal colectomy with an ileal-rectal anastomosis, and a total colectomy with an endorectal pull-through. At the present time, we prefer the total colectomy with an endorectal pull-through because the entire colonic mucosa is removed, but an ileostomy is avoided. In those patients in whom the rectum has been left in, sigmoidoscopy must be carried out every six months.

Gardner's syndrome is associated with multiple adenomatous polyps of the colon and is inherited as a Mendelian autosomal dominant. In addition, osteomas, epidermoid cysts and desmoid tumors are also found. These polyps are again premalignant and the surgical therapy is the same as that recommended for familial polyposis. There is an increased incidence of carcinoma of the ampulla of Vater in this syndrome. Turcot's syndrome consists of multiple adenomatous colonic polyps inherited as an autosomal recessive. It is associated with central nervous system tumors, specifically medulloblastoma and glioblastoma.

Lymphoid Nodular Hyperplasia

Lymphoid nodular hyperplasia consists of an overgrowth of submucosal lymphoid nodules as a response to either infection or allergy. There is an associated deficiency of IgA. The condition is often associated with minimal amounts of rectal bleeding and usually is resolved with steroid therapy. This abnormality is occasionally seen in a colon distal to a colostomy stoma and usually resolves after the colostomy has been closed.

Miscellaneous Causes

Arteriovenous malformations and hemangiomas. Arteriovenous malformations of the intestine can result in chronic blood loss or massive gastrointestinal bleeding. They are often associated with cutaneous hemangiomas and can occur in any portion of the gastrointestinal tract. One of the classic examples of vascular malformations of the gastrointestinal tract is the Rendu-Osler-Weber syndrome. These lesions are often difficult to diagnose but can occasionally be visualized with arteriography. If arteriography is unsuccessful in delineating the malformation, then colonoscopy for colonic lesions and operative endoscopy with transillumination are helpful. Recently, use of the Doppler intraoperatively has been helpful in detecting these lesions. The general approach is extreme conservatism in as much as repeated intestinal resections can result in the short bowel syndrome and an intestinal cripple. These patients are admitted to the hospital during an acute hemorrhage and must be well-stabilized with transfusions. In the case of chronic bleeding with a typical blood loss anemia, intermittent hospital admission for transfusions constitutes appropriate therapy.

Infectious gastroenteritis. Bacterial, viral, fungal, and parasitic infections of the intestinal tract result in significant gastrointestinal bleeding. Typical examples of this are shigellosis, typhoid fever, amebiasis, and tuberculosis. In addition, pseudomembranous enterocolitis, as a result of antibiotic therapy, can also result in major gastrointestinal blood loss.

Henoch-Schonlein purpura. Henoch-Schonlein purpura usually follows a streptococcal infection, often leads to bleeding into the wall of the small intestine with the development of intestinal wall hematomas. This can result in irritation of the intestinal mucosa with subsequent gastrointestinal bleeding. Clinically, the patient often develops abdominal cramps secondary to the bowel wall hematomas. Occasionally, the intramural hematoma of the intestine can act as a lead point for a small bowel intussusception. It is often difficult to distinguish the hematomas alone from an actual intussusception. In most cases, the abdominal cramps decrease once steroid therapy has been started. At this same time, the gastrointestinal bleeding usually stops.

Hemolytic-uremic syndrome. Hemolytic-uremic syndrome is an unusual vasculitis of childhood which is usually associated with hematuria, renal failure and colonic ischemia. The colonic ischemia is often manifested by moderate gastrointestinal bleeding. On rare occasions, the colonic ischemia can result in total necrosis of the bowel with perforation and peritonitis.

Other causes of gastrointestinal bleeding in infants and children include nonspecific ulceration of the ileum and colon, iron ingestion and the presence of a foreign body in the intestinal tract.

Peptic Ulcer

A detailed discussion of peptic ulcer disease in infants and children is beyond the scope of this chapter; nevertheless, a few pertinent comments should be included. Ulcer disease in infants and children is rare, but not unheard of. In fact, a registry in Bismarck, North Dakota, collects all the cases of ulcer disease in children throughout the United States and to date has listed over 750 cases. The symptoms in infants and young children are quite different than those in adults. After the age of 10 years, the clinical picture becomes closer to that of the adult. In the newborn, the ulcer crater is often very superficial, whereas in the older child, it becomes deeper as it does in the adult.

There are four distinct clinical patterns to peptic ulcer disease in infants and children. If an ulcer is present during the first two weeks of life, it usually presents with hemorrhage or perforation. Quite often at this age, the diagnosis is overlooked. The bleeding is usually minimal, but can be massive and usually presents as both hematemesis and melena. The picture with perforation is similar to that of spontaneous perforation of the stomach in the newborn. Peptic ulcer during the period of infancy to 2 years of age is quite rare and is usually secondary to a stressful situation such as sepsis, shock, or severe respiratory insufficiency. When it occurs as an isolated entity during this age period, it usually presents a clinical picture of feeding difficulty with frequent vomiting. Occasionally vague abdominal pain is associated with this symptom complex. During the age period 2 years to 6 years, the incidence of peptic ulceration is extremely rare. Hemorrhage and perforation are the characteristic symptoms when it does occur; however, pain is also a prominent feature. After the age of 9 years, the clinical picture of peptic ulcer disease becomes quite similar to that seen in adults.

The management of the neonate with bleeding from a peptic ulcer consists of Vitamin K administration, gastric lavage, and transfusion as needed. Surgery is rarely indicated. Perforation requires surgical closure. The older child with bleeding or perforation is handled in a similar fashion. In the older child, pain from ulcer disease is usually managed medically with either antacids or, more frequently, with cimetidine. However, occasionally medical management is totally unsuccessful and a definitive ulcer operation is required. This is especially true in the case of the adolescent and teenager. At the present time, the operations of choice for the definitive management of ulcer disease in childhood are antrectomy and vagotomy, and pyloroplasty and vagotomy.

Esophageal Varices

Once again, a discussion of esophageal varices and portal hypertension in childhood is beyond the scope of this chapter. However, a few comments are in order. Most cases of esophageal varices are secondary to extrahepatic portal hypertension. This usually results from portal vein thrombosis in the newborn period following such episodes as omphalitis, exchange transfusions, severe dehydration and trauma. A much smaller percentage of cases of portal hypertension are secondary to intrinsic liver disease such as posthepatitis cirrhosis, biliary cirrhosis secondary to biliary atresia, Wilson's disease, cystic fibrosis, congenital hepatic fibrosis and alpha 1 antitrypsin deficiency. Most children with extrahepatic portal hypertension do not develop gastrointestinal bleeding until they are at least 3 years of age. They usually present with hematemesis and melena and rarely develop hypovolemic shock. An enlarged spleen is usually palpable on physical examination. It is extremely important for the physician to warn the parents that aspirin administration may precipitate bleeding from esophageal varices in these children. Therefore, during periods of fever and upper respiratory tract infections, aspirin must be avoided and other antipyretic agents should be utilized.

When bleeding occurs, these children are admitted to the hospital and are placed at bedrest with sedation. A nasogastric tube is inserted and blood transfusions are given as needed. Occasionally, a Pitressin infusion is required to slow down the bleeding. It is rare to have to use a Sengstaken tube. Once the child has stabilized and stopped bleeding, diagnostic studies should be carried out to definitively determine the etiology of the portal hypertension. This is best done with a superior mesenteric arteriogram with particular attention paid to the venous phase. These children often return to the hospital on several occasions over the subsequent years with repeated bouts of gastrointestinal hemorrhage. However, these episodes are easily managed with the program just outlined. Two-thirds of children with extrahepatic portal hypertension and bleeding esophageal varices will not require any major operative therapy. Occasionally, a child may not stop bleeding and may require emergency surgical intervention. If the child is small and the size of the splenic vein is less than a centimeter in diameter, then a transesophageal ligation of varices is an effective way to immediately stop the bleeding. In those children that do require portal decompression, the portal-systemic shunt can usually be done under elective conditions. The various shunts used for the management of extrahepatic portal hypertension in children are the mesocaval shunt, the splenorenal shunt and the H-graft interposition shunt. We prefer the central splenorenal shunt for the management of this condition.

PRINCIPLES OF MANAGEMENT

Most children with rectal bleeding present with minimal amounts of bright red blood. If only 1 or 2 episodes of this nature have occurred, examination of the anus and sigmoidoscopy are the only studies necessary even if no lesion is found. If this type of minimal rectal bleeding becomes recurrent, then an air-contrast barium enema and possible colonoscopy should be carried out.

Major bleeding per rectum requires more extensive evaluation after the patient has been resuscitated and stabilized. A nasogastric tube should be passed and the aspirate should be checked for the presence of blood. The presence of blood in the gastric aspirate almost always indicates bleeding above the ligament of Treitz, whereas the absence of blood in the gastric aspirate, and the presence of blood in the stool, usually means bleeding distal to the fourth portion of the duodenum. A complete coagulation profile should be performed to rule out any coagulation abnormalities. Further diagnostic studies should include gastroduodenoscopy when blood is present in the stomach, colonoscopy, radiological contrast studies of the stomach, small bowel, and colon, and a pertechnetate scan to detect ectopic gastric mucosa. If all of the above studies are normal, then arteriography should be considered as a final diagnostic step. In addition, arteriography is often useful in the acute bleeding situation to detect the exact site of bleeding.

In 90% of infants and children with rectal bleeding, the hemorrhage usually abates spontaneously or a cause is found. If all of the diagnostic studies do not reveal a cause for the bleeding, then an exploratory laparotomy can be carried out as a last resort in the case of major gastrointestinal hemorrhage, even though, in most cases, the laparotomy will not reveal the source of bleeding [6]. The laparotomy should be considered, however, only after a significant period of watchful waiting.

REFERENCES

1. Apt L, Downey WS Jr: Melena neonatorum: the swallowed blood syndrome. J Pediatr 47:6, 1955
2. Berman WM, Holtzapple PG: Gastrointestinal hemorrhage. Pediatr Clin N Am 22:885, 1975
3. Boley SJ, Daum F: Rectal bleeding. In Ravitch MM (ed): Pediatric Surgery. Chicago, Yearbook, 1979
4. Grand RJ, Point W: Evaluation of gastrointestinal bleeding during adolescence. Postgrad Med 56:87, 1974
5. Jewett TC, Duszynski DO, Allen JE: The visualization of Meckel's diverticulum with 99m Tc-pertechnetate. Surgery 68:567, 1970
6. Shandling B: Laparotomy for rectal bleeding. Pediatrics 35:787, 1965
7. Sherman NJ, Clatworthy HW Jr: Gastrointestinal bleeding in neonates: a study of 94 cases. Surgery 62:614, 1967
8. Spencer R: Gastrointestinal hemorrhage in infancy and childhood: 467 cases. Surgery 55:718, 1964
9. Wagner, ML: Acute gastrointestinal bleeding in infants and children. Pediatr Ann 4:663, 1975

Jean-Pierre Raufmann, M.D.
William O. Dobbins, III, M.D.

Evaluation of Chronic Gastrointestinal Blood Loss

ABSTRACT

The patient who presents with recurrent iron deficiency anemia as the result of chronic or recurrent gastrointestinal (GI) bleeding either develops symptoms of chronic anemia or may be found to be anemic when an hematocrit is performed. Hemoccult slide tests of stools for blood is the most effective way to detect occult GI bleeding with an acceptably low rate of false positive tests. Diagnostic evaluation of patients with chronic GI bleeding requires a careful history and physical followed by routine laboratory tests. Studies should proceed from those of low cost and noninvasiveness to the more expensive and invasive ones. Sigmoidoscopy tends to be a high yield procedure and should be "routine" in chronic bleeders. Nasogastric aspiration may occasionally distinguish upper from lower intestinal bleeding. Air contrast barium enema followed by air contrast upper GI series and small bowel x-rays should be followed by colonoscopy and upper endoscopy, generally in this order until a likely bleeding source has been identified. Angiography is very helpful in identifying both bleeding and nonbleeding vascular lesions missed by the preceding diagnostic studies. If the bleeding source has not been identified by the thorough diagnostic approach outlined, it is not likely that exploratory laparotomy will be helpful. Surgery is often the appropriate therapeutic approach once a diagnosis has been established.

Gross gastrointestinal (GI) bleeding is frequently the most life-threatening patient problem to confront the physician. However, the patient with recurrent iron deficiency anemia, the result of chronic GI blood loss, often presents a

---

Jean-Pierre Raufmann, M.D.: Fellow in Gastroenterology, Department of Internal Medicine, University of Michigan Medical Center; William O. Dobbins, III, M.D.: Associate Chief of Staff for Research, Ann Arbor Veterans Administration Medical Center, and Professor of Internal Medicine, University of Michigan Medical Center, Ann Arbor, Michigan.

more challenging, if not as dramatic, problem. These patients may be referred to the gastroenterologist or general surgeon after multiple previous GI evaluations for source of blood loss have been negative. Occasionally, a patient will have had a presumably corrective surgical procedure, only to experience once again anemia secondary to chronic GI bleeding. Recognizing that the site of bleeding in up to 25% of chronically bleeding patients remains undetected [10, 18, 25, 28, 33], we have outlined a diagnostic approach that should significantly decrease this high failure rate.

PRESENTATION OF CHRONIC BLOOD LOSS

The initial manifestations vary. Fatigue and malaise due to anemia should prompt studies to establish the GI tract as the source of bleeding. A positive test for occult blood may be discovered upon routine physical examination. Another group of patients may present with a complaint referable to the bleeding lesion, e.g., heartburn in esophagitis or altered stool caliber and constipation in colonic malignancy.

A man or postmenopausal woman with a fall in hematocrit and a peripheral smear or indices demonstrating microcytosis and hypochromasia (evidence of iron deficiency) should be evaluated for GI blood loss. Repeated stool tests for occult blood may be negative since many GI lesions are known to bleed intermittently [21], including colon cancer. Occult GI bleeding, evidenced by the presence of blood in the stool on chemical analysis, may be discovered in a patient with a normal hematocrit and indices. In either case, it is necessary to determine the source of blood loss.

A major goal is to establish adequate criteria for determining the presence of blood in the stool. Three basic tests are available for this purpose, the guaiac test, Hematest tablets, and Hemoccult slides. Ostrow et al [21, 23] evaluated these 3 tests in patients given chromium-51 labeled red blood cells through a nasogastric tube. Using fecal losses of chromium-51 as a reference, guaiac and Hematest tablets gave very few false positive reactions, but did have a 50% false negative rate when the stool concentration of hemoglobin was less than 10 mg/g stool [21]. This higher degree of false negative reactions may be secondary to in transit loss of peroxidase activity as blood passes through the GI tract. Interpretation of Hematest tablet results shows substantial observer variability. However, agreement on the results of Hemoccult slide testing is almost 100% and the percentage of false negatives can be decreased significantly if the patient tests 2 different parts of a stool daily for 3 days, a total of 6 slides, while on a meat-free, high-bulk diet [21]. A meat-free diet (chicken and fish allowed) decreases the chance of exogenous blood yielding a false positive reaction. High bulk theoretically increases the contact of stool with the bleeding lesion. Using these precautions, one positive Hemoccult slide signifies GI blood loss and warrants further investigation. Patients should avoid vitamin C which may result in false negative Hemoccult slide tests as well as horseradish and turnips which contain peroxidase and result in false positive reactions. Oral iron therapy does not affect results. The stool concentration of hemoglobin normally ranges from 0 to 2 mg/g stool.

IMPORTANCE OF FINDING SOURCE OF CHRONIC BLEEDING

Colonic carcinoma remains the most common visceral malignancy in the United States, causing over 50,000 deaths annually. Each year 100,000 new cases of colonic cancer are discovered. Prognosis is clearly related to the extent of cancer at the time of diagnosis. Approximately 40% of colonic cancers are localized to the colon without lymph node metastases at the time of detection. Localized disease results in a 67% 10 year survival compared to 37% survival with nonlocalized disease [36]. In fact, in asymptomatic patients, who have localized disease (Duke's A and B), 15 year survival approaches 80% in some studies. Therefore, discovery of colonic cancer as an asymptomatic cause of chronic blood loss is of clear benefit to the patient.

Tracing occult blood loss to a colonic polyp, and removing that polyp, may prevent the later development of malignancy. Gilbertsen [13] has shown in an uncontrolled series that removal of polypoid lesions from the rectum decreased the incidence of subsequent rectal carcinoma by over 85% in 18,000 patients undergoing annual proctosigmoidoscopy. It has been estimated that approximately 5% of all adenomatous polyps are associated with colonic cancer. Of these, 75% are tubular and 10% are villous, the remainder being of the mixed tubulovillous variety. Villous adenomas, which are proportionally rarer than tubular adenomas, carry a far higher risk of associated malignancy. Invasive cancer has been reported in almost 50% of villous adenomas over 2 cm in diameter.

Finally, defining the source of chronic blood loss will often allow definitive therapy. An aggressive diagnostic approach and appropriate corrective treatment remove the requirement for chronic iron therapy and repeat laboratory determinations. Furthermore, should a benign lesion be detected as the blood source, therapeutic measures may be more rapidly instituted in the face of a major bleeding episode in the future.

CONDITIONS ASSOCIATED WITH CHRONIC BLOOD LOSS

The major causes of chronic GI blood loss are listed in Table 1.

Drugs

Several studies have shown that aspirin ingestion leads to chronic blood loss. Croft and Wood [8] showed that 70% of 226 subjects on aspirin therapy had positive tests for occult blood. In a study of 89 volunteers and 58 patients

Table 1
Major Causes of Chronic GI Blood Loss

Drugs (aspirin, alcohol, anticoagulants, indomethacin)

Genetic disorders (hereditary hemorrhagic telangiectasia, Peutz-Jehgers syndrome, familial polyposis, connective tissue disorders)

Bleeding diathesis (leukemia, polycythemia vera, hemophilia)

Colon cancer/polyps

Vascular malformations

Colitis (inflammatory bowel disease, ischemia, radiation injury)

Gastric cancer

Esophagitis/gastritis

Asymptomatic peptic ulcer disease

Miscellaneous (hemorrhoids, anal fissure, Meckel's diverticulum, swallowed blood, small bowel tumors, blue rubber bleb nevus syndrome, hookworm, hemobilia, factitious bleeding)

---

without GI disease, 108 (73%) lost more than 1.5 ml of blood per day during a 7 day period of ingestion of 2400 mg/day of aspirin. The mean control blood loss was 0.5 ml/day and increased to 4.7 ml/day during aspirin administration. Importantly, buffered aspirin or aspirin taken with food or milk was also associated with this degree of blood loss. The newer nonsteroidal antiinflammatory agents apparently do not have this effect on the GI tract [24]. Thus, it is prudent to discontinue all nonessential medications and alcohol when testing for occult blood.

Genetic Disorders

Under this listing we include the following: (1) Hereditary hemorrhagic telangiectasia (HHT, Rendu-Osler-Weber syndrome) which should be considered particularly in the patient with telangiectatic lesions of the face or body and recurrent epistaxis. A family history of this condition (autosomal dominant trait) may be helpful but is not always apparent as skipped generations have been reported. (2) Peutz-Jehgers syndrome of familial (autosomal dominant) gastrointestinal polyposis and mucocutaneous pigmentation. (3) Familial polyposis coli consisting of colonic polyposis with an almost universal (59% by age 30, 65% by age 40) incidence of colonic malignancy [36]. Cysts of the skin and osteomas may be seen in the Gardner's syndrome variant of familial colonic polyposis. The association of central nervous tumors with colonic polyposis is called Turcot's syndrome. (4) Connective tissue disorders, e.g., Ehlers-Danlos syndrome (skin hyperelasticity, blood vessel fragility, blue sclerae, and retinal angioid streaks transmitted as an autosomal dominant trait) and pseudoxanthoma elasticum (yellow-orange skin papules, laxity of skin in neck and axillae), and degenerative vascular changes associated with retinal angioid streaks.

Bleeding Diathesis

Various dysproteinemias, polycythemia vera, leukemias, and other lesions which cause defects in clotting function (hemophilia, Christmas disease) may be associated with occult blood loss [10].

Colon Cancer

Several risk factors may suggest colon cancer as the cause of chronic blood loss: (1) Age — usually the patients are forty years or older with a peak incidence in the seventies. (2) Polyps — there appears to be an increased rate of colonic carcinoma in patients with adenomatous (tubular) polyps of the colon greater than 1 cm in size. Villous adenomas are clearly associated with an increased risk of colonic cancer and familial polyposis coli invariably terminates with colonic cancer. (3) Previous colon cancer — there is a three-fold likelihood in developing an additional colonic cancer when compared to the normal population. (4) Genetic predisposition — i.e., a family history of colon cancer or a high number of malignancies involving any organ system increases the risk of colon cancer three-fold; (5) Inflammatory bowel disease — ulcerative colitis patients have 10-20 times the risk of developing colonic cancer when compared to the general population. The patient with total colitis is at risk of cancer developing only after 7-10 years of disease. Crohn's disease carries less risk of malignancy.

Colon Polyps

Bleeding from these lesions as well as the risk of malignant degeneration is discussed above.

Vascular Malformations

Vascular lesions of the GI tract appear to be uncommon in the population as a whole. However, in considering the source of chronic blood loss, especially in those patients over 60 years of age, they take on added significance [12]. Classifying vascular malformations of the GI tract is not easy and has resulted in a confusing terminology (angiodysplasia, ectasia, a-v malformation, telangiectasia). As far as diagnosis and treatment are concerned, the nomenclature is of little import, save to differentiate those patients with hereditary hemorrhagic telangiectasia [2]. The majority of lesions do not produce symptoms and the extent of bleeding can run the gamut from intermittent oozing to exsanguination [5].

Several features of vascular malformations are of major clinical importance: (1) The patients are usually older than 60 years of age. (2) Although apparently most common in the cecum and proximal ascending colon [3, 5, 15], these lesions can be found anywhere in the GI tract including the stomach [29] and duodenum [32]. (3) The lesions are usually less than 5 mm in size [2]. (4) They cannot be seen by contrast x-rays and require either angiography or endoscopy for diagnosis. Rarely, routine x-rays of the abdomen may reveal those vascular abnormalities that are prone to calcification, such as large hemangiomas. These calcifications, when present in an unusual location, should alert the physician to the possibility of a vascular malformation [39]. (5) There is a significant association between vascular lesions of the GI tract and aortic stenosis [9, 10, 29, 34, 35]. Of patients with aortic stenosis, 2.5% have GI bleeding related to vascular malformations. The pathogenesis of the vascular malformations in relationship to aortic stenosis remains unexplained. Baum et al [3] suggested that these lesions may be a response to mucosal ischemia secondary to chronic submucosal arteriovenous shunting resulting from increases in intraluminal pressure. Boley et al [5], postulated alternatively that these lesions formed secondary to chronic, intermittent obstruction of submucosal veins with resulting dilatation and tortuosity of the mucosal blood vessel. Although Boley found these lesions to be the commonest cause of major lower GI bleeding in the elderly, the frequency with which they cause chronic or occult GI bleeding in all age groups remains to be determined.

Colitis

Rarely, inflammatory bowel disease (ulcerative colitis and Crohn's disease) and ischemic colitis manifest themselves as chronic GI blood loss in an otherwise asymptomatic patient [10]. Especially in the elderly patient, a localized segment of ischemic colitis with predominantly mucosal involvement can cause low grade bleeding without other symptoms. Any low cardiac output state (congestive heart failure or cardiac arrhythmias) in an elderly patient with chronic low grade bleeding should suggest the possibility of ischemic colitis. Radiation enterocolitis can result in chronic blood loss many years after radiotherapy.

Gastric Cancer, Esophagitis/Gastritis, and Asymptomatic Peptic Ulcers

These lesions sometimes present with chronic GI blood loss and are detected by barium study of the upper GI tract or by endoscopy [10].

Miscellaneous Lesions

(1) Hemorrhoids or anal fissures should be apparent on the initial examination. (2) Meckel's diverticulum should be suspected in young patients with chronic GI blood loss [31]. Occult bleeding from this lesion is rare [4]. (3)

Swallowed blood, from nasopharyngeal tumors or pulmonary lesions may be overlooked initially. (4) Small bowel tumors. (5) Blue rubber bleb nevus syndrome is a very rare vascular cause of chronic blood loss [10]. (6) Hookworm infestation (*Ancylostoma duodenale, Necatur americanus*) can cause chronic blood loss without gross blood in the stool although occult blood is readily found [7]. (7) Factitious GI bleeding should be considered as a possibility in the patient with chronic or recurrent GI bleeding in whom repeated evaluations fail to reveal an obvious etiology for the blood loss.

LESIONS PROBABLY NOT ASSOCIATED WITH CHRONIC GI BLOOD LOSS

Hiatus Hernia

Hiatus hernia is a common disorder (present in over 30% of patients older than 55 years) that is usually an incidental finding. In the age of endoscopy, these lesions cannot usually be blamed for chronic GI blood loss. An associated esophagitis with clearly friable mucosa must be documented in order to implicate hiatus hernia in blood loss [10].

Diverticular Disease

Again, this is a common finding in older patients and should not be labeled the cause of chronic bleeding unless blood is clearly seen to be oozing from a diverticulum at the time of colonoscopy [6, 10, 27]. Previous assessments of right colonic diverticula as causes of chronic blood loss were probably in error, the blood loss being due to vascular malformations missed in the preangiography, preendoscopy era [5, 17, 20].

Varices

These have not been reported to cause chronic blood loss.

DIAGNOSTIC METHODS IN EVALUATING BLOOD LOSS

A listing of diagnostic methods for evaluation of chronic blood loss is given in Table 2.

History and Physical Examination

A history and a physical examination are the cornerstones of diagnosis and should detect the source of chronic blood loss in a majority of patients. General features such as weight loss or abdominal pain or more specific features such as

Table 2
Methods for Evaluating Chronic Blood Loss

Diagnostic Method	Discernible Lesion
History, physical examination	Drugs, genetic disorders, rectal cancer
Routine laboratory tests	Bleeding diathesis, hemobilia
Nasogastric aspirate	Gastric cancer, esophagitis, gastritis
Sigmoidoscopy	Hemorrhoids, anal fissure, colon cancer/polyps, colitis
Air contrast barium enema	Colon cancer/polyps
Colonoscopy	Vascular malformations, colon cancer/polyps, colitis
Air contrast GI series and small bowel x-rays	Peptic ulcers, gastric cancer, small bowel tumors/diverticuli
Upper endoscopy	Esophagitis/gastritis, peptic ulcer, gastric cancer, hemobilia, vascular malformations
Angiography	Vascular malformations, small bowel tumors/diverticuli, colon cancer, colitis

heartburn or familial history of GI bleeding will allow the physician to concentrate initial diagnostic efforts on the likeliest source of bleeding. The physical examination, including an adequate rectal examination, may detect an obvious abnormality such as a firm, non-tender cecal mass or a palpable polyp or mass in the rectum. Characteristic mucocutaneous pigmentation of Peutz-Jehgers syndrome or the facial telangiectasias of Rendu-Osler-Weber syndrome, although not excluding the presence of other lesions, should lead immediately to consideration of GI polyps or intestinal telangiectasias, respectively. The presence of aortic stenosis suggests the possibility of a vascular malformation. Clues that a good history and physical examination can yield are too exhaustive to be listed here.

Routine Laboratory Tests

Tests may be helpful in suggesting the source of bleeding and include liver chemistries (SGOT, SGPT, alkaline phosphatase, bilirubin), calcium, creatinine, and serum electrolyte studies. An elevated serum bilirubin and alkaline phosphatase may suggest a periampullary neoplasm while an elevated serum calcium may be secondary to a metastatic GI cancer just to cite a few examples. A coagulation profile (prothrombin time, platelet count) may give the first clue to the presence of a bleeding diathesis.

Nasogastric Aspirate

Passing a tube into the upper GI tract may help distinguish upper versus lower GI bleeding, allowing one to tailor the diagnostic work-up appropriately. Beware of misleading Hemoccult positive nasogastric aspirates secondary to trauma from the tube alone. Only the detection of gross blood or "coffee grounds" in the stomach can be taken as clear evidence of upper GI bleeding.

Sigmoidoscopy

Sigmoidoscopy is an extremely high yield procedure that should be part of any work-up for chronic GI blood loss. It has been estimated that approximately 55% of colon cancers occur within the range of the 25 cm sigmoidoscope [13, 14, 36]. The prevalence of polyps on proctosigmoidoscopy in patients over 40 years of age is reported to vary from 4.7 to 9.7% in several studies [13, 14]. Newer flexible fiberoptic sigmoidoscopes may be expected to improve on the detection of colonic polyps. However, patients with chronic blood loss should have a complete colonoscopic examination when sigmoidoscopy and barium enema have failed to reveal the site of bleeding. The longer reach of the flexible sigmoidoscope may be important in screening examinations, especially considering the apparent "left to right" shift in the location of colonic cancers noted in recent years [14, 37].

Air Contrast Barium Enema

This test is extremely important in the orderly evaluation of chronic blood loss. The standard barium enema without good air contrast techniques can miss up to 40% of polypoid lesions and 20% of carcinomas compared to a good air contrast barium enema [38]. An air contrast barium enema should precede colonoscopic examination. Colonoscopically blind areas in the rectosigmoid colon, the splenic and hepatic flexures, and in the cecum may be better examined by air contrast barium enema. Additionally, a good air contrast barium enema can guide the colonoscopist to areas of mucosal disease for biopsy or to areas where a diligent search for a lesion should be made.

Colonoscopy

This modality has become a necessity in the adequate evaluation of chronic blood loss. In the face of a positive barium enema, colonoscopy may be used to biopsy the lesion seen or, if a polyp is seen, perform the curative polypectomy. In the event of a negative barium enema, colonoscopy is used to seek a missed lesion. Experienced colonoscopists reach the splenic flexure in approximately 90%, the hepatic flexure in 85% and the cecum in 80% of patients examined [10]. Morbidity for this procedure should be less than 0.5% [36]. Colonoscopy detects large numbers of small polyps (less than 1.0 cm) not seen on, barium enema and modest numbers of polyps greater than 1.0 cm when missed by barium enema (Table 3). Further, in the same study colonoscopy uncovered 2 colon cancers totally missed on barium enema, as well as excluding 9 cancers falsely implicated by barium enema [38]. Hunt et al [17] studied 868 patients with either anemia or rectal bleeding. In 652 patients with rectal bleeding and negative barium enema and sigmoidoscopic studies, a causative lesion was found at colonoscopy in 295 patients (45%) (66 cancers, 136 polyps, and 61 cases of inflammatory bowel disease). In 157 patients with rectal bleeding and diverticular disease on barium enema, colonoscopy revealed 15 cancers and 63 additional lesions. Finally, in 59 patients with recurrent anemia who had negative barium enema/upper GI series, and upper endoscopy, colonoscopy revealed 8 cancers (14%) and 20 unspecified disorders. Vascular malformations, which are not seen on air contrast barium enema, can be readily seen by the diligent colonoscopist. At least one group [30], has treated these lesions by colonoscopic electrocoagulation with limited success. Colonoscopic biopsies can establish the diagnosis of cancer and in the case of chronic ulcerative colitis with dysplastic changes, may even predict the presence of carcinoma elsewhere in the colon [36].

Air Contrast GI Series and Small Bowel X-Rays

If both the barium enema and colonoscopy have been negative, attention should then be directed to the upper GI tract in order to make sure a lesion has not been missed there. Some physicians might argue against doing a GI series because we are likely to recommend gastroscopy as well. However, we feel that small bowel x-rays need to be done to detect tumors or diverticuli and the GI series can be useful in ruling out esophageal diverticuli or webs which might cause difficulty in passing the endoscope, and directing endoscopic examination to suspicious areas of the upper GI tract.

Table 3
Radiographically Missed Polyps Seen With Colonoscopy

Diameter (cm)	X-Ray Diagnosed	Colonoscopy Diagnosed
Less than 1.0	36	133
1.0–1.9	84	101
2.0–2.9	43	47
More than 3.0	3	3
Total – greater than 1.0	130	151

Adapted from Wolff et al [38].

Upper Endoscopy

Endoscopy is necessary to detect mucosal lesions (esophagitis, gastritis) and vascular malformations which sometimes cause chronic blood loss. In addition, a fair number of lesions may be missed on air contrast GI series. In one study of 226 consecutive patients, upper endoscopy detected 7 gastric ulcers, 2 polyps, 3 duodenal ulcers, and 1 esophageal carcinoma that were missed with air contrast upper GI series [40]. In other words, 5% of patients had an endoscopically detected lesion that was missed radiographically. Caution should be used in ascribing chronic blood loss to esophagitis or gastritis unless bleeding is actually seen at the time of endoscopy.

Angiography

It is likely that many cases of chronic GI bleeding reported in older series that escaped diagnosis despite extensive evaluation would have benefited from angiography. Undoubtedly many of the undiagnosed patients were bleeding from vascular malformations. The reason for this relates to the difficulty in detecting vascular lesions at the time of surgical exploration or at necropsy. Baum and coworkers [3] did much of the early work which established vascular malformations as a significant cause of acute and chronic bleeding. They were even able to define blood vessels as small as 50 to 90 microns by serial magnification of visceral angiography. Alfidi et al [1], performed angiography in 12 chronic bleeders who had remained undiagnosed despite adequate radiographic and endoscopic studies. All 12 patients had vascular lesions of the bowel. It is not likely that evidence of actual bleeding can be seen in chronic bleeders by this technique because this would assume a bleeding rate of at least 0.5 cc/min. Nevertheless, in one study of 88 patients who were not actively bleeding at the time of angiography, Sheedy et al [32] were able to establish a likely source of bleeding in 41 (45%). These sources included 22 vascular malformations, 5 GI neoplasms, 4 visceral artery aneurysms, 3 GI polyps, 2 Meckel's diverticula, 2 cases of gastritis and 1 case each of regional enteritis, ileal ulcer, and pancreatic islet cell tumor. Half of the lesions were located in the cecum or ascending colon.

Miscellaneous

In this category we place diagnostic techniques which are either of unproven benefit or have such a high false negative rate that their use is severely limited: (1) Colonic lavage for cytology requires an expert cytologist and is of value only when obtained from gross lesions or where the colonoscopist cannot reach radiologically suspicious areas (e.g. strictures, fixation of bowel secondary to radiation, adhesions or diverticulosis). (2) Carcinoembryonic antigen is of no value in the diagnosis of carcinoma but may be helpful following resection of colonic cancer, particularly when recurrence is suspected and early postoperative levels are known [36]. (3) Meckel's scans using radioactive technetium, which concentrates in ectopic gastric mucosa, may suggest presence of Meckel's diverticuli as a source of chronic blood loss in the adolescent and young adult. The high rate of false positive and negative results detracts from the usefulness of this procedure [4, 11]. (4) Fluorescein string tests and the injection of chromium labeled red blood cells with multilevel GI aspiration have not been extensively tested, are difficult to perform and may give ambiguous or frankly misleading results [10]. (5) Scanning following injection of technetium-labeled autologous erythrocytes may identify highly vascular lesions of the gastrointestinal tract and deserves further clinical evaluation [16].

Laparotomy

Laparotomy without a clearly defined preoperative objective does not help either to diagnose or treat chronic GI bleeding in most cases [10, 22, 26]. Retzlaff et al [25] reviewed 100 chronic GI bleeders who underwent exploratory laparotomy. In 70%, no lesion was found that could definitely account for the bleeding. Over half of these patients continued to bleed after operation. The surgeon usually cannot feel a polyp in the small intestine, an ectasia in the colon, or a lesion causing hemobilia, all of which may be the cause of bleeding missed by an exhaustive diagnostic investigation. The presence of intraabdominal adhesions from prior laparotomy or previous infections may make a thorough examination of the bowel difficult or impossible. Inability to identify the site of bleeding at laparotomy has at times led to blind bowel resection, which often proves to be therapeutically ineffective as did blind subtotal gastrectomy, a procedure frequently practiced just 20 years ago. In one study of 22 patients with angiographically and pathologically proven vascular malformations, 6 of the 16 (37%) who underwent right hemicolectomy still had recurrent melena, rectal bleeding, or chronic iron deficiency following the presumably curative surgical procedure [19]. Therefore, when a lesion that is not actively bleeding is identified and removed surgically, there is a strong possibility that the operation will not be curative.

DIAGNOSTIC APPROACH TO THE CHRONICALLY BLEEDING PATIENT

Diagnostic studies should proceed from those of low cost and low invasiveness to the more expensive and invasive (Fig. 1). Although this sequence should be followed in most patients with chronic gastrointestinal blood loss and often yields a diagnosis, clinical judgement should always dictate the order in which testing should be done. For example, the patient with negative air contrast x-rays and sigmoidoscopy who returns passing gross blood per rectum should probably have immediate angiography, which is likely to detect the bleeding site when the bleeding rate is greater than 0.5 cc/min. Finding the

CHRONIC GASTROINTESTINAL BLOOD LOSS

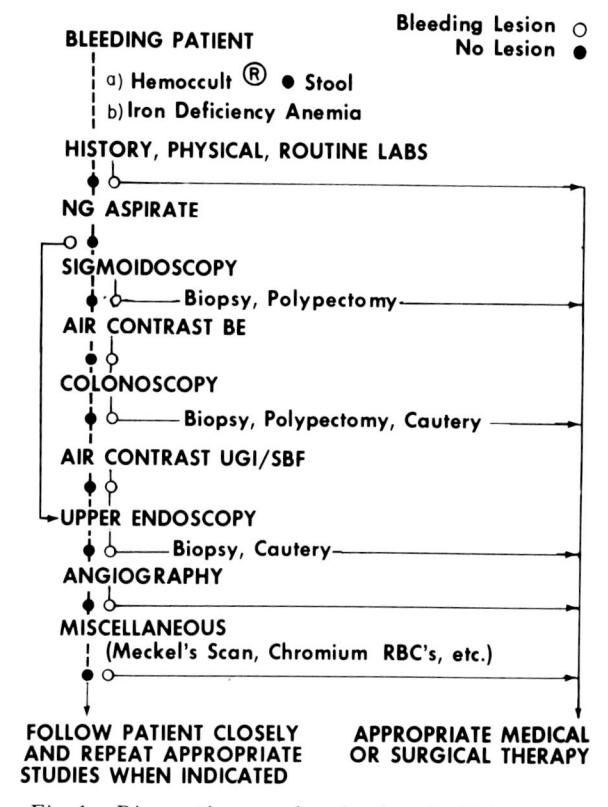

```
                                    Bleeding Lesion ○
         BLEEDING PATIENT              No Lesion    ●
           a) Hemoccult ®  ● Stool
           b) Iron Deficiency Anemia
         HISTORY, PHYSICAL, ROUTINE LABS
         NG ASPIRATE
         SIGMOIDOSCOPY
              ─── Biopsy, Polypectomy ───
         AIR CONTRAST BE
         COLONOSCOPY
              ─── Biopsy, Polypectomy, Cautery ───
         AIR CONTRAST UGI/SBF
         UPPER ENDOSCOPY
              ─── Biopsy, Cautery ───
         ANGIOGRAPHY
         MISCELLANEOUS
           (Meckel's Scan, Chromium RBC's, etc.)

   FOLLOW PATIENT CLOSELY         APPROPRIATE MEDICAL
   AND REPEAT APPROPRIATE         OR SURGICAL THERAPY
   STUDIES WHEN INDICATED
```

Fig. 1. Diagnostic procedure in chronic GI bleeding.

bleeding site in these patients is often an art, timing is critical, and the procedure requires an expert angiographer. For this reason, patients with chronic gastrointestinal blood loss of unknown etiology should be evaluated at a tertiary medical center which has expert endoscopy and radiology techniques readily available. We emphasize that more than one possible bleeding lesion may exist in the same patient. This is especially true in the population over 60 years of age. For example, the small cecal carcinoma should not be overlooked when a nonbleeding vascular malformation is found in the transverse colon. Studies should therefore be as complete as possible in each case, unless bleeding can definitely be ascribed to the lesion at hand.

During the diagnostic evaluation, precautions should be taken to ensure that the clinical status of the patient does not deteriorate. Hematocrits and other clinical indices should be followed so that an adequate blood volume is maintained. Multiple enemas, laxatives and liquid diets can clearly take their toll on patient nutrition. Precautions should be taken not to weaken the patient further who may be already anemic and debilitated from his/her underlying disease. Tests should be scheduled as efficiently and humanely as possible so as not to add to the misery of chronic illness, especially in elderly patients. Patience is a virtue, and a calm unhurried approach to these patients without resort to blind laparotomy or other unproven diagnostic modalities should reveal the bleeding site without adding further risks to the patient.

REFERENCES

1. Alfidi RF, Esselstyn CD, Tarar R, et al: Recognition and angio-surgical detection of arteriovenous malformations of the bowel. Ann Surg 174:573, 1971
2. Baer JW, Ryan S: Analysis of cecal vasculature in the search for vascular malformations. Am J Roentgenol 126:394, 1976
3. Baum S, Nusbaum M, Blakemore WS: The preoperative radiographic demonstration of intra-abdominal bleeding from undetermined sites by percutaneous selective celiac and superior mesenteric arteriography. Surgery 58:797, 1965
4. Berquist TH, Nolan NG, Adson MA, et.al.: Diagnosis of Meckel's diverticulum by radioisotope scanning. Mayo Clin Proc 48:98, 1973
5. Boley SJ, Sammartano R, Adams A, et al: On the nature and etiology of vascular ectasias of the colon. Gastroenterology 72:650, 1977
6. Broders CW: Bleeding from diverticula of the colon. Surg Clin N Am 52:315, 1972
7. Brown HW: Basic Clinical Parasitology (ed. 3). New York, Appleton-Century-Crofts, 1969, pp 121-129
8. Croft DN, Wood PHN: Gastric mucosa and susceptibility to occult gastrointestinal bleeding caused by aspirin. Br Med J 1:137, 1967
9. Cody MC, O'Donovan PB, Hughes RW Jr: Idiopathic gastrointestinal bleeding and aortic stenosis. Am J Dig Dis 19:393, 1974
10. Douvres PA, Glass GBJ: Cryptogenic gastrointestinal bleeding. In Jerzy GBJ (ed): Progress in Gastroenterology, Vol II. New York, Grune and Stratton, 1970, pp 466-493
11. Eisenberg D, Sherwood CE: Bleeding Meckel's diverticulum diagnosed by arteriography and radioisotope imaging. Am J Dig Dis 20:573, 1975
12. Galloway SJ: Vascular malformations of the right colon as a cause of bleeding in patients with aortic stenosis. Radiology 113:11, 1974
13. Gilbertsen VA: Proctosigmoidoscopy and polypectomy in reducing the incidence of rectal cancer. Cancer 34:936, 1974
14. Gilbertsen VA, Nelms JM: The prevention of invasive cancer of the rectum. Cancer 41:1137, 1978
15. Hagihara PF, Chuang VP, Griffin WO: Arteriovenous malformations of the colon. Am J Surg 133:681, 1977
16. Heyman S: Localization of bleeding small intestinal lesions using scanning techniques. Surgery 85:372, 1979

17. Hunt RH, Swarbrick ET, Teague RH, et al: Colonoscopy for unexplained rectal bleeding. (Abstr) Gastroenterology 76:1158, 1979
18. Jones FA, Read AE, Stubbe JL: Alimentary bleeding of obscure origin. Br Med J 2:1138, 1959
19. Meyer CT, Sheagren DG, Galloway S, et al: The incidence of recurrent bleeding following right hemicolectomy for colonic arteriovenous malformations (AVM's). (Abstr) Gastroenterology 76:1202, 1979
20. Meyers MA, Volberg F, Katzen B, et al: The angioarchitecture of colonic diverticula. Radiology 108:249, 1973
21. Morris DW, Hansell JR, Ostrow D, et al: Reliability of chemical tests for fecal occult blood in hospitalized patients. Am J Dig Dis 21:845, 1976
22. Moore RH: Massive melena. Ann Surg 136:167, 1952
23. Ostrow JD, Mulvaney CA, Hansell JR, et al: Sensitivity and reproductivity of chemical tests for fecal occult blood with an emphasis on false-positive reactions. Am J Dig Dis 18:930, 1973
24. Pemberton RE, Stand LJ: A review of upper gastrointestinal effect of the newer nonsteroidal anti-inflammatory agents. Dig Dis Sci 24:53, 1979
25. Retzlaff JA, Hagedorn AB, Bartholomew LG: Abdominal exploration for gastrointestinal bleeding of obscure origin. JAMA 177:104, 1961
26. Reuter SR, Bookstein JJ: Angiographic localization of gastrointestinal bleeding. Gastroenterology 54:876, 1968
27. Rigg BM, Ewing MR: Current attitudes on diverticulitis with particular reference to colonic bleeding. Arch Surg 92:321, 1966
28. Rives JD, Emmet RO: Melena: A survey of 206 cases. Am J Surg 20:458, 1954
29. Robertson RH, Zander RE, Colcher H, et al: Gastric telangiectasia associated with recurrent major gastrointestinal bleeding in patients with aortic valve disease. (Abstr) Gastroenterology 76:1227, 1979
30. Rogers BHG, Adler F: Hemangiomas of the cecum. Gastroenterology 71:1079, 1976
31. Rutherford RB, Akers DR: Meckel's diverticulum. Surgery 59:618, 1966
32. Sheedy PF, Fulton RE, Atwell DT: Angiographic evaluation of patients with chronic gastrointestinal bleeding. Am J Roentgenol 132:338, 1975
33. Stone HB: Large melena of obscure origin. Ann Surg 120:582, 1944
34. Weaver GA, Alpern HD, David JS, et al: Gastrointestinal angiodysplasia associated with aortic valve disease: Part of a spectrum of angiodysplasia of the gut. Gastroenterology 77:1, 1979
35. Williams RC: Aortic stenosis and unexplained gastrointestinal bleeding. Arch Int Med 108:859, 1961
36. Winawer SJ, Sherlock P, Schottenfeld D, et al: Screening for colon cancer. Gastroenterology 70:783, 1976
37. Winawer SJ, Leidner SD, Boyle C, et al: Comparison of flexible sigmoidoscopy with other diagnostic techniques in the diagnosis of rectocolon neoplasia. Dig Dis Sci 24:277, 1979
38. Wolff WI, Shinya H, Geffen A, et al: Comparison of colonoscopy and the contrast enema in five hundred patients with colorectal disease. Am J Surg 129:181, 1975

39. Wolff WI, Grossman MB, Shinya H: Angiodysplasia of the colon: Diagnosis and treatment. Gastroenterology 72:329, 1977
40. Wu WC, Ott DJ, Shiflett DW, et al: Is UGI series obsolete? (Abstr) Gastroenterology 76:1271, 1979

Thomas L. Dent, M.D.

Diagnostic Endoscopy

ABSTRACT

The recent development of flexible fiberoptic gastroscopes and colonoscopes has permitted the direct visualization and precise identification of bleeding lesions of the entire upper gastrointestinal tract and of the lower gastrointestinal tract from the terminal ileum to the anus. A vigorous diagnostic approach to the bleeding patient is advocated. Experienced endoscopists with a modern, well-equipped endoscopic unit will provide a precise diagnosis of over 90% of actively bleeding upper gastrointestinal lesions and 40% of the intermittently bleeding lower gastrointestinal lesions. Complications of endoscopy are rare. Careful timing of the endoscopic examination and intelligent selection of patients to be examined will minimize the hazards of the procedure and maximize the diagnostic yield.

Flexible fiberoptic endoscopy has revolutionized the evaluation of patients suffering from gastrointestinal hemorrhage. Only 15 years ago, direct visualization of the stomach, duodenum, and colon was impossible. Patients with gastrointestinal hemorrhage had to be treated on the basis of a clinical impression aided by imprecise barium radiologic studies which resulted in a diagnosis as often incorrect as it was correct [3, 4, 27]. Exploratory laparotomy, subtotal colectomy, and "blind" gastrectomy, with the surgeon having little or no idea of the true source of the hemorrhage, were performed frequently. The application of fiberoptics to visual inspection of the gastrointestinal tract began in 1958 [12], was refined and improved during the 1960's, and reached broad clinical use in the early 1970's [34]. Bleeding lesions of the gastrointestinal tract can now be directly visualized and treatment can be based on a precise diagnosis. Flexible fiberoptic endoscopes (aided in the more difficult cases by visceral arteriography whose development paralleled that of endoscopy) have practically eliminated the need for barium x-ray studies. Exploratory laparotomy and blind intestinal resection for bleeding are now extremely rare events.

Thomas L. Dent, M.D.: Professor of Surgery, Chief, Division of Gastrointestinal Surgery, Section of General Surgery, University of Michigan Medical Center, Ann Arbor, Michigan.

I will discuss endoscopy in the evaluation of patients with gastrointestinal hemorrhage as it is used at the University of Michigan in 1980. Present endoscopic techniques and technology allow the rapid, precise, and safe evaluation of patients with active, recent, or chronic bleeding lesions of the upper gastrointestinal tract, while endoscopic evaluation of the colon is best performed for patients whose bleeding is recent or chronic, but not acute.

UPPER GASTROINTESTINAL ENDOSCOPY

Using an endoscope, the entire mucosal surface of the upper gastrointestinal tract from the mouth to the duodenal-jejunal junction can be directly visualized and mucosal biopsies can be taken when indicated. Recent advances in instrumentation and techniques now permit rapid, accurate, and relatively safe inspection to determine the source and nature of bleeding lesions. The timing of the examination is important in order to minimize the risk of the examination to the patient and to maximize the diagnostic yield. Complications do occur and must be recognized and treated promptly. It is hoped that an improvement in mortality and morbidity of patients suffering from gastrointestinal hemorrhage will follow the improvement in diagnostic accuracy that endoscopy has produced, although this has yet to be demonstrated [8].

Facilities and Equipment

Most early or urgent endoscopy should be performed in the regular endoscopy unit where all of the equipment is available. It is occasionally necessary to perform upper gastrointestinal endoscopy in the intensive care unit because the patient cannot be moved or, rarely, in the operating room because of the need for immediate operation. Resuscitation equipment and personnel experienced in its use should be immediately available. We have been impressed that the advantages of the new, thin, endviewing panendoscopes (greater tip deflection, less need for sedation, less possibility of traumatizing varices [19]) outweigh their disadvantages (smaller field of vision, need for higher power illumination, easily blocked suction port) and we routinely use these to examine most patients with upper gastrointestinal hemorrhage. Only if they fail, or if the bleeding is massive do we resort to the standard 1.5 cm diameter endoscopes. The procedure should be performed or directly supervised by an experienced endoscopist. Endoscopic examination of a patient bleeding acutely from the upper gastrointestinal tract can be difficult, and interpretation of what is seen through the endoscope will determine further diagnosis and therapy for a patient whose life is unquestionably in great danger [33].

Advances in endoscopic equipment are permitting more rapid, more accurate, more comfortable, and safer evaluation of bleeding patients.

Technique

An exact description of the technical details of performing upper gastrointestinal panendoscopy is outside the scope of this paper, but several important principles of the procedure should be mentioned.

Usually patients with acute upper gastrointestinal hemorrhage can be examined without any sedation. They are generally tired and cooperative. If sedation is required, one should use as little as possible. Topical anesthetics are avoided in order to maintain the cough reflex and prevent aspiration. The newer pencil-thin panendoscopes have allowed us to examine patients more comfortably and efficiently, and sedation is rarely required [19].

The examination is performed in the lateral decubitus position to allow rapid evacuation of blood and debris from the mouth and oropharynx if vomiting occurs. The left lateral position is used initially because blood and debris will pool in the fundus, the least likely source of hemorrhage, and it allows rapid visualization of the esophagus, the gastric cardia, body and antrum, and the entire duodenum. Even if a patient was hemorrhaging massively, initial gastric lavage with a large tube and rapid passage of the endoscope through the esophagus, stomach, and duodenum combined with rapid air insufflation of these organs has allowed visualization of the bleeding lesions before they were obscured by blood. It is important to try to see all areas of the upper gastrointestinal tract because multiple lesions are not uncommon [4].

The examination should be performed slowly enough to establish a firm diagnosis and rapidly enough to minimize the discomfort and dangers of the procedure. It should rarely exceed 15 min.

Accuracy

For many years, patients with upper gastrointestinal hemorrhage were treated on the basis of a clinical diagnosis made from a history and physical examination, sometimes supported by the results of a barium meal x-ray examination. Unfortunately, a clinical diagnosis is wrong at least 50% of the time [3, 4, 27]. A barium study of the upper gastrointestinal tract is indirect and inaccurate, missing 40% of gastric ulcers and carcinomas [3], and is useless in identifying mucosal lesions such as gastritis and esophagitis.

It it logical that once the entire mucosal surface of the upper gastrointestinal tract could be visualized directly by the flexible fiberoptic panendoscope, the diagnostic accuracy of this method would approach 100%. Many recently reported series of bleeding patients evaluated with endoscopy do, in fact, demonstrate a diagnostic accuracy in excess of 90% [4, 14, 27]. Cotton, et al [4] showed that of all patients admitted with hematemesis or melena whose bleeding was later proven to have come from the upper gastrointestinal tract, the exact cause and site of the bleeding was identified by endoscopy in 96%.

When compared with barium upper gastrointestinal radiography in prospective, randomized studies, endoscopy is a clearly superior diagnostic study [7, 16, 20]. Even radiologists agree that endoscopy is the diagnostic procedure of choice in the initial evaluation of patients with upper gastrointestinal hemorrhage [2, 27]. For a patient who has had prior gastric surgery, endoscopy has an even greater advantage over barium radiologic studies [22]. Marginal ulcers, as well as gastritis and esophagitis, can be seen despite the postsurgical deformity of the upper gastrointestinal tract. Even a patient with gastrointestinal hemorrhage in the early postoperative period may be examined safely and accurately by a careful, experienced endoscopist.

Visceral arteriography has a comparable diagnostic accuracy to endoscopy only if the lesion is bleeding massively at the time of the study [19]. Since most patients with upper gastrointestinal hemorrhage bleed intermittently and also because of the additional time, expense, personnel commitment, and potential complications associated with arteriography, endoscopy should be the initial diagnostic study. Arteriography is reserved for endoscopic failures, most of which are due to excessive hemorrhage obscuring the view or, rarely, when endoscopy is contraindicated.

It has been well demonstrated that many patients have multiple potential bleeding sites, and that only direct visualization can determine which lesion is bleeding or has recently bled. Cotton et al [4] reported a 15.4% incidence of multiple potential bleeding sites, and pointed out that 26% of his patients with duodenal ulcers were actually bleeding from sites other than the ulcer. Foster, et al [9] has described signs associated with lesions (fresh bleeding, adherent clot, or a protruding vessel) which not only localize the bleeding site but predict the need for urgent surgical therapy. Several authors [5, 31, 32] have suggested that when patients with known portal hypertension and esophagogastric varices develop gastrointestinal hemorrhage, 50% or fewer will be bleeding from the varices, and that most will be bleeding from other lesions (e.g., gastritis, ulcers). Our experience, however, is different and agrees with that of Mitchell and Jewell [19] who found that under early endoscopy 88% of such patients were bleeding from their varices.

For patients with active, or recently active, massive upper gastrointestinal hemorrhage, endoscopy is the most accurate diagnostic study and should be performed before any other study. For patients with chronic upper gastrointestinal hemorrhage, the more conventional barium studies should be employed first, and endoscopy used only if these are negative.

Timing

Upper gastrointestinal panendoscopy is the first diagnostic study performed for patients with upper gastrointestinal hemorrhage, but should not be performed until the bleeding patient has been resuscitated and a rapid history and physical examination have been completed.

First, a nasogastric tube is passed and the stomach is aspirated if there has been recent (within previous 48 hours) massive gastrointestinal hemorrhage. If there is blood or guaiac-positive material in the stomach or a history of hematemesis, upper gastrointestinal endoscopy is the logical study. We prefer to wait a few hours (early or urgent endoscopy as opposed to emergent endoscopy), if possible, for several reasons. The acute bleeding frequently slows or stops and endoscopic visualization of the upper gastrointestinal tract is then easier, the patient is more stable following adequate fluid resuscitation, and the presence of an experienced, senior endoscopist for this frequently demanding examination is assured [33]. One should not delay longer than 24-48 hours because the diagnostic accuracy of endoscopy is significantly decreased after this time [18, 19], and prolongs the time needed for diagnosis if rebleeding occurs before endoscopy can be performed. If the bleeding is truly massive and an urgent operation is being considered, emergent endoscopy is performed. Sometimes this examination is best performed in the operating room following the placement of a cuffed endotracheal tube to prevent aspiration of stomach contents.

If the nasogastric tube returns clear bile from a patient who is *unquestionably* actively bleeding from the gastrointestinal tract, a lower gastrointestinal evaluation (sigmoidoscopy, arteriography, barium enema) is begun immediately. If, however, the gastric aspirate contains no blood but the patient may have ceased bleeding temporarily, we feel strongly that an urgent upper gastrointestinal endoscopy should precede any lower gastrointestinal evaluation for several reasons. The great majority of lesions of the gastrointestinal tract which bleed massively are in the upper tract. Symptoms suggestive of lower gastrointestinal bleeding (red blood per rectum) are frequently upper gastrointestinal in origin. If a lesion of the upper gastrointestinal tract is diagnosed, treatment can begin immediately. If a lesion is absent, little time has been lost, and a time-consuming, less accurate lower gastrointestinal evaluation can begin.

For patients with chronic or intermittent gastrointestinal hemorrhage, endoscopy is reserved until and if the conventional barium studies are unrewarding. There is no need to subject a patient even to the mild discomfort and minor risk of endoscopy if a barium study can demonstrate the lesion.

Causes of Bleeding

Now that highly accurate and specific diagnoses of both the site and nature of bleeding lesions of the upper gastrointestinal tract can be made using flexible fiberoptic endoscopy, large series of bleeding patients have been published (Table 1). It is interesting to note the wide range in the frequency of each diagnosis. Esophageal varices account for only 2% of the bleeding lesions in one series but 16% in another. Esophagitis ranges from 0 to 8%, peptic ulcer from 24 to 50%, mucosal erosions from 17 to 45%, and Mallory-Weiss tear from 1 to 15% [17] in the various series. This variability has several possible explanations.

Table 1
Incidence of Diagnoses in Patients With
Upper Gastrointestinal Hemorrhage

	Cotton (1973) [4]	Katz (1976) [15]	Himal (1978) [11]	Iglesias (1979) [14]
Number of patients	208	1429	334	789
Esophagogastric varices	2%	16%	6%	4%
Mallory-Weiss tears	1%	3%	1%	0.8%
Peptic ulcer	50%	25%	62%	24%
Mucosal erosions	17%	44%	18%	45%

The most obvious is variation in patient population. Institutions providing secondary and tertiary care see fewer patients with acute alcoholic gastritis and more with bleeding esophageal varices. Bleeding esophagitis is more common in hospitals, like our own, with immunosuppressed patients following renal transplantation. Less obvious, but more interesting reasons for this variability were pointed out by Graham and Davis [10] when they demonstrated that the incidence of bleeding from acute mucosal lesions (gastritis, duodenitis, and esophagitis) was only 9% in patients presenting to the hospital because of acute major gastrointestinal bleeding, but was 28% in patients whose major bleeding began after being hospitalized for other diseases. They also pointed out that some endoscopic series have not included the truly massive bleeder because endoscopy was not performed or failed, thereby excluding the patients more likely to have gastric or duodenal ulcers from the incidence calculations.

Finally, enthusiasm of endoscopists seems to play a role in the variability of the diagnoses. Most series [4, 14, 15] report an incidence of Mallory-Weiss tears of 0.8 to 2%. A report by Knauer [17] described acute hemorrhage due to Mallory-Weiss tears in 11% of 528 patients with upper gastrointestinal hemorrhage. However, 26% of these 58 patients with an endoscopic diagnosis of Mallory-Weiss tears had a history of neither vomiting nor retching, 20% had esophagogastric varices, 20% had acute esophagitis, and although the average blood loss was 3.4 units, only 3 patients required surgical therapy. It would seem that at least some of these patients would not fit the classical definition of Mallory-Weiss hemorrhage.

Complications and Contraindications

Most of the major series of endoscopic evaluations of gastrointestinal hemorrhage report extremely low complication rates or do not mention the problem at all. A survey of the British Society for Digestive Endoscopy [24] revealed 77 (0.3%) complications and 6 (0.03%) deaths in 23,563 diagnostic examinations, but only 25% were performed with modern forward-viewing panendoscopes. A survey of the American Society for Gastrointestinal Endoscopy [25] reported 275 (0.1%) complications and 10 (0.004%) deaths in 211,410 examinations. Neither of these surveys separated out the complication for emergent or urgent endoscopy which is certainly higher than for elective endoscopy. Stadelman [26] reported 92 serious complications in 99,426 examinations. At least 15 of these complications occurred during emergent examinations, which probably constituted only 5% of the total. A large, prospective survey of endoscopy for patients bleeding from the gastrointestinal tract is now being tabulated by the Research Committee of the American Society for Gastrointestinal Endoscopy. This should provide more precise information about the complications of urgent endoscopy for bleeding.

In general, there are several groups of complications which can occur as a result of diagnostic endoscopy: misleading diagnosis, medication reactions, perforation, pulmonary aspiration, cardiac arrhythmias, hemorrhage, and miscellaneous [24]. Although not, strictly speaking, a complication, a misleading diagnosis can have significant effect upon the subsequent treatment of the bleeding patient. It can delay therapy or initiate inappropriate therapy. Obviously, the procedure should be performed by experienced endoscopists, but endoscopy, despite its accuracy, is just another diagnostic test. And like any test, if the results obtained do not fit with the overall clinical picture, the test results must be ignored or the test repeated.

Medication reactions, both to the topical anesthetic and to intravenous sedation can occur. We do not use topical anesthetics for emergency endoscopy, and try to use as little intravenous sedation as possible. We routinely use the newer pencil-thin panendoscopes which are much more comfortable for patients had have markedly decreased the need for sedation.

Perforation of the esophagus, stomach, and duodenum can occur and usually is the result of "blind" passage of the endoscope when no lumen can be seen. Deep ulcers can perforate with air insufflation of the upper gastrointestinal tract. Although immediate operation is usually required for acute perforation, this complication can sometimes be successfully treated nonoperatively [24].

Pulmonary aspiration and eventual pneumonia is probably more common following urgent or emergent endoscopy than is generally realized or reported. The incidence of aspiration can be minimized by the avoidance, whenever possible, of topical anesthetics and intravenous sedation.

Cardiovascular complications occur and because routine cardiac monitoring is not usually employed, minor arrhythmias are missed [21], but emergency drugs and resuscitation equipment must be available when endoscopy is performed.

Bleeding undoubtedly can be restarted by manipulation of the clot or lesion by the endoscope or biopsy instrument. Although, theoretically, hemorrhage from esophagogastric varices can be restarted by endoscopic trauma, this is very unusual in our experience and is further minimized by the newer pencil-thin instruments [19].

Miscellaneous complications have been reported and include endoscope impaction, swallowed mouthguard, small bowel volvulus, and subparotid swelling.

In our view, there are no absolute contraindications to upper gastrointestinal endoscopy in the evaluation of gastrointestinal hemorrhage just as there are no absolute contraindications to operative therapy of the bleeding patient. There are, however, three relative contraindications: signs or symptoms of perforation of the gastrointestinal tract, recent myocardial infarction, and severe cardiac arrhythmia. Several other situations require special precautions during the endoscopy but are not contraindications to the examination: exsanguinating hemorrhage, extremely uncooperative patient, comatose patient, recent postoperative patient, and acute viral hepatitis.

Usefulness

Flexible fiberoptic upper gastrointestinal panendoscopy is the most rapid and reliable diagnostic examination presently at our disposal in the evaluation of upper gastrointestinal hemorrhage. It has been enthusiastically accepted by clinicians frustrated by previously inaccurate diagnostic methods. In a recent survey, endoscopy was the first specific investigation for bleeding requested in 82% of hospitals [23]. Although there are hazards in its application, these can be minimized by its careful and appropriate use in patients with acute and chronic hemorrhage of the gastrointestinal tract.

LOWER GASTROINTESTINAL ENDOSCOPY

Endoscopy of the lower gastrointestinal tract can be useful in the diagnosis of patients with gastrointestinal hemorrhage. It should be remembered, however, that upper gastrointestinal hemorrhage occurs much more frequently (and can simulate lower gastrointestinal hemorrhage) and is limited to the upper 3 feet of the gastrointestinal tract. Lower gastrointestinal hemorrhage, conversely, is uncommon and can occur over the distal 35 feet of the gastrointestinal tract. With present endoscopes, only the colon and terminal ileum can be directly visualized, and because evacuation of intestinal contents and blood presents much more of a problem than for upper gastrointestinal endoscopy, only patients with mild or intermittent hemorrhage can be adequately examined with flexible fiberoptic instruments. The distal 25 cm of the colon, however, can be examined quite adequately during massive hemorrhage with the standard rigid proctosigmoidoscope.

Flexible Fiberoptic Sigmoidoscopy

It is our view, despite literature and advertising to the contrary, that the 65 cm flexible fiberoptic sigmoidoscope is merely a short colonoscope. It is subject to the same limitations as colonoscopy, requires the same amount of technical training, and will have the same or greater complication rate. Certainly, there are indications for a colonoscopic examination of only the left colon, but this should be performed by an experienced colonoscopist. Specifically, in a search for a lower gastrointestinal bleeding site, total colonoscopy is indicated if the barium enema does not show a colonic lesion. If a left colonic lesion has been demonstrated, the colonoscopist may choose the length colonoscope best suited to the individual situation.

Colonoscopy

Despite occasional reports of success [1, 6], we do not recommend colonoscopy for the evaluation of acute active lower gastrointestinal hemorrhage. Evacuation of blood and feces is extremely difficult and most massive bleeding comes from small non-mucosal sources (diverticulosis, angiodysplasia), generalized colonic disease (ulcerative colitis), or large infiltrative lesions (colon carcinoma) which are more rapidly and safely diagnosed by rigid proctosigmoidoscopy, visceral arteriography, or barium enema.

Colonoscopy can be helpful in the localization of lower gastrointestinal hemorrhage which is intermittent and can be occasionally helpful in the evaluation of the chronic bleeder.

Prior to evaluation of the colon, potential bleeding sites in the upper gastrointestinal tract must be eliminated by upper gastrointestinal endoscopy unless there is very specific evidence that the bleeding is coming from the colon (fresh red blood in small amounts coming from above the proctosigmoidoscope). Proctosigmoidoscopy and air contrast barium enema should precede colonoscopy. If these conditions have been met, 40% of such patients will have "significant" lesions demonstrated by colonoscopy [28-30] (Table 2). The yield was less (20%) in the few patients who were examined for occult gastrointestinal

Table 2
Colonoscopy for Unexplained Rectal Bleeding

	Swarbrick et al [28] (1978)	Teague et al [29] (1978)	Tedesco et al [30] (1978)
Number of patients	239	215	258
Significant lesion	40%	41%	42%
Polyps	16%	14%	16%
Carcinoma	10%	13%	11%
Inflammatory bowel disease	10%	7%	8%
Vascular malformation	2%	1%	7%

hemorrhage. Other important findings from these three reports were unsuspected colon carcinoma in 12% and previously undiagnosed inflammatory bowel disease in 7-10%. The 7% incidence of cecal telangiectasia in the American series as opposed to 1% and 2% in the British series suggests a difference in philosophy as to the role of arteriovenous malformations in lower gastrointestinal hemorrhage.

Hunt [13] has suggested that all patients with known diverticular disease who present with rectal bleeding should be examined by colonoscopy because of the difficulty in making a radiological diagnosis. In his series, as well as others, 15% of such patients will have colon carcinoma despite a negative barium enema.

Colonoscopy is a useful diagnostic aid when intermittent rectal bleeding, a very significant symptom, cannot be explained by proctosigmoidoscopy or air contrast barium enema. It is, at present, only occasionally useful for acute active hemorrhage.

REFERENCES

1. Beychok IA: Precise diagnosis in severe hematochezia. Arch Surg 113:634, 1978
2. Burwood RJ, Ross FGM: A radiologist's viewpoint. In Schiller KFR and Salmon PR (eds): Modern topics in gastrointestinal endoscopy. London, Heinemann, 1976, p 199
3. Chandler GN, Walls WD, Glanville JN: Hematemesis and melena. In Schiller KFR and Salmon PR (eds): Modern topics in gastrointestinal endoscopy. London, Heinemann, 1976, p 109
4. Cotton PB, Rosenberg MT, Waldram RPL, et al: Early endoscopy of oesophagus, stomach, and duodenal bulb in patients with hematemesis and melena. Br Med J 2:505, 1973
5. Dagradi AE, Mehler R, Tan DTD, et al: Sources of upper gastrointestinal bleeding in patients with cirrhosis and large oesophagogastric varices. Am J Gastroenterol 54:458, 1970
6. Deyhle P, Blum AL, Nuesch HJ, et al: Emergency colonoscopy in the management of acute peranal hemorrhage. Endoscopy 6:229, 1974
7. Dronfield MW, McIllmurray MB, Ferguson R, et al: A prospective, randomized study of endoscopy and radiology in acute upper-gastrointestinal-tract bleeding. Lancet 1:1167, 1977
8. Eastwood GL: Does early endoscopy benefit the patient with active upper gastrointestinal bleeding? Gastroenterology 72:737, 1977
9. Foster DN, Miloszewski KJ, Losowsky MS: Stigmata of recent hemorrhage in diagnosis and prognosis of upper gastrointestinal bleeding. Br Med J 1:1173, 1978
10. Graham DY, Davis RE: Acute upper gastrointestinal hemorrhage. New observations on an old problem. Am J Dig Dis 23:76, 1978
11. Himal HS, Perrault C, Mzabi R: Upper gastrointestinal hemorrhage. Surgery 84:448, 1978

12. Hirschowitz BI, Curtiss LE, Peters CW, et al: Demonstration of a new gastroscope—the fiberscope. Gastroenterology 35:50, 1958
13. Hunt RH: Rectal bleeding. Clin Gastroenterol 7:719, 1978
14. Iglesias MC, Dourdourekas D, Adomavicius J, et al: Prompt endoscopic diagnosis of upper gastrointestinal hemorrhage. Ann Surg 189:90, 1979
15. Katz D, Petchumoni CS, Thomas E, et al: The endoscopic diagnosis of upper gastrointestinal hemorrhage. Am J Dig Dis 21:182, 1976
16. Keller RT, Logan GM Jr: Comparison of emergent endoscopy and upper gastrointestinal series radiology in acute upper gastrointestinal hemorrhage. Gut 17:180, 1976
17. Knauer CM: Mallory-Weiss syndrome. Gastroenterology 71:5, 1976
18. Leinicke JA, Shafer RD, Hogan WJ, et al: Emergency endoscopy in acute gastrointestinal bleeding: Does timing affect the significance of diagnostic yield? Gastrointest Endosc 22:228, 1976
19. Mitchell CJ, Jewell DP: The diagnosis of the site of upper gastrointestinal hemorrhage in patients with established portal hypertension. Endoscopy 9:131, 1977
20. Morris DW, Levin GM, Soloway RD, et al: Prospective, randomized study of diagnosis and outcome in acute upper-gastrointestinal bleeding. Am J Dig Dis 20:1103, 1975
21. Pyorala K, Salmi HJ, Jussila J, et al: Electrocardiographic changes during gastroscopy. Endoscopy 5:186, 1973
22. Rosenberg MT: The operated stomach. In Schiller KFR and Salmon P (eds): Modern topics in gastrointestinal endoscopy. London, Heinemann, 1976, p 131
23. Schiller KFR, Cotton PB: Acute upper gastrointestinal hemorrhage. Clin Gastroenterol 7:595, 1978
24. Schiller KFR, Prout BJ: Hazards. In Schiller KFR and Salmon PR (eds): Modern topics in gastrointestinal endoscopy. London, Heinemann, 1976, p 147
25. Silvis SE, Nebel O, Rogers G, et al: Endoscopic complications. JAMA 235:928, 1976
26. Stadelman O as quoted in Schiller KFR and Prout BJ; Hazards. In Schiller KFR and Salmon PR (eds): Modern topics in gastrointestinal endoscopy. London, Heinemann, 1976, p 147
27. Stevenson GW, Cox RR, Roberts CJ: Prospective comparison of double-contrast barium meal examination and fiberoptic endoscopy in acute upper gastrointestinal hemorrhage. Br Med J 2:723, 1976
28. Swarbrick ET, Feure DI, Hunt RR, et al: Colonoscopy for unexplained rectal bleeding. Br Med J 2:1685, 1978
29. Teague RH, Thornton JR, Manning AP, et al: Colonoscopy for investigation of unexplained rectal bleeding. Lancet 1:1350, 1978
30. Tedesco FJ, Waye JD, Raskin JB, et al: Colonoscopy evaluation of rectal bleeding. Ann Int Med 89:907, 1978
31. Teres J, Bordas JM, Bru C, et al: Upper gastrointestinal bleeding in cirrhosis. Gut 17:37, 1976

32. Waldram RM, Davis M, Nunnerley H, et al: Emergency endoscopy after gastrointestinal hemorrhage in 50 patients with portal hypertension. Br Med J 5:94, 1974
33. Winans CS: Emergency upper gastrointestinal endoscopy: does haste make waste? Am J Dig Dis 22:536, 1977
34. Wolf WI, Shinya H: Modern endoscopy of the alimentary tract. Curr Prob Surg, New York, 1974

Kyung J. Cho, M.D.
Douglass F. Adams, M.D.

Diagnostic Angiography in Gastrointestinal Hemorrhage

ABSTRACT

Selective angiography has assumed a central role in localizing and defining the underlying pathologic process responsible in cases of gastrointestinal hemorrhage. Endoscopy remains a primary diagnostic step in suspected upper gastrointestinal hemorrhage, while selective angiography plays a primary role in acute rectal hemorrhage. Angiography is indicated for both diagnostic and therapeutic purposes in patients with unremitting, severe upper gastrointestinal hemorrhage. Unfortunately, conventional diagnostic tests (endoscopy and barium examination) are frequently negative in patients with chronic, recurrent gastrointestinal hemorrhage, forcing the physician to consider angiography even though the yield may be low.

Common causes of upper gastrointestinal hemorrhage include peptic ulcers, hemorrhagic gastritis, Mallory-Weiss tears and gastroesophageal varices. Colonic diverticula and vascular ectasia are the most common causes of acute rectal hemorrhage in the elderly. Diagnostic angiography in gastrointestinal hemorrhage is an essential element in the proper management of patients.

Since the introduction of the Seldinger percutaneous catheterization technique in 1953 [34], angiography has become a powerful diagnostic tool. Nearly a decade passed, however, before the explosive expansion of this technique was first applied to the diagnosis of gastrointestinal hemorrhage [2, 3, 24]. The use of selective angiography has permitted both the precise localization of a bleeding point and the definition of the nature of the basic pathology responsible for acute or chronic recurrent gastrointestinal hemorrhage [7, 10, 13, 18, 28, 35].

Kyung J. Cho, M.D.: Associate Professor, Department of Radiology, and Director, Division of Cardiovascular Radiology, University of Michigan Medical Center; Douglass F. Adams, M.D.: Professor and Chairman, Department of Radiology, University of Michigan Medical Center, Ann Arbor, Michigan.

In recent years, one of the most important applications of selective angiographic technique has been for therapy of massive hemorrhage in the gastrointestinal tract. Several angiographic techniques including infusion of vasoconstrictive agent, selective embolization and other occlusive methods have evolved.

The role of selective angiography in patients with gastrointestinal hemorrhage will be described in two steps: diagnostic and therapeutic. The importance of angiography in the diagnosis of gastrointestinal hemorrhage will be reviewed in this chapter and the current status of therapeutic angiography in the management of gastrointestinal hemorrhage will be described in the following chapter.

INDICATIONS FOR ANGIOGRAPHY IN GASTROINTESTINAL HEMORRHAGE

Gastrointestinal hemorrhage may cease spontaneously or following conventional therapy or, rarely, during an angiographic procedure. Patients with persistent bleeding should undergo special diagnostic examinations and may require specific therapy. Barium examinations in patients with acute hemorrhage are not recommended as they are often unrewarding due to interference by blood clot and the patients being generally uncooperative. Additionally, the barium in the gastrointestinal tract may make the angiographic identification of bleeding impossible.

Endoscopy plays a primary role in the diagnosis and localization of upper gastrointestinal bleeding but it is obviously not valuable for acute rectal hemorrhage. When endoscopy fails to localize the bleeding or is contraindicated or sometimes even when it does identify a potential bleeding site, angiography may also be indicated because of uncertainty of the relationship between the demonstrated pathology and the bleeding site. Additionally, therapy using interventional technique may be indicated. In severe, continuous rectal hemorrhage, angiography should be the initial diagnostic procedure [7, 10]. Conventional diagnostic examinations including endoscopy and barium study are performed in chronic or recurrent gastrointestinal hemorrhage before angiography. Angiography may identify the lesion responsible for bleeding in as many as 45% of patients with chronic bleeding in whom conventional diagnostic tests are negative [35].

ANGIOGRAPHIC TECHNIQUE

Angiographers, endoscopists, referring physicians and nurses should function as a team to achieve prompt diagnosis and successful management of patients

DIAGNOSTIC ANGIOGRAPHY

with massive gastrointestinal hemorrhage. Thus the angiographer's commitment to the 24-hour availability of angiographic services is essential.

The celiac, superior mesenteric or inferior mesenteric arteries are selectively catheterized using a percutaneous transfemoral approach or transaxillary approach if femoral pulses are absent. If endoscopy or nasogastric aspiration indicates upper gastrointestinal hemorrhage, selective celiac and superior mesenteric angiography is performed. If extravasation of contrast medium is demonstrated on these angiograms, selective catheterization of the bleeding artery is performed to institute appropriate angiographic treatment. If bleeding is not demonstrated, subselective angiography of left gastric, gastroduodenal and splenic arteries is performed. If these subselective angiographies are negative, the degree of hemorrhage should be reassessed. Continuous hemorrhage documented in patients with a negative arteriogram may suggest mucosal or variceal bleeding. Varices may or may not be present on angiogram or endoscopy.

When colonic bleeding is suspected, selective inferior mesenteric angiography is performed initially to avoid a distended and opacified bladder and is followed by a superior mesenteric angiogram. Two injections of each mesenteric artery may be required to allow filming of the entire mesenteric circulation. When both superior and inferior mesenteric angiograms are negative, a celiac angiogram should be performed.

Superior and inferior mesenteric arteriography following intraarterial injection of a vasodilator, such as tolazoline, may improve visualization of the portal venous system. A balloon occlusion mesenteric angiographic technique may accomplish the same goal. Rectosigmoid varices secondary to either portal hypertension or inferior mesenteric vein occlusion have been implicated as a rare cause of occult rectal hemorrhage.

ANGIOGRAPHIC DIAGNOSIS OF GASTROINTESTINAL HEMORRHAGE

The diagnosis of bleeding is made angiographically through the extravasation of contrast agent during the arterial phase which persists throughout the entire filming sequence. Extravasated contrast medium may outline mucosal folds (see Fig. 6B, p 218) or occasionally demonstrate a diverticulum or ulcer crater. Frequently the contrast medium appears as a tubular structure due to surrounding clot simulating a venous structure. This "pseudovein" is a sign of arterial hemorrhage [29]. Experimental studies indicate that a bleeding rate of over 0.5 ml per minute can be identified by selective angiography [24]. Only such brisk arterial hemorrhage is likely to be demonstrated using angiography. Mucosal or venous bleeding is usually not demonstrable on the angiogram because of rapid dilution of intraarterially injected contrast medium.

Occasionally an adrenal stain or a small hemangioma of the left hepatic lobe may mimic bleeding. An adrenal stain should have a typical triangular appearance. Repeat angiography in the oblique projection or following the introduction of air into the stomach should distinguish bleeding from either an adrenal stain or a tumor stain.

Bleeding Mallory-Weiss Tears

Bleeding due to Mallory-Weiss tears is usually treated conservatively or may stop spontaneously [14]. Fiberoptic endoscopy is the diagnostic procedure of choice; however, selective angiography may be performed for therapeutic reasons in patients with unremitting hemorrhage. The extravasated contrast medium appears as a linear or rounded collection at or near the gastroesophageal junction on selective celiac and/or left gastric angiograms (Fig. 1). A bleeding ulcer of the high lesser curvature of the stomach or in the hiatus hernia may be angiographically indistinguishable from a Mallory-Weiss tear.

Bleeding Peptic Ulcers

Peptic ulcer disease accounts for 60% of all upper gastrointestinal hemorrhage and documented causes. Gastric bleeding can be demonstrated by either celiac or left gastric arteriogram. Short gastric, inferior phrenic, right gastric and right gastroepiploic arteries are the rare sources of bleeding. The gastroduodenal artery usually supplies bleeding sites in the pyloric and duodenal areas. Extravasated contrast medium may here also outline mucosal folds or an ulcer crater. A pseudoaneurysm, due to erosion of an artery at the base of an ulcer crater, may be demonstrated.

Acute Gastric Mucosal Hemorrhage and Stress Ulcers

The diagnosis of acute gastric mucosal hemorrhage or hemorrhagic gastritis is usually established by endoscopic examination. Angiography is performed principally for the transcatheter intraarterial infusion of the vasoconstrictor, vasopressin. The angiographic findings are nonspecific. Celiac or left gastric angiogram may demonstrate a dilated left gastric artery with increased staining of the stomach wall. Multiple discrete points of contrast agent extravasation may also be seen.

Bleeding Marginal Ulcers

As they are typically located on the jejunal side of the anastomosis, superior mesenteric angiography is performed to demonstrate bleeding from marginal ulcers (Fig. 2). Bleeding usually occurs from the first or second jejunal branch of the superior mesenteric artery [32].

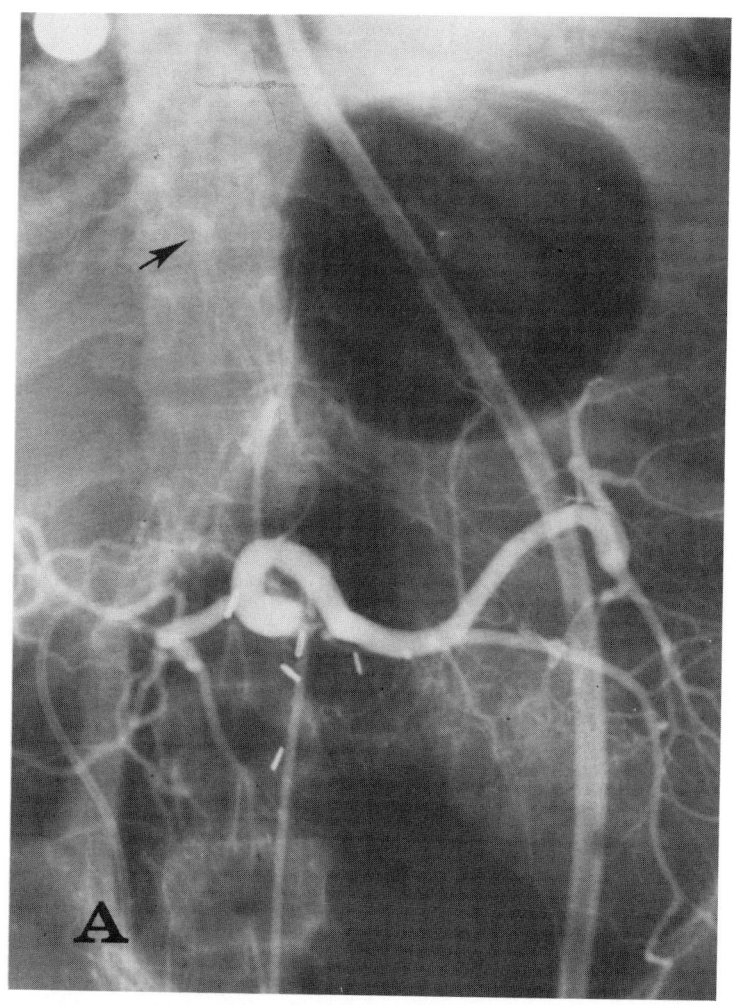

Fig. 1A. Celiac angiogram in 37-year-old man with bleeding Mallory-Weiss tears shows extravasation of contrast medium (arrow) near cardioesophageal junction.

Bleeding Neoplasms

Gastrointestinal tract neoplasms may cause mild or massive, acute, chronic or recurrent hemorrhage. Angiography, when performed during an episode of brisk hemorrhage, may demonstrate extravasation of contrast medium (Fig. 3). Gastrointestinal tumors can usually be diagnosed by barium studies or endoscopy prior to angiography. Localization of gastrointestinal myomatous

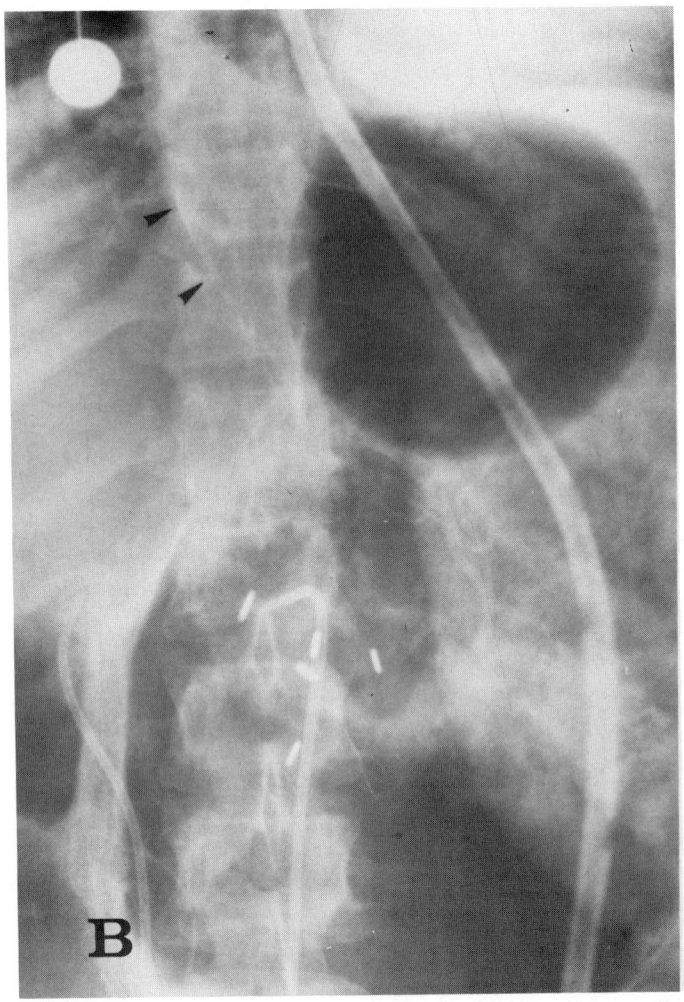

Fig. 1B. Capillary phase of same angiogram demonstrates linear collection of contrast medium between torn mucosa (arrowheads).

tumors may best be accomplished by angiography, however, because they are generally hypervascular and because barium studies are frequently negative.

Other Causes of Upper Gastrointestinal Hemorrhage

Bleeding into the biliary tree (hemobilia) and into the pancreatic duct (hemosuccus pancreaticus) is rare, but can be an important cause of massive gastrointestinal hemorrhage [19]. Hemobilia clinically presents with recurrent attacks of biliary colic, jaundice and recurrent gastrointestinal hemorrhage.

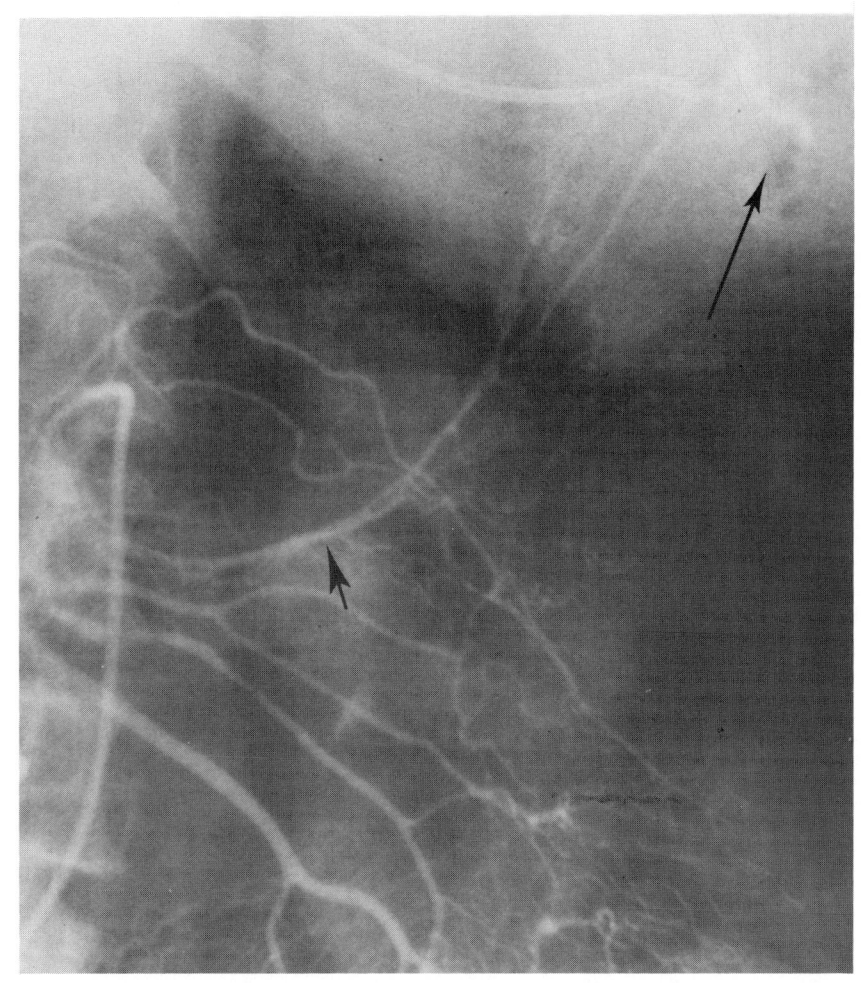

Fig. 2. Superior mesenteric angiogram in patient with marginal ulcer demonstrates extravasation of contrast medium (long arrow) from the first jejunal artery (short arrow).

Hepatic hematoma or an arteriovenous fistula may be demonstrated by hepatic angiography. Direct visualization of the biliary tree by extravasated contrast medium rarely occurs on the angiogram unless the study is performed at the time of brisk bleeding.

Massive gastrointestinal hemorrhage is a serious complication of chronic pancreatic inflammation with a reported incidence of 1.4%-41% [12, 37, 38]. Hemorrhage often results from the creation of pseudoaneurysm by pancreatic enzyme action on walls. The pseudoaneurysm may rupture directly into the

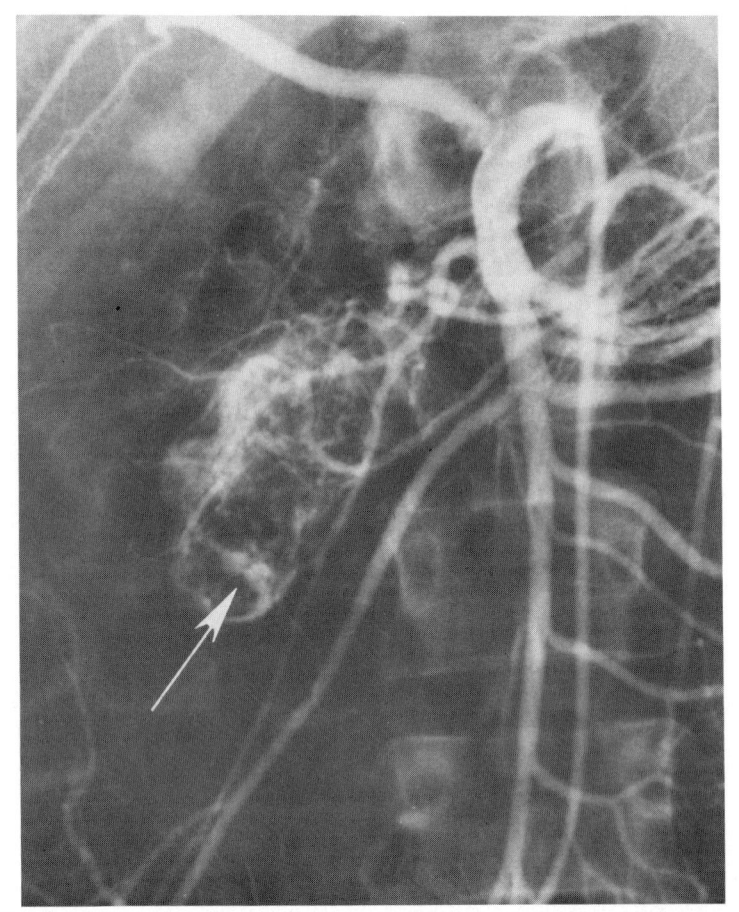

Fig. 3. Superior mesenteric angiogram in 27-year-old woman with recurrent gastrointestinal hemorrhage shows cystic, vascular leiomyoma in distal duodenum. Extravasation of contrast medium from tumor is present (arrow).

gastrointestinal tract, a pseudocyst or the pancreatic duct. The presence of pancreatic or peripancreatic aneurysms on celiac or splenic angiogram in patients with acute gastrointestinal hemorrhage should suggest pancreatitis as the cause for the hemorrhage [39]. Rarely, the pancreatic duct has been visualized by extravasated contrast medium [38].

Aortoenteric fistulas usually present with massive gastrointestinal hemorrhage with a reported incidence of 1%-10% following abdominal aortic surgery [11, 17, 33, 36]. Approximately 80% of the fistulas occur in the duodenum [36]. Angiographic studies should be performed early in all patients with gastrointestinal hemorrhage following an abdominal aortic operation. A flush biplane prone abdominal aortography should be performed prior to

DIAGNOSTIC ANGIOGRAPHY 59

selective visceral angiography. Direct extravasation is infrequently demonstrated on this aortogram. The presence of a false aneurysm at the proximal anastomotic site suggests the presence of an aortoenteric fistula and warrants operation.

Massive upper gastrointestinal hemorrhage is considered to be variceal in origin when gastroesophageal varices are demonstrated in the absence of extravasation elsewhere on the angiogram. Angiographic studies may demonstrate the cause of varices when it is other than cirrhosis. Hepatomas or pancreatic neoplasms may present with gastrointestinal hemorrhage due to portal hypertension resulting from invasion of the extrahepatic portal vein (Fig. 4).

Isolated gastric varices secondary to splenic vein occlusion is a well known cause of massive gastric hemorrhage (Fig. 5). The condition is commonly caused

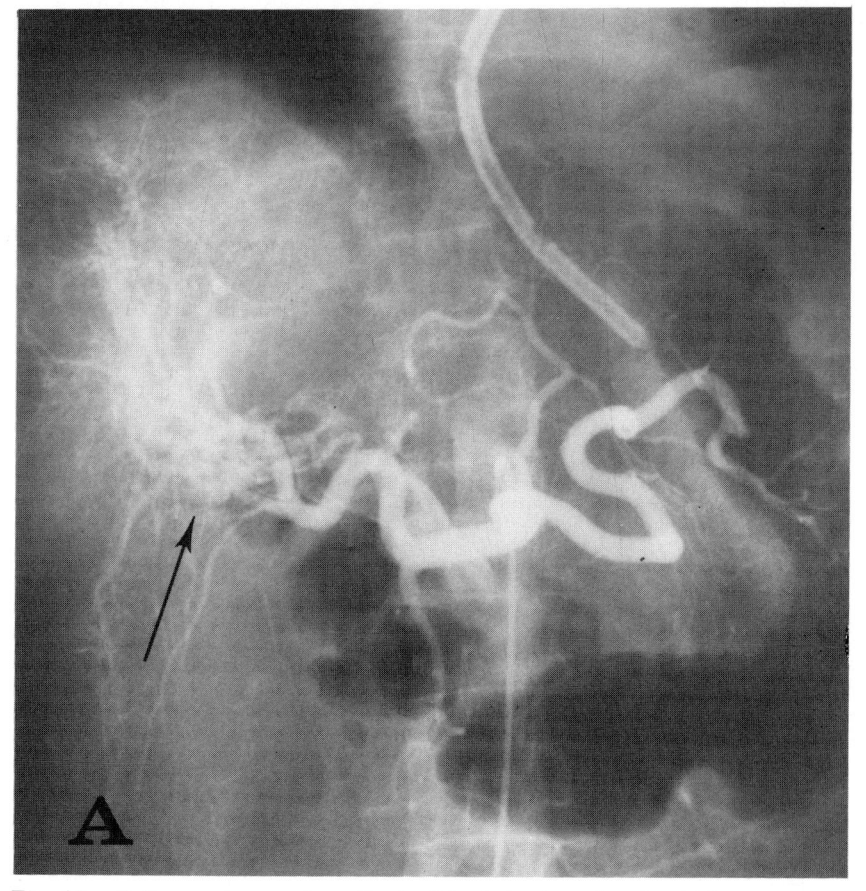

Fig. 4A. Celiac angiogram in patient with cirrhosis and variceal bleeding shows tumor cast in the portal vein (arrow). Linear neovascularity ("thread and streaks" sign) is characteristic of hepatoma.

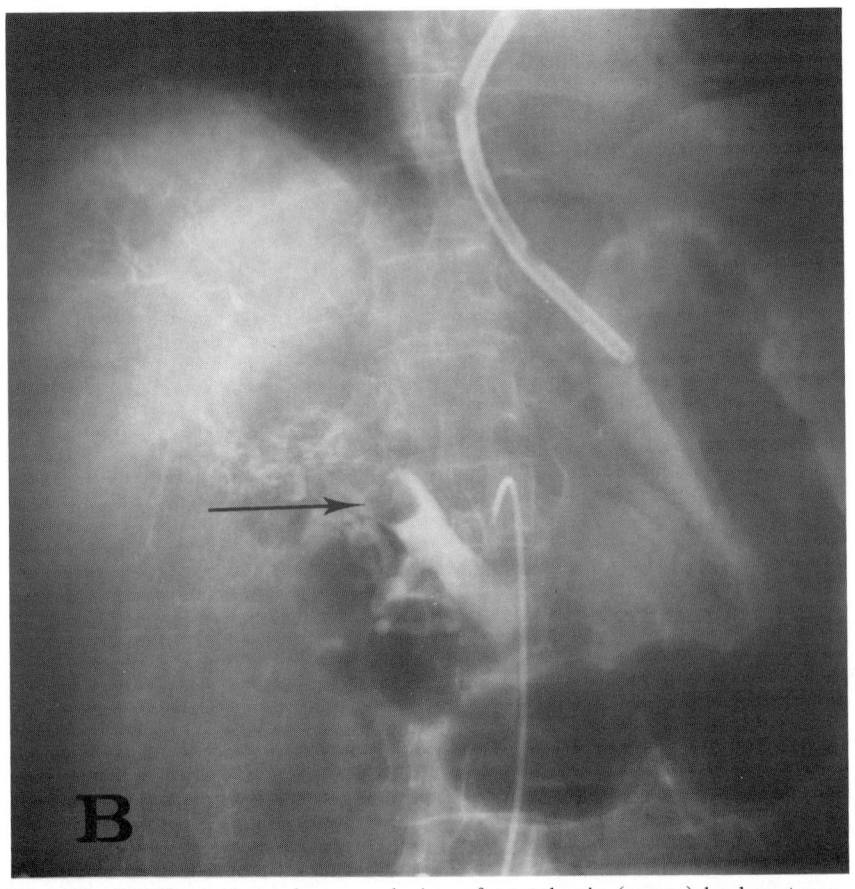

Fig. 4B. Capillary phase shows occlusion of portal vein (arrow) by hepatoma.

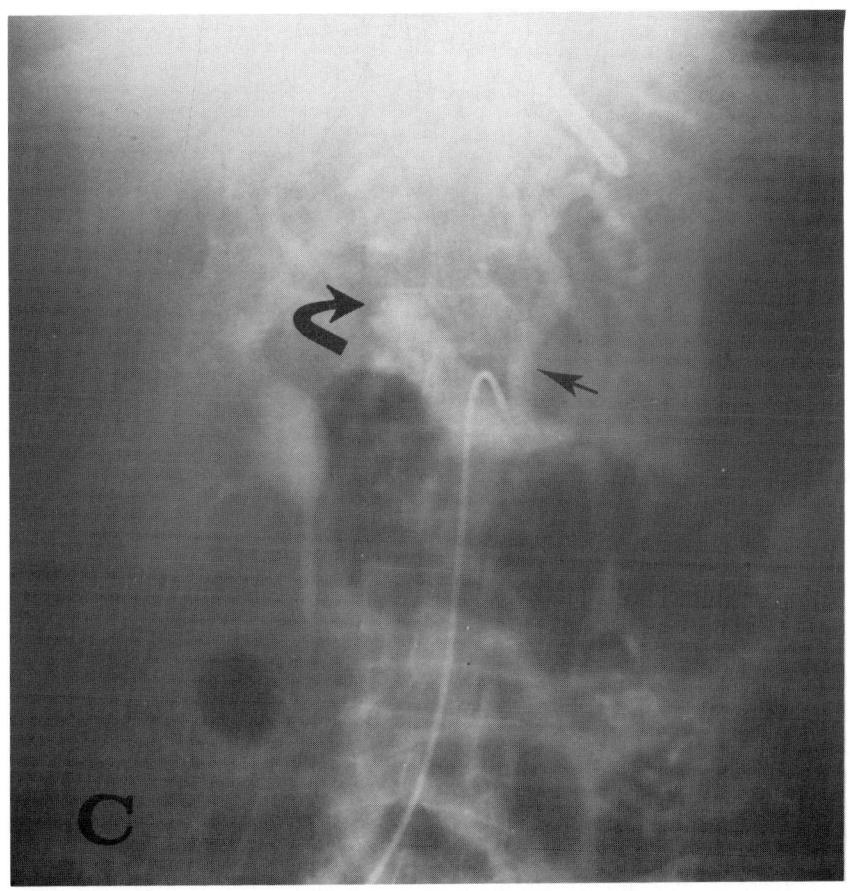

Fig. 4C. Venous phase of superior mesenteric angiogram shows an occlusion of the portal vein (curved arrow) and varices (straight arrow).

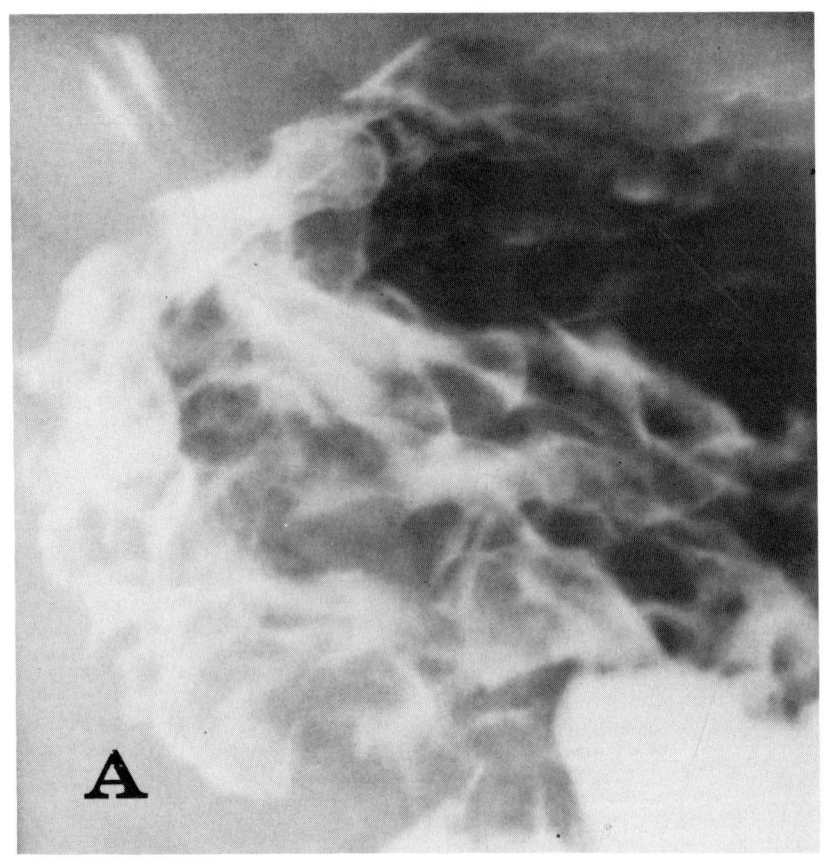

Fig. 5A. Barium study of stomach with double contrast technique in 51-year-old man with pancreatitis and gastric hemorrhage shows polypoid and serpentine defects in proximal part of stomach.

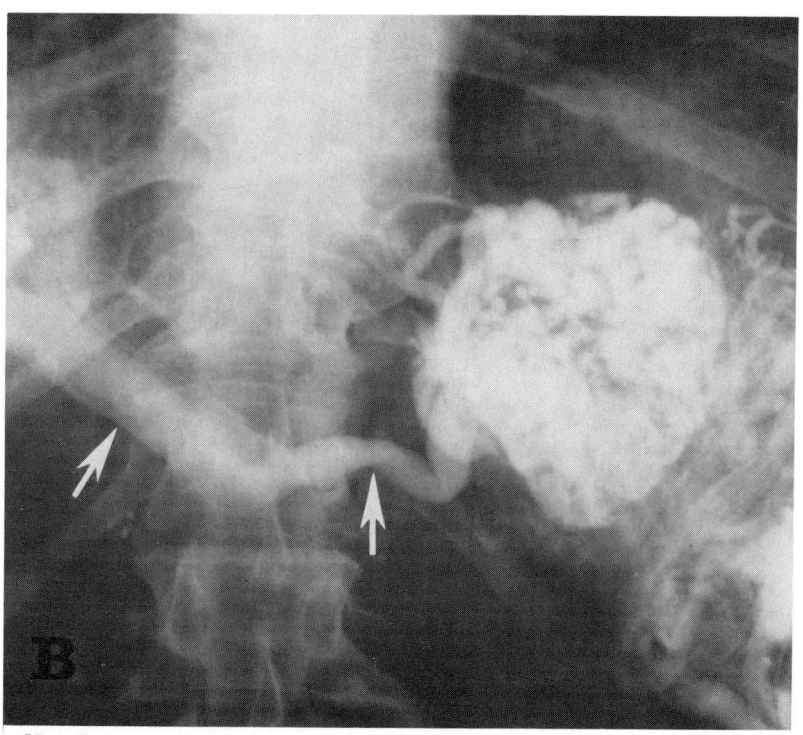

Fig. 5B. Splenoportogram shows large gastric varices filling coronary and portal veins (arrows). Splenic vein is occluded and no esophageal varices are seen. [From Cho KJ, Martel W: Recognition of splenic vein occlusion. Am J Roentgenol 131:439, 1978. Reproduced with permission, ©1978, American Roentgen Ray Society.]

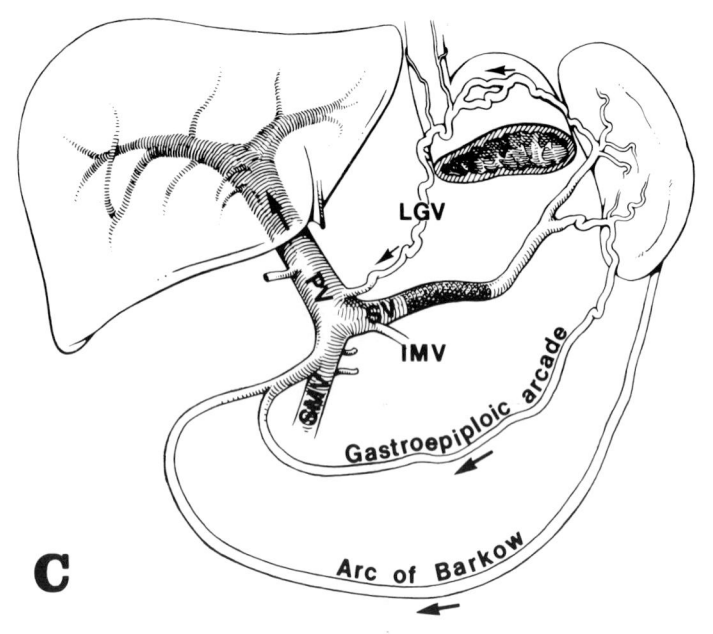

Fig. 5C. Venous collaterals in splenic vein occlusion. In isolated splenic vein occlusion, preferential direction of collateral flow is toward portal vein. Gastric varices are formed by short gastric-coronary and gastroepiploic collateral circulation. Arrows indicate venous flow direction. LGV, left gastric vein (or coronary vein); SV, splenic vein occlusion; PV, portal vein; SMV, superior mesenteric vein.

by pancreatic disease or retroperitoneal fibrosis [9]. This type of segmental portal hypertension can be relieved by splenectomy.

ANGIOGRAPHIC DIAGNOSIS OF LOWER GASTROINTESTINAL HEMORRHAGE

Several pathologic processes may be responsible for acute and chronic rectal hemorrhage [5]. In a review of 60 consecutive patients with lower gastrointestinal hemorrhage [7], colonic diverticula were found to be the most common cause (42%). Arteriovenous malformation, duodenal ulcer, carcinoma of the colon, Meckel's diverticulum, jejunal diverticulum, rectal trauma, inflammatory bowel disease and intestinal varices are additional causes [1, 7, 10, 23, 31, 35, 40]. Conventional diagnostic studies fail to disclose the source of bleeding in half of the patients with chronic melena [30]. Even exploratory laparotomy has been negative in up to 70% of those patients [27]. Angiography is helpful not

DIAGNOSTIC ANGIOGRAPHY

only in localization of bleeding but also in defining the underlying pathologic processes in cases of chronic rectal hemorrhage.

Diverticular Bleeding

Colonic diverticula are the most common cause of acute rectal hemorrhage, especially in elderly patients [8] (Fig. 6). Despite a preponderance of diverticula in the left colon, bleeding diverticula are encountered in the right-sided colon in 60%-80% of the cases. Neither clinical nor histologic evidence of diverticulitis has been found in most cases of bleeding diverticula [20, 25]. Angiographically, bleeding diverticula appear as dense, rounded extravasations of contrast medium during the early arterial phase which persist throughout the venous phase. Colonic haustra may be outlined during massive extravasation.

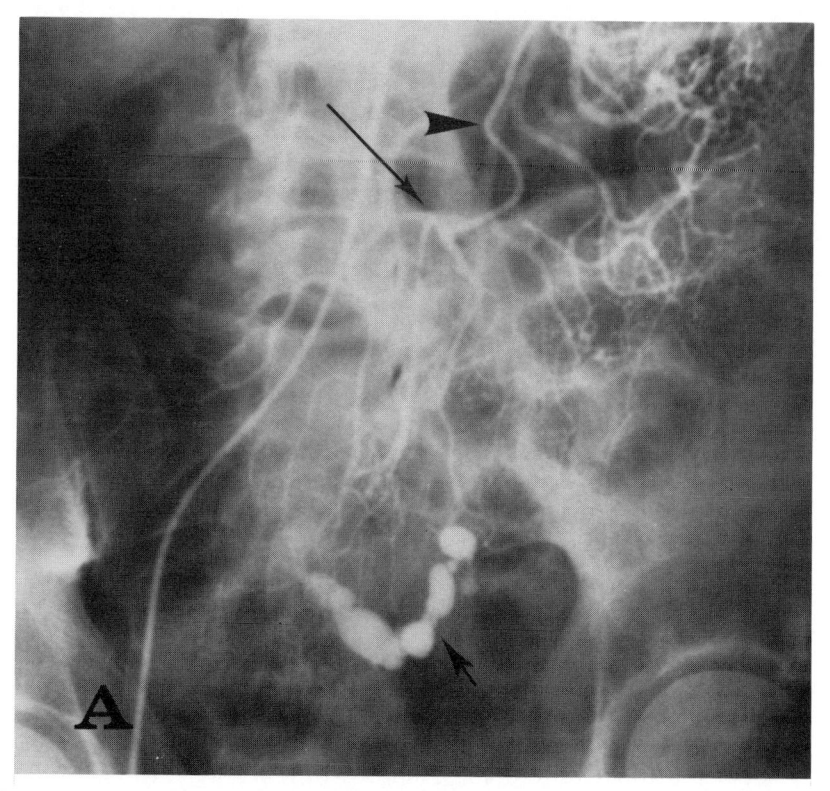

Fig. 6A. Late arterial phase of superior mesenteric angiogram in elderly man with bleeding diverticulum (centered over the pelvis) shows active bleeding in the sigmoid colon (short arrow). Hemorrhage is visualized on superior mesenteric angiogram because of occlusion of inferior mesenteric artery (long arrow). Left colic artery (arrowhead) filled from the middle colic branch of superior mesenteric artery (shown in B).

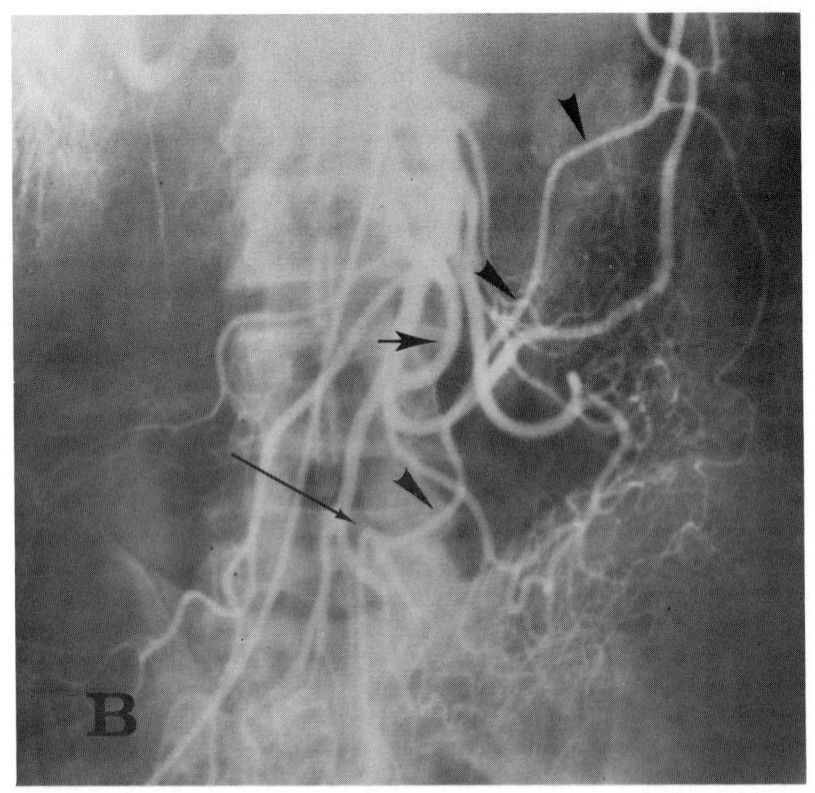

Fig. 6B. Superior mesenteric angiography shows dilated middle colic (arrow) and left colic arteries (arrowheads) because of inferior mesenteric artery occlusion (long arrow). [Courtesy of Robert Elwood, M.D., William Beaumont Hospital, Royal Oak, Michigan.]

Arteriovenous Malformations

Half of the lesions found in patients with chronic gastrointestinal bleeding are arteriovenous malformations [35]. Half of these malformations are located in the cecum or ascending colon. Angiography is the diagnostic method of choice for localizing arteriovenous malformations. They are usually not visible at operation and may remain unrecognized even at histologic examination unless the lesion is localized by specimen angiography.

Three forms of arteriovenous malformations have been recognized [4, 22]. The most common form, vascular ectasia, predominantly involves patients over the age of 55. The angiographic findings of this lesion have been well established [1]: (1) abnormal clusters of small arteries along the antimesenteric border of the right colon seen during the late arterial phase of the angiogram; (2) accumulations of contrast material in vascular spaces during the capillary phase; (3) early and dense opacification of enlarged draining veins; and (4) simultaneous visualization of both supplying artery and vein (Fig. 7). Colonic vascular ectasia causes intermittent as well as acute episodes of massive rectal hemorrhage. Extravasation of contrast medium may be identified on the angiogram when it is performed during acute bleeding. In one-fourth of the 33 patients with colonic angiodysplasia reported by Miller et al [21] the lesions were located in the left colon and one-third of his patients were younger than 60. Miller emphasized that the entity occurs in the left colon more frequently than generally appreciated and advocated a complete angiographic survey of the entire gastrointestinal tract.

The second form of arteriovenous malformations is of congenital origin and usually affects people before the age of 50 years. They are generally larger and may involve a short segment of bowel. Angiographically, they have tortuous prominent arteries with a dense accumulation of contrast medium in the capillary phase of the angiogram (Fig. 8). A dense early opacification of veins may also be seen.

The third form is small capillary angiomata which may be associated with Rendu-Osler-Weber syndrome. These angiomata are small telangiectasia scattered throughout the bowel. The angiographic abnormality includes punctate areas of contrast medium accumulation in late arterial and capillary phases of angiogram without early draining veins.

Inflammatory Bowel Disease

Inflammatory bowel disease is a rare cause of acute rectal hemorrhage [16]. Ulcerative colitis, ischemic colitis and Crohn's disease have been reported as the causes for massive lower gastrointestinal hemorrhage. The bleeding may be the initial presentation of the disease. The diagnosis is generally made by barium examination or endoscopy. The angiographic findings of inflammatory bowel disease are nonspecific but include mucosal and submucosal hypervascularity, dilated vasa recta and dense opacification of the draining veins. Superior mesenteric or inferior mesenteric angiograms are performed to define the site of bleeding, and the same catheter can be used for vasopressin therapy.

Bleeding Colonic Carcinoma

Colonic carcinoma is a common cause of occult gastrointestinal hemorrhage. Angiography may demonstrate extravasation of contrast medium in addition to the tumor vessels and the encasement of intestinal arteries. Barium enema and endoscopy are the diagnostic procedures of choice.

Duodenal Ulcer

In patients with clinical signs of massive hemorrhage, in whom superior mesenteric and inferior mesenteric angiography fail to reveal hemorrhage, celiac

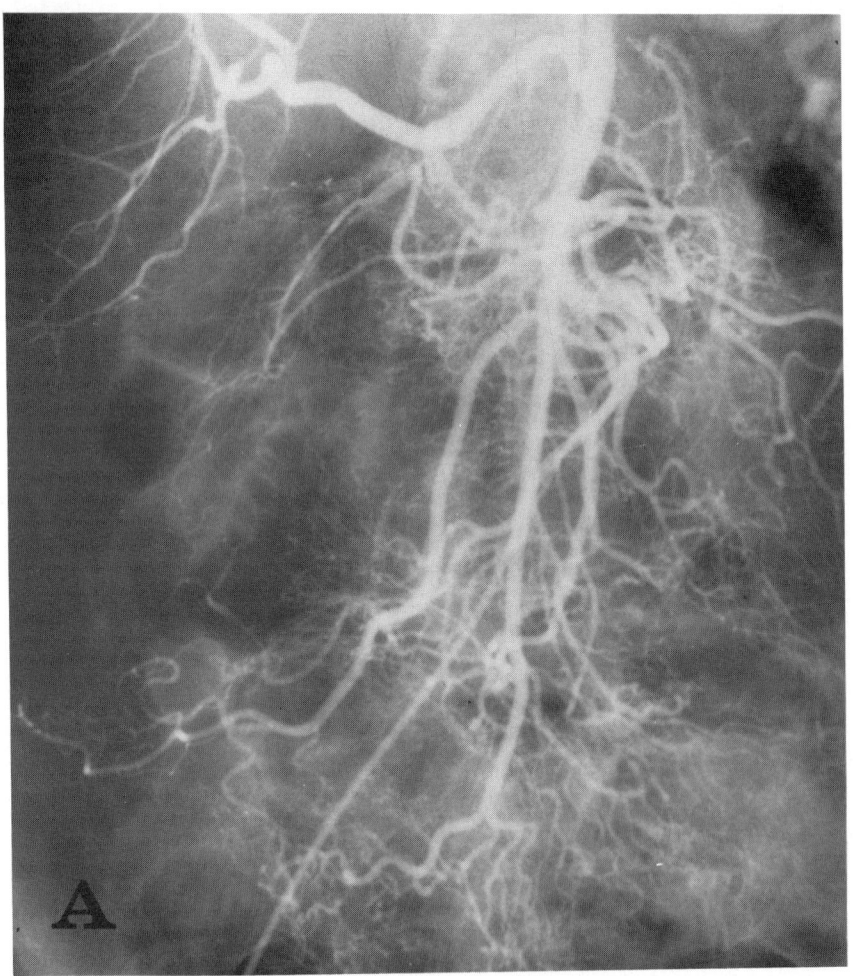

Fig. 7. A 65-year-old woman with 7-year history of recurrent lower gastrointestinal bleeding and multiple episodes of blood transfusion. (A) Arterial phase of superior mesenteric arteriograms shows no abnormality. (B) Early venous phase of same angiogram shows early, dense opacification of a vein from the cecum (arrow). (C) Magnification angiogram of cecum and ascending colon after introduction of air shows small area of contrast accumulation (arrow) at antimesenteric border of ascending colon. Both supplying artery and vein are seen simultaneously (arrowhead). (D) Specimen angiogram of resected colon in another patient with recurrent lower gastrointestinal bleeding shows vascular ectasia (arrow) at the antimesenteric border of the cecum.

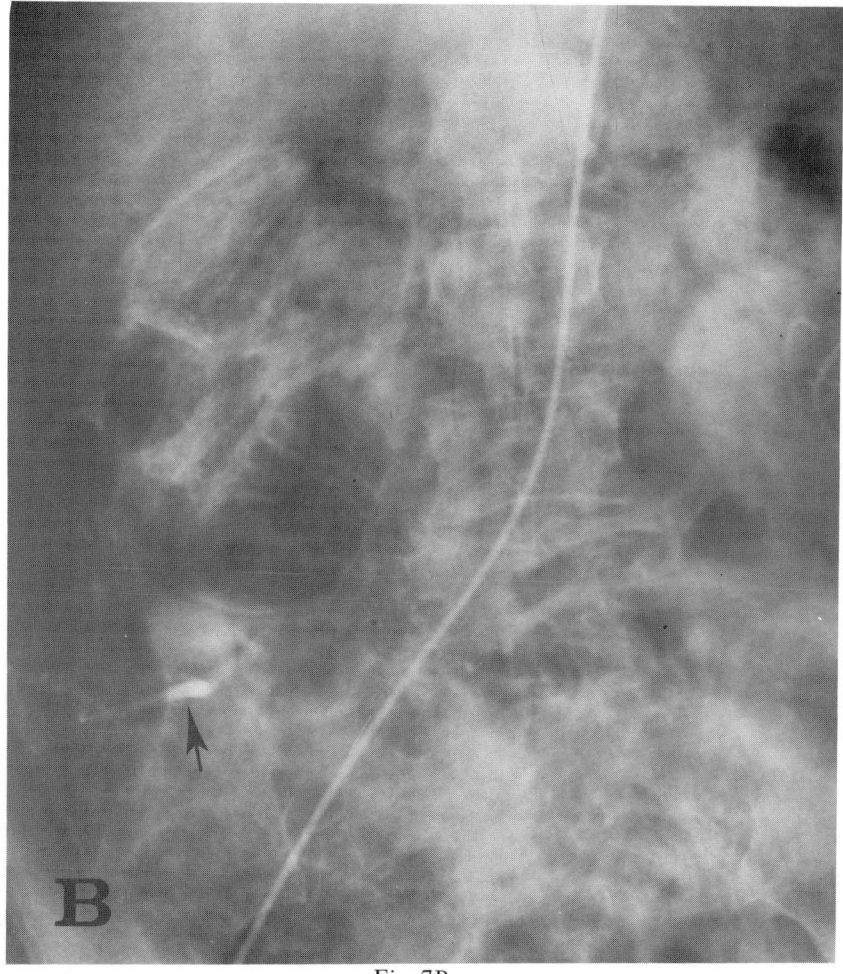

Fig. 7B.

arteriography should be performed. Additional subselective catheterization of the gastroduodenal artery should accompany it since duodenal pathology may present as apparent lower gastrointestinal hemorrhage.

Meckel's Diverticulum

Peptic ulceration of the ileal mucosa secondary to ectopic gastric mucosa within Meckel's diverticulum is a rare cause of lower gastrointestinal hemorrhage. Barium examination frequently has been negative. Isotopic scan with Tc-99m has occasionally been useful in demonstrating ectopic gastric mucosa of Meckel's diverticulum. The angiographic abnormality includes an abnormal

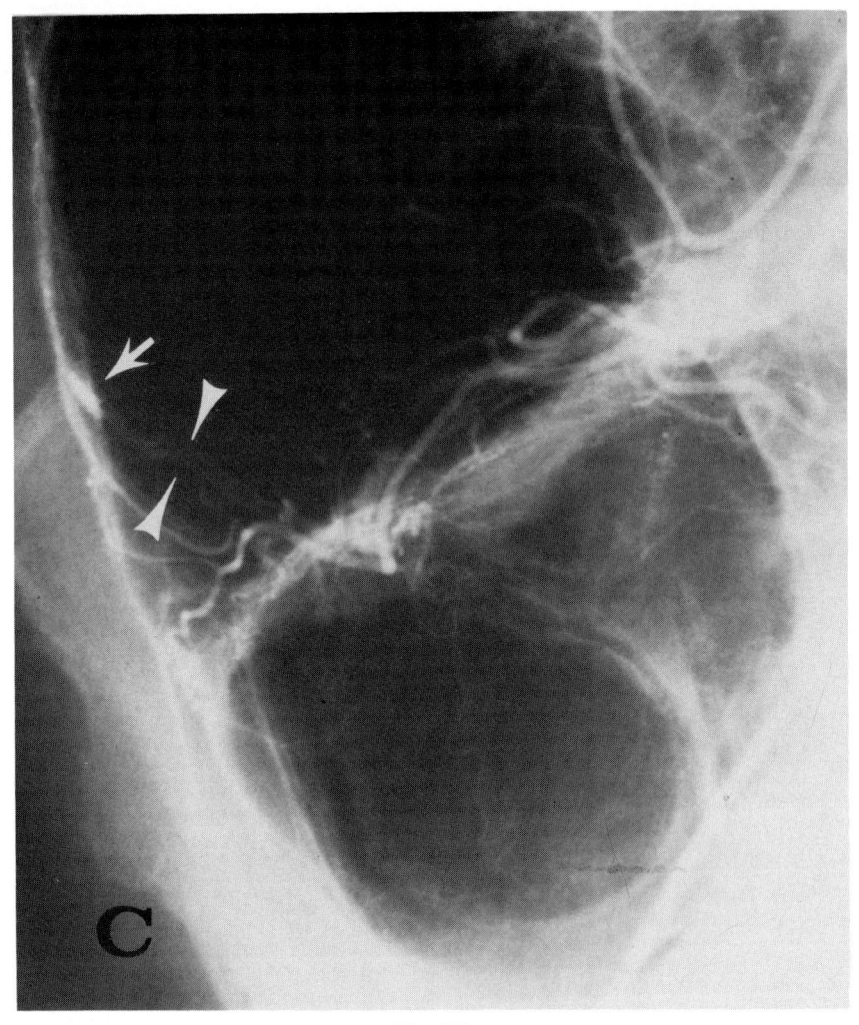

Fig. 7C.

branch of the superior mesenteric artery supplying a hypervascular area in the lower abdomen (Fig. 9). Superior mesenteric angiography has localized active hemorrhage in Meckel's diverticulum in 2 patients [6, 26].

Jejunal Diverticula

Jejunal diverticula have been known to cause massive hemorrhage [7]. Angiography is normal unless it is performed at the time of brisk bleeding. The involved segment of bowel is localized by identifying an intestinal branch supplying the bleeding site. Jejunal diverticulum can be visualized by small bowel study with barium.

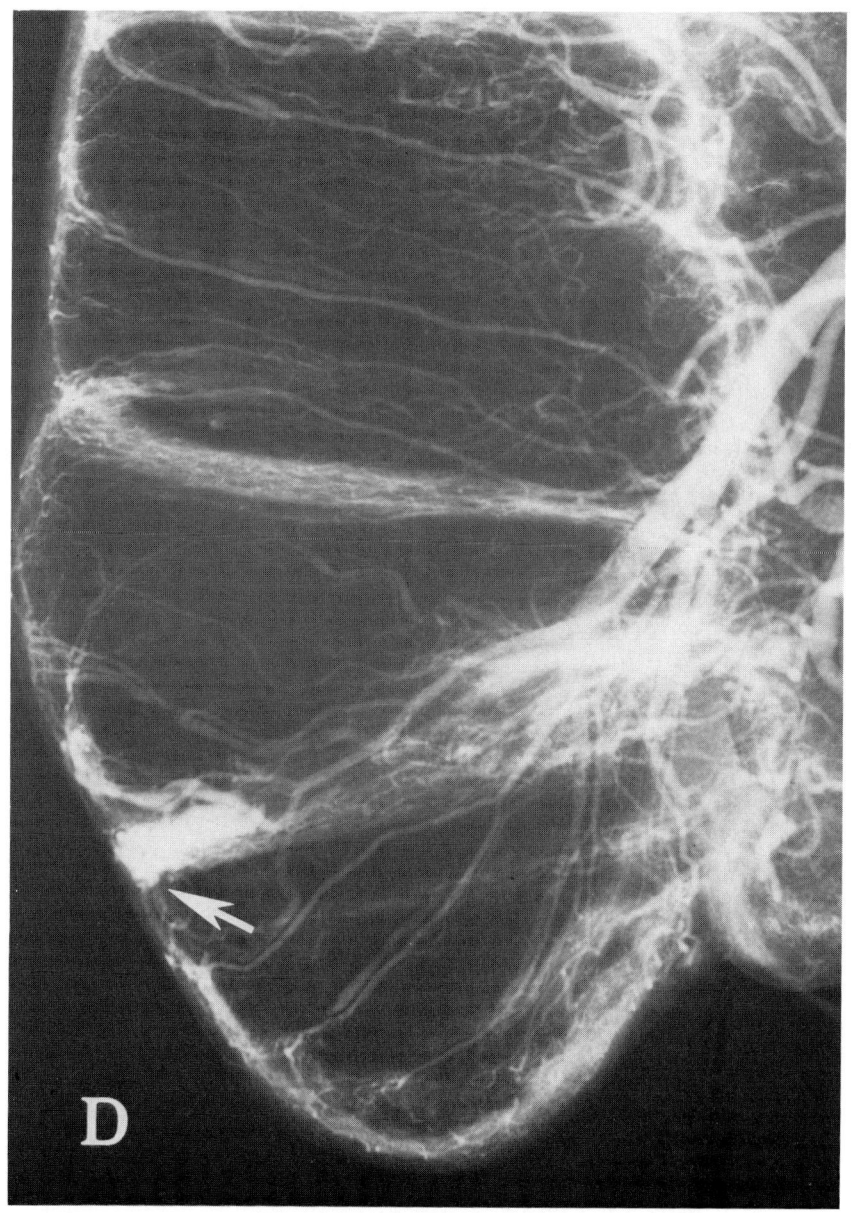

Fig. 7D.

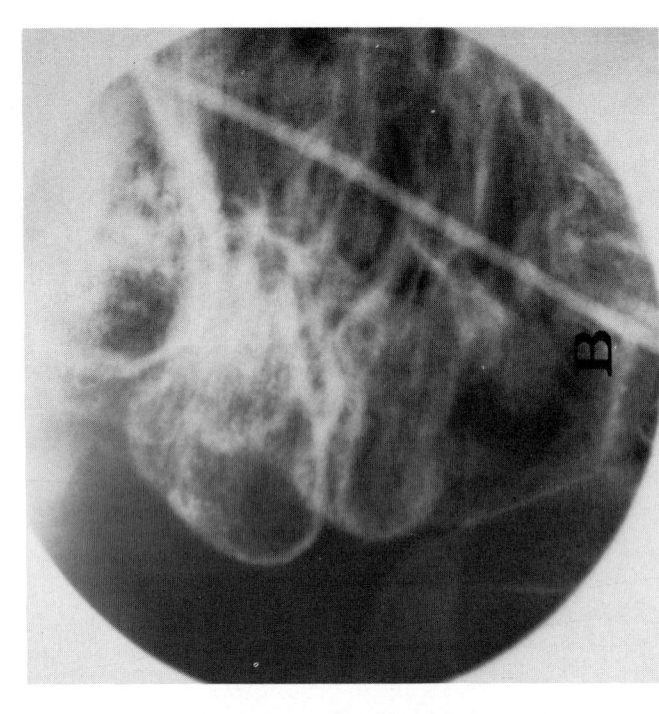

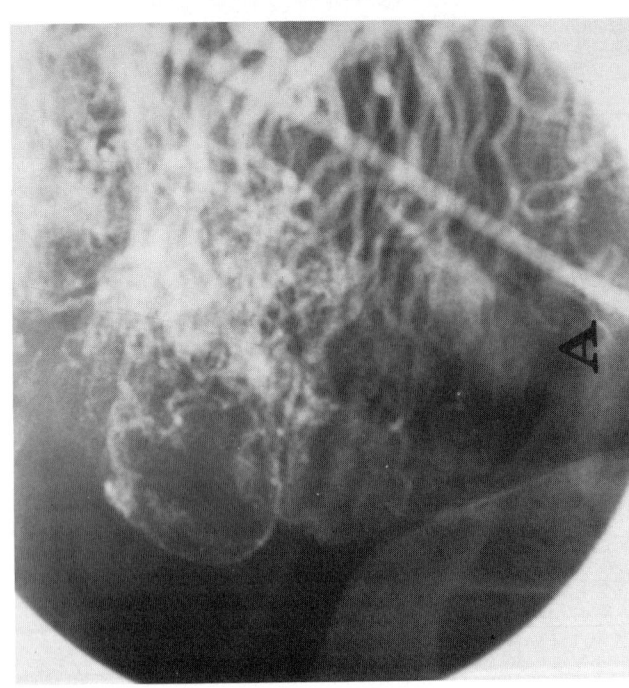

Fig. 8. Jejunal arteriovenous malformation in 40-year-old man with anemia and multiple episodes of melena. (A) Magnification mesenteric angiogram of jejunum shows tortuous abnormal vascular malformations. (B) Capillary phase of same angiogram shows dense contrast accumulation in the bowel wall and prominent draining veins.

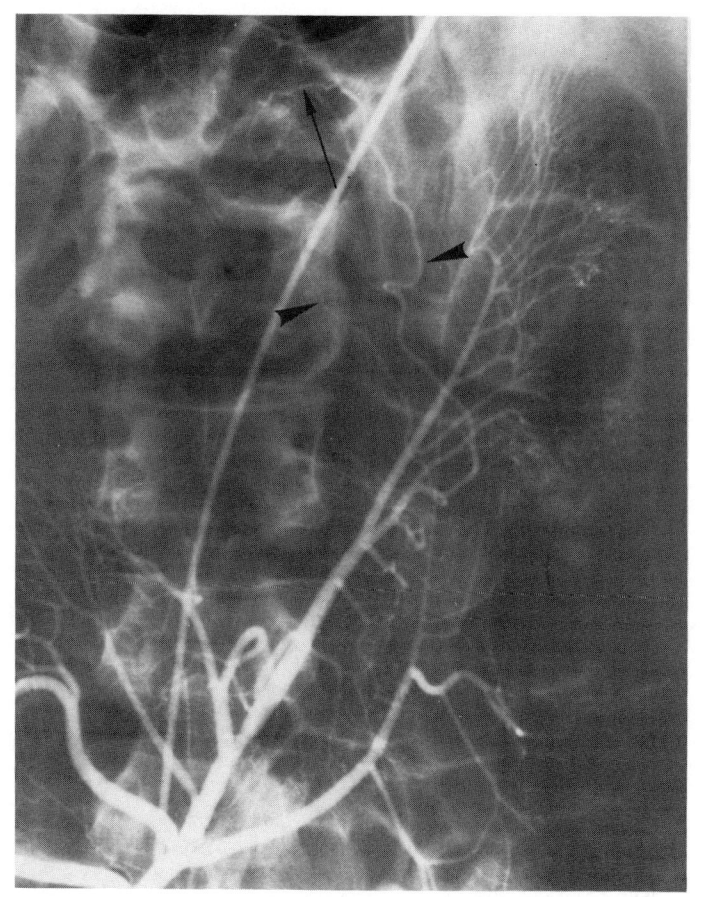

Fig. 9. Superior mesenteric angiogram in young man with recurrent gastrointestinal bleeding shows 2 anomalous arterial branches (arrows) originating from the right colic artery, supplying a Meckel's diverticulum. Distal end of artery (arrow) is irregular due to inflammatory scar associated with ulceration found at pathologic examination.

Colonic Trauma

Penetrating injury, fecal disimpaction and polypectomy are among traumatic causes of rectal hemorrhage [23, 31]. Endoscopic polypectomy of the colon has been complicated by hemorrhage in 1.9% of the cases [31].

Intestinal Varices

Intestinal varices are rare causes of massive lower gastrointestinal bleeding [15, 40]. The presence of adhesions from previous operative procedure may

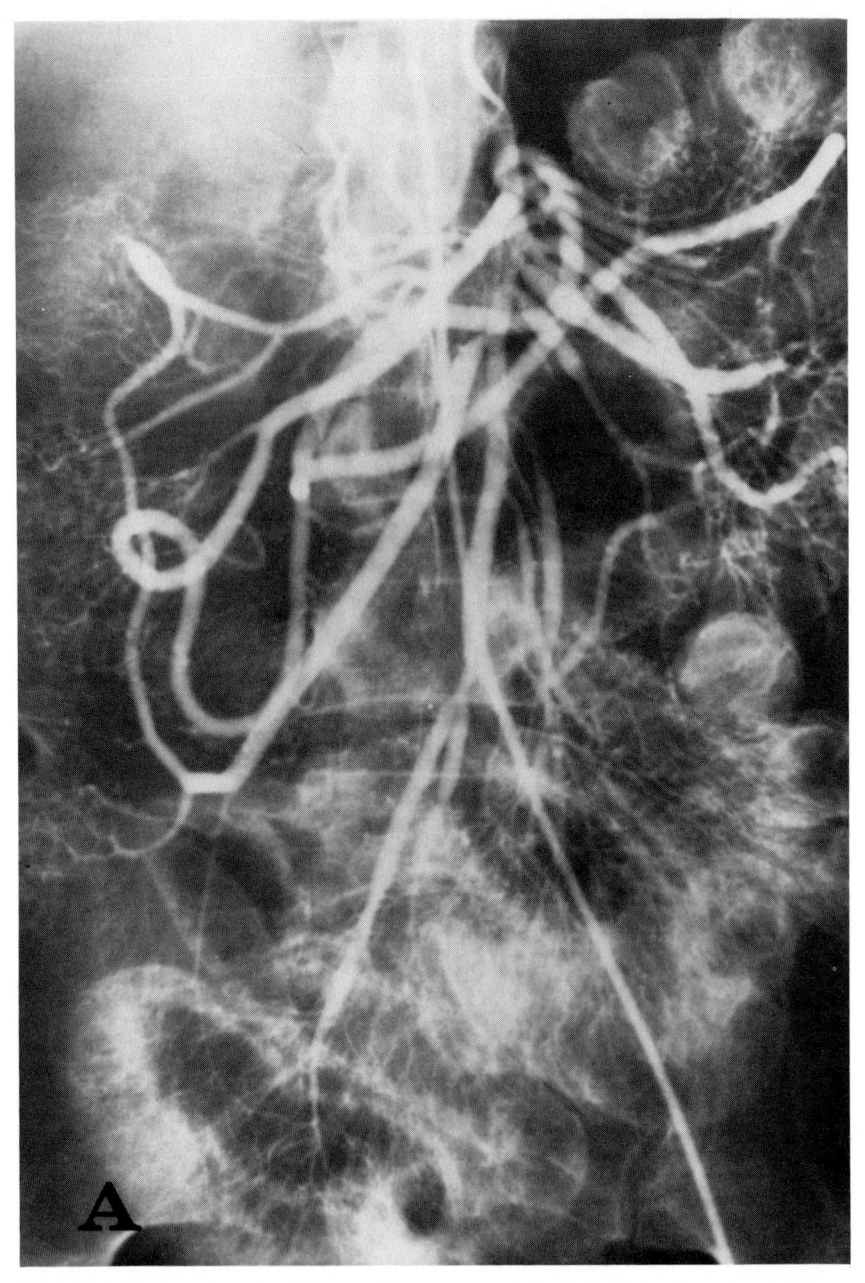

Fig. 10. Ileal varices in 45-year-old woman with cirrhosis and recurrent lower gastrointestinal bleeding. (A) Superior mesenteric angiogram (arterial phase) shows vasoconstriction of distal mesenteric arteries due to systemic vasopressin infusion made before this angiogram. (B, right) Venous phase of the same angiogram shows large varices filled from the ileocolic vein. Ileal resection and portacaval shunt were performed.

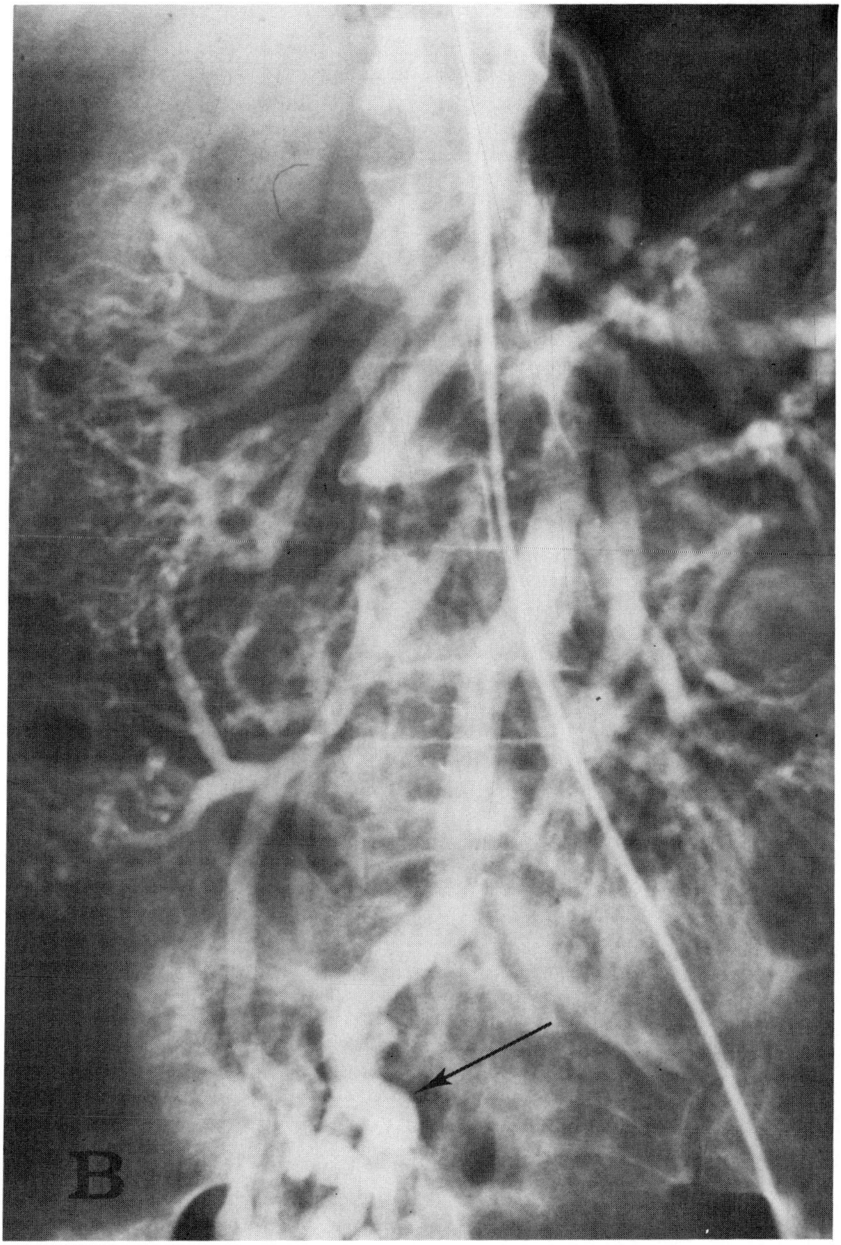
B

predispose to development of varices at unusual locations. Portasystemic collaterals between superior mesenteric and right gonadal vein in portal hypertension produce ileocecal varices and may cause lower gastrointestinal bleeding [15]. The recognition of intestinal varices on a superior mesenteric angiogram is essential for proper management of the patient. A portasystemic shunt or resection of the involved segment of bowel can cure the hemorrhage (Fig. 10). Rectosigmoid varices secondary to an occlusion of inferior mesenteric vein or splenic vein is a rare cause of low-grade rectal hemorrhage. Inferior mesenteric angiography with intraarterial injection of tolazoline is performed for the diagnosis, and vasopressin infusion into inferior mesenteric artery should control the hemorrhage.

REFERENCES

1. Baum S, Athanasoulis CA, Waltman AC, et al: Angiodysplasia of the right colon: a cause of gastrointestinal bleeding. Am J Roentgenol 129:789, 1977
2. Baum S, Nusbaum M, Blakemore WS, Finkelstein AK: The preoperative radiographic demonstration of intraabdominal bleeding from undetermined sites of percutaneous selective celiac and superior mesenteric arteriography. Surgery 58:797, 1965
3. Baum S, Nusbaum M, Clearfield HR, et al: Angiography in the diagnosis of gastrointestinal bleeding. Arch Intern Med 119:16, 1967
4. Boley SJ, Sammartano R, Adams A, et al: On the nature and etiology of vascular ectasias of the colon. Gastroenterology 72:650, 1977
5. Boijsen E, Reuter SR: Angiography in diagnosis of chronic unexplained melena. Radiology 89:413, 1967
6. Bree RL, Reuter SR: Angiographic demonstration of a bleeding Meckel's diverticulum. Radiology 108:287, 1973
7. Casarella WJ, Galloway SJ, Taxin RN, et al: "Lower" gastrointestinal tract hemorrhage: new concepts based on arteriography. Am J Roentgenol 121:357, 1974
8. Casarella WJ, Kanter IE, Seaman WB: Right-sided colonic diverticula as a cause of acute rectal hemorrhage. N Engl J Med 286:450, 1972
9. Cho KJ, Martel W: Recognition of splenic vein occlusion. Am J Roentgenol 131:439, 1978
10. Clark RA, Rösch J: Arteriography in diagnosis of large bowel bleeding. Radiology 94:83, 1970
11. Elliott JP Jr, Smith RF, Szilagy DE: Aorto-enteric and paraprosthetic-enteric fistulas. Arch Surg 108:479, 1974
12. Erb WH, Grimes EL: Pseudocysts of the pancreas. Am J Surg 100:30, 1960
13. Frey CF, Reuter SR, Bookstein JJ: Localization of gastrointestinal hemorrhage by selective angiography. Surgery 67:548, 1970
14. Graham DY, Schwartz JT: The spectrum of the Mallory-Weiss tears. Medicine (Baltimore) 57:307, 1978

15. Gray RK, Grollman JH Jr: Acute lower gastrointestinal bleeding secondary to varices of the superior mesenteric venous system. Angiographic demonstration. Radiology 111:559, 1974
16. Homan WP, Tang CK, Thorbjarnarson B: Acute massive hemorrhage from intestinal Crohn's disease. Report of seven cases and review of the literature. Arch Surg 111:901, 1976
17. Humphries AW, Young JR, de Wolfe VG, et al: Complications of abdominal aortic surgery. Arch Surg 86:43, 1963
18. Klein HJ, Alfidi, RJ, Meaney TF, et al: Angiography in diagnosis of chronic gastrointestinal bleeding. Radiology 98:83, 1971
19. Koehler PR, Nelson JA, Berenson MM: Massive extra-enteric gastrointestinal bleeding: angiographic diagnosis. Radiology 119:41, 1976
20. Meyers MA, Alonso DR, Baer JW: Pathogenesis of massively bleeding colonic diverticulosis: new observations. Am J Roentgenol 127:901, 1976
21. Miller KD Jr, Tutton RH, Bell KA, et al: Angiodysplasia of the colon. Radiology 132:309, 1979
22. Moore JD, Thompson NW, Appelman HD, et al: Arteriovenous malformations of the gastrointestinal tract. Arch Surg 111:381, 1976
23. Naderi MJ, Bookstein JJ: Rectal bleeding secondary to fecal disimpaction: angiographic diagnosis and treatment. Radiology 126:387, 1978
24. Nusbaum M, Baum S: Radiographic demonstration of unknown sites of gastrointestinal bleeding. Surg Forum 14:374, 1963
25. Olsen WR: Hemorrhage from diverticular disease of the colon. The role of emergency subtotal colectomy. Am J Surg 115:247, 1968
26. Ostergaard HA, Fredens M: Arteriographic demonstration of bleeding from Meckel's diverticulum: report of a case. Scand J Gastroenterol 6:109, 1971
27. Retzloff JA, Hagedorn AB, Bartholomew LG: Abdominal exploration for gastrointestinal bleeding of obscure origin. JAMA 177:104, 1961
28. Reuter SR, Bookstein JJ: Angiographic localization of gastrointestinal bleeding. Gastroenterology 54:876, 1968
29. Ring EJ, Athanasoulis CA, Waltman AC, et al: The pseudo-vein: an angiographic appearance of arterial hemorrhage. J Canad Assoc Radiologists 24:242, 1973
30. Rives JD, Emmett RO: Massive melena: survey of 129 cases seen at Charity Hospital from March 1950 to December 1952. J Louisiana Med Soc 105:293, 1953
31. Rogers BHG, Silvis SE, Nebel OT, et al: Complications of flexible fiberoptic colonoscopy and polypectomy. Gastrointest Endosc 22:73, 1975
32. Rosenbaum A, Siegelman SS, Sprayregen S: The bleeding marginal ulcer: catheterization, diagnosis and therapy. Am J Roentgenol 125:812, 1975
33. Schramek A, Weisz GM, Erlik D: Gastrointestinal bleeding due to arterioenteric fistula. Digestion 4:103, 1971
34. Seldinger SI: Catheter replacement of the needle in percutaneous arteriography: a new technique. Acta Radiol 39:368, 1953
35. Sheedy PF, Fulton RE, Atwell DT: Angiographic evaluation of patients with chronic gastrointestinal bleeding. Am J Roentgenol 123:338, 1975

36. Thompson WM, Jackson DC, Johnsrude IS: Aortoenteric and paraprosthetic-enteric fistulas: radiologic findings. Am J Roentgenol 127:235, 1976
37. van Heerden JA, ReMine WH: Pseudocysts of the pancreas. Arch Surg 110:500, 1975
38. Walter JF, Chuang VP, Bookstein JJ, et al: Angiography of massive hemorrhage secondary to pancreatic disease. Radiology 124:337, 1977
39. White AF, Baum S, Buranasiri S: Aneurysms secondary to pancreatitis. Am J Roentgenol 127:393, 1976
40. Wilson SE, Stone RT, Christie JP, et al: Massive lower gastrointestinal bleeding from intestinal varices. Arch Surg 114:1158, 1979

Peptic Ulcer Disease

Timothy T. Nostrant, M.D.
Jean-Pierre Raufmann, M.D.

The Natural History of Bleeding Peptic Ulcers

ABSTRACT

Our current approach to the management of patients with bleeding ulcers, both in the urgent and elective situation, is outlined.

Since both surgery and newer methods to arrest bleeding prevent death by stopping hemorrhage, the patient population studied should be at substantial risk of death from bleeding if valid comparisons are to be made. Although advanced age and increased transfusion requirements are associated with increased mortality, this mortality is rarely secondary to bleeding itself. Markers, such as the visible vessel or active bleeding at the time of endoscopy may predict a patient population at risk of bleeding death.

In the elective situation, treatment is aimed at preventing recurrent hemorrhage. In contrast to mortality, the age of the patient, the severity of blood loss, the pattern of in-hospital bleeding, and a previous history of hemorrhage cannot predict which patient will have recurrent bleeding. Problems in interpreting past studies, such as diagnostic accuracy and variable surgical technique are used to illustrate the need for homogeneous risk populations, both for mortality and recurrent bleeding. Valid comparisons between medical and surgical treatment to prevent recurrent bleeding cannot be made at this time, since the factors determining recurrent bleeding are not known.

Bleeding from acute and chronic peptic lesions of the stomach and duodenum constitutes 75% of all upper-gastrointestinal hemorrhage [20, 31]. It has been estimated to occur in 25% of patients hospitalized for ulcer disease [19, 31, 45], and in 10% of all patients with radiologically defined peptic ulcers [19, 31, 58]. The objective of this chapter is to analyze what is known about the natural history of bleeding from these lesions. This is necessary if we are to

---

Timothy T. Nostrant, M.D.: Instructor, Section of Gastroenterology, Department of Internal Medicine, University of Michigan Medical Center; Jean-Pierre Raufmann, M.D.: Fellow in Gastroenterology, Department of Internal Medicine, University of Michigan Medical Center, Ann Arbor, Michigan.

determine the proper role of conservative management vs. aggressive treatment of patients with bleeding ulcers in the light of recent endoscopic [34, 37], angiographic [30, 57] and pharmacologic advances [3, 18].

BACKGROUND

Treatment directed at patients with ulcer bleeding attempts to save life and prevent recurrent hemorrhage. However, saving life and decreasing recurrence rate are two independent treatment objectives. Oversewing a bleeding ulcer may save the patient's life, but it will not prevent either recurrent ulceration or bleeding. Similarly, although vagotomy and antrectomy may prevent recurrent hemorrhage, they may also leave the patient with more disabling symptoms than blood loss, let alone take his life. Thus to delineate the populations at risk for death or recurrent hemorrhage, we require an understanding of the factors which influence mortality and which determine recurrence. Unfortunately, these cannot be defined unequivocally, despite the voluminous literature dealing with this topic. Problems in defining risk factors stem from the diagnostic inaccuracy of earlier studies [25, 36], the range of ages of patients studied [1, 25], the variable definition of bleeding and recurrence [5, 8, 9, 25] and the differences in surgical technique [21, 29, 48, 49]. Discussion of these problems will illustrate the difficulties encountered in interpreting past studies to answer the question about what is optimal therapy for bleeding.

The ability to diagnose the location and the type of lesion causing hemorrhage was limited before the use of gastrointestinal endoscopy. Initial studies during the early years of upper gastrointestinal radiology used symptoms exclusively to define the location and type of gastroduodenal abnormality antemortem [1, 25, 58]. Midepigastric pain occurring just before the next meal and relieved by food or antacids was considered a sufficient definition of uncomplicated chronic duodenal ulcer. Complicated duodenal ulcers or gastric ulcers were thought to produce continuous or intermittent pain, frequently increased by eating. Horrocks, however, showed that less than 50% of patients with uncomplicated duodenal ulcers had pain coming on before meals or relieved by food intake [28]. Likewise, most patients with meal-produced pain had uncomplicated duodenal ulcer disease. Thus, those studies using symptoms alone to define the source of upper gastrointestinal hemorrhage are subject to serious error. Similarly, the efficacy of treatment based on relief of symptoms alone may not be interpretable.

When the patient is actively bleeding, barium radiology cannot determine the source of blood loss. False positive or false negative results have occurred in 10% to 50% of radiologically diagnosed cases when compared prospectively with endoscopic findings [13, 20, 23, 43]. The actual percentage of false results depends on the bleeding lesion (chronic ulcers vs acute erosive disease). This error is compounded by the 25% incidence of multiple lesions [20]. Thus, treatment success or failure based on radiological criteria is hard to interpret. Similarly, risk of death or recurrent hemorrhage cannot be defined on radiological grounds alone.

In addition to the problems of defining the source of bleeding, the population of patients with bleeding ulcers was composed of different age groups [1]. Younger patients are known to be at less risk of death than older patients, even when matched for severity of bleeding [1, 46, 58]. The risk of recurrent bleeding, however, has either been the same for both groups or greater in the younger population [2, 4, 8, 9, 56]. The higher risk of death in the older patients has been due, in part, to the presence of complicating disease [1, 58]. Longer life expectancy increases the recurrence rate in the younger population [56, 58]. Thus, combining populations of different age will invalidate the results of treatment, unless these results are stated separately for mortality and recurrence rate and compared with matched controls.

Timing of treatment is partly determined by the degree and rapidity of bleeding. This should be described for each bleeding episode. When bleeding was defined as any manifest blood loss, i.e., hematemesis, melena, shock, or occult blood in the stools, recurrence rate is very high (50%-90%) [4, 8, 9, 56], but the mortality is low (0-3%) [2, 4, 8, 9, 56]. However, if only patients with "clinically significant" bleeding were studied, i.e., patients requiring transfusions to maintain stable vital signs or hematocrit, mortality was much higher than for patients with lesser degrees of bleeding but recurrence rate was much less (10%-20%) [32, 35, 44, 53, 55]. In addition, the treatment course chosen did not affect the recurrence rate [25, 32]. Therefore, the definition of "bleeding" must be known before the effects of treatment can be interpreted.

The lack of homogeneous populations at risk is only part of the problem. Even if this could be eliminated, comparison of medical vs. surgical treatment in preventing death or recurrent bleeding would still be difficult. Rapid changes in surgical technique, without concurrent controlled studies to compare possible benefits, have made it impossible to select optimal surgical treatment [4, 12, 16, 21, 48, 49, 51, 52, 53, 55]. In the 1940s to early 1960s, immediate or urgent subtotal gastrectomy was the treatment for all patients with "serious peptic ulcer bleeding" [51, 52, 53]. The rationale for this operation equated "serious" bleeding with continuous bleeding [51, 52, 53]. Patients with "serious" bleeding were believed to have an increased risk for death and recurrent hemorrhage. Therefore, removal of the bleeding source would simultaneously decrease mortality and recurrence rate. These assumptions have proven to be wrong. Severe bleeding does not necessarily correlate with continued bleeding or recurrent in-hospital hemorrhage [5, 12, 45, 46]. Most bleeding secondary to peptic ulcers stops spontaneously and few patients die from exsanguination [1, 40, 54]. In addition, recurrence rate need not be decreased by removal of the bleeding source since recurrent bleeding after discharge may come from lesions not present at the time of operation [17]. Thus, it is not surprising that the recurrence rate of bleeding was high (15-32%) [4, 12, 53] and the mortality of gastric resection disconcerting (20% emergent [1, 51, 52], 10% elective [21, 48, 49]).

In rapid succession, vagotomy and drainage, vagotomy and antrectomy, and proximal gastric vagotomy, have been proposed as the operation of choice for bleeding peptic ulcers. Again, the objective of the operation is important. None of the above listed operations has been compared prospectively in the emergency setting to safe life. Where elective treatment for the prevention of recurrent bleeding is desired, prospective trials comparing vagotomy and drainage, vagotomy and antrectomy, and subtotal gastrectomy have shown little to favor one operation over another, based on decreased mortality or morbidity [21, 29, 48, 49]. Recurrence rate of hemorrhage, severity of bleeding, and the source of blood loss were not stated. Thus, as with medical treatment, a study designed to test the efficacy of surgical treatment in patients with bleeding ulcers must incorporate three points: The objective of the operation, i.e., saving life or preventing recurrent bleeding, must be clearly stated; the study population should be at substantial risk for this complication, since only in this patient group can success or failure be easily appreciated; and any treatment to prevent complications must be tested against appropriate controls without treatment to assess the overall benefit of treatment.

TENETS OF ULCER BLEEDING

Despite the above considerations dealing with the design and interpretation of past studies, much dogma about the management of ulcer patients who are bleeding has emerged. A critical examination of some commonly held beliefs may help to define populations at risk for mortality of recurrent bleeding:

1. Older Patients (Over 50 Years) Bleed More Severely and More Frequently Than Younger Patients (Below 50 Years) and Thus Require Earlier Operation

Three questions need to be answered: (1) Do older patients bleed more severely? (2) Are older patients less likely to stop bleeding? (3) Do older patients have a higher recurrence rate of bleeding after discharge?

When severity was defined by the number of transfusions required to maintain vital signs or a stable hematocrit, Wenchert showed no significant difference in severity of bleeding between older and younger patients [59]. This similarity was maintained when the source of bleeding was subdivided by the type of lesion (gastric, duodenal, both). Likewise, the chances of a favorable course, i.e., the patient survived, had no recurrent bleeding, and was not operated on, were identical in all age groups [59]. These observations were confirmed by other studies [2, 4, 5, 8, 9]. When the pattern of in-hospital bleeding was studied, Northfield found no significant difference between age groups in the recurrence rate of hemorrhage. However, mortality increased twenty-fold in patients who bled again while in the hospital regardless of their age [45, 46].

If older patients do not bleed more severely or more continuously, do they have an increased recurrence rate of bleeding after discharge? Chinn studied a group of 310 patients with radiologically defined peptic ulcer disease, who came to a city hospital with their first episode of gastrointestinal hemorrhage [8, 9]. He found that age had no bearing on the recurrence rate of bleeding when these patients were followed for up to 10 years (approximately 50% in both groups) [8, 9]. Again, the type of bleeding lesion did not change the outcome of the age analysis. The initial mortality of 9% reported in this study is similar to that of other studies with clearly defined severe bleeding [1, 51, 52]. In conclusion, age did not seem to influence the severity of initial bleeding, the risk of early in-hospital bleeding, or the likelihood of recurrent hemorrhage after discharge. However, the risk of death while in the hospital increased with age and with recurrent blood loss.

2. Rate of Recurrence Increases With Each Bleeding Episode

When recurrence was defined as presence of blood in gastric contents or stool, Stolte and others [12, 56], have shown a 60-90% incidence of recurrent bleeding from peptic ulcers during a 10-30 yr follow up period. The probability of recurrent hemorrhage increased after the second bleeding episode. If, however, decreasing hematocrit or overt shock were required to establish recurrence, the incidence of recurrence decreased and was not affected by the previous history of bleeding [35, 44, 52, 53, 55]. The incidence of recurrent "significant bleeding" was the same in operated and nonoperated patients [32]. In the large cooperative Veteran's Administration study of gastric ulcer, the recurrence rate of bleeding was 30% after each bleeding episode [38]. Thus, the literature does not support an increased rate of recurrence of "significant bleeding" in the patient with multiple bleeding episodes.

3. The Severity of Initial Bleeding Influences the Risk of Recurrent Hemorrhage or the Severity of Bleeding in the Future

Severity of bleeding, although it may influence initial mortality from hemorrhage, bears no relation to the recurrence rate or severity of subsequent bleeding episodes. Borland showed that patients who required 7 to 9 units of blood had the same recurrence rate as those patients who required only zero to three units of blood [5]. Likewise, the number of patients requiring less than six units of blood during subsequent bleeding episodes did not differ substantially between the two groups (82% vs 87%) [5]. Therefore, severity of index hemorrhage cannot be used as an argument favoring elective surgery to prevent recurrent bleeding.

4. Urgent or Immediate Surgery is the Best Treatment for Bleeding From Peptic Ulcer

Prevention of death from bleeding is the crucial issue. This benefit must be weighed against the chance of surgical mortality. The important determinants of operative risk are age and fitness for operation. Patients selected for emergency surgery have a higher mortality than those operated on electively because this group of patients is usually older and has more serious bleeding. Medical therapy is seldom continued in those with heavy or continuous bleeding, thus, increasing the number of poor risk patients treated surgically. Enquist compared patients treated by three different methods after an episode of upper gastrointestinal hemorrhage [15]. The first involved strict dietary therapy, with minimal transfusion and no operation. The latter two methods differed only in the timing of emergency surgery (less than 24 hours), vs delayed surgery (more than 48 hours). Groups did not differ substantially in terms of age, severity of bleeding as measured by transfusion requirements, or the type of bleeding lesion. The authors were unable to find a difference in mortality favoring any of the methods of treatment. This was true even if the patients were subdivided by type of lesion, age, fitness for operation, or severity of bleeding. This was confirmed by Dronfield who reviewed operative policies at two regional British hospitals [14]. In addition, Schiller found a higher recurrence rate after emergency operations than after elective procedures, even if the type of operation was the same [52]. Thus, a policy of "watchful waiting" and "judicious transfusion" does not appear to increase mortality or recurrence rate.

5. Surgery Prevents Recurrence of Hemorrhage

This tenet is entrenched in the minds of most physicians. Unfortunately, the evidence for this is tenuous. Despite its usefulness in some complications of peptic ulcer disease [58], partial gastrectomy may be followed by recurrent bleeding [4, 12, 53]. This is particularly true for patients who have significant rebleeding [4, 12, 32, 53]. The reasons for this have been discussed above. Two points need to be made. No prospective study of recurrence rate for bleeding has compared all the major operations used to stop recurrent bleeding. Secondly, recurrent ulceration has not always been separated from recurrent bleeding. Thus, long-term evaluation of both ulceration and bleeding using endoscopy in the postsurgical patient is needed.

6. Mortality and Morbidity in Patients With Bleeding From Peptic Ulcers is Mainly Due to the Hemorrhage

Allan and Dykes' study was the first major retrospective and prospective work to determine the causes of mortality in patients with upper gastrointestinal bleeding [1]. Retrospective analysis showed that mortality has not changed over the past 30 years, despite advances in surgical and critical care management. However, a significant decrease in mortality since 1950 was found when patients 60 years or older were compared (9% vs 25%). Thus, the lack of change in mortality figures was due to an increase in the percentage of patients older than 60 years of age in the newer studies (from 10% to 40%).

Prospectively, 300 consecutive patients with upper gastrointestinal hemorrhage were studied to determine the risk factors of mortality. This study was not randomized. Mortality was 9.7%. Of these 29 deaths, 14 were considered inevitable because of advanced malignancy or end stage cardiovascular disease. Of the remaining 15 deaths, only 1 was considered to be secondary to bleeding. The remaining 14 deaths occurred either postoperatively (11) or after intensive medical therapy (3). Ten of these 14 deaths were due to thrombosis or postoperative infection. All of the patients with potentially preventable deaths were older than 70 years. These findings reiterate that bleeding itself rarely causes death. Although surgery may be successful in stopping hemorrhage, it is not as successful in preventing death. Thus, new therapy must be aimed both at stopping hemorrhage and preventing postoperative death.

7. There Is No Effective Medical Therapy for Bleeding From Peptic Ulcers

Once again, prevention of death during the initial hemorrhage must be separated from prevention of recurrent bleeding. To date, there are no convincing data to suggest that medical therapy will modify mortality or stop bleeding during an acute episode. Studies with cimetidine, although initially promising, have not been confirmed, although more extensive work with endoscopically defined bleeding sources are needed [18, 47]. In the prevention of bleeding from stress induced lesions, however, both antacids and cimetidine have been shown to decrease mortality from bleeding and prevent recurrence [3, 11, 18, 39]. No controlled studies have yet examined the problem of decreasing recurrent bleeding from chronic peptic ulcers. Cimetidine has been shown to decrease ulcer recurrence [2, 7, 17, 18]. This effect, however, only lasts as long as the medication is being taken [2, 18, 47]. Long-term toxicity studies are thus needed before cimetidine can be used for this purpose, since therapy may be for life. Initial one to two year studies have shown minimal or absent toxicity from full dose cimetidine.

SUMMARY OF TENETS ABOUT BLEEDING ULCERS

It appears, therefore, that the age of the patient, the pattern of bleeding while in the hospital (single episode vs recurrent or continuous bleeding) and the presence of co-existent disease (i.e., fitness for operation), are the major features determining mortality, regardless of treatment. Until studies are available to define the optimal therapeutic regimen, subjective decision making must suffice. The recurrence rate, on the other hand, is not determined by the age of the patient, the severity or pattern of bleeding, the previous bleeding history, or the treatment used. Therefore, arguments used favoring early operation in decreasing mortality while the patient is actively bleeding cannot be used in the elective situation where prevention of bleeding recurrence is desired.

ENDOSCOPY IN DETERMINING THE RISK OF MORTALITY

Since recurrent hemorrhage within the hospital adversely affects mortality, can we predict this event before it occurs? As it has been repeatedly shown that recurrent bleeding usually occurs within the first 48-72 hours after an acute bleeding episode, endoscopy must be used early if it is to useful as a predictor of recurrent in-hospital bleeding [45, 46, 58]. Initial endoscopic studies have determined a population at risk for recurrent or continuous bleeding [20, 23]. In one study, all of the patients who had visible vessels in ulcer craters, bled again and required operation [23]. This group constituted 10% of all bleeding episodes but one-third of all patients who did not spontaneously stop bleeding. Active bleeding seen at the time of endoscopy may carry a prognosis similar to the presence of a visible vessel but further study is necessary [20].

Another major subgroup of patients at increased risk of death and recurrent bleeding are those patients with the Zollinger-Ellison syndrome [50]. This group of patients can be identified by an increased fasting serum gastrin concentration. This determination should be obtained prior to any elective operation for peptic ulcer disease because more than 70% of Z-E patients have uncomplicated peptic ulcers initially [50]. Basal and maximal acid secretion coupled with secretin tests may then be necessary to exclude other hypergastrinemic states, which do not require total gastrectomy to control the ulcer diathesis. Cimetidine has been used to prevent recurrent ulceration and may eliminate the need for extensive operation unless resectable lesions are present [18, 50].

POTENTIAL PROSPECTIVE STUDIES IN ULCER BLEEDING

Based on the above considerations, the time to replace conservative medical therapy by more vigorous attempts to stop bleeding is still unknown. A prospective trial involving the populations at high risk for death could be designed to answer this question. A group of patients greater than 50 years of age and having clinically significant bleeding could be chosen. This group of patients would then undergo endoscopy and those with visible vessels or bleeding at the time of endoscopy could be randomized into specific groups. These groups would undergo conservative medical therapy with angiographic or endoscopic control of hemorrhage, conservative treatment with medical or angiographic arrest of bleeding, followed by definitive surgery, or conservative treatment followed by immediate operation. These patients could be followed to determine the rate of recurrent hemorrhage and ulceration post-treatment. An adjunct to the study would be the addition of a group of patients in each treatment regimen who would also receive H_2 receptor antagonists after the initial mortality study. This group compared to the placebo group would then give information about recurrence (bleeding and ulceration) after using long-term antisecretory therapy. The potential of the ASGE study group in this regard is obvious [20].

CURRENT MANAGEMENT

Since a proven optimal management for patients with bleeding ulcers is not available, what is our approach to the patient with upper gastrointestinal hemorrhage? We believe that patients with "clinically significant" bleeding (i.e., the patient requires transfusion to maintain stable vital signs and hematocrit) require endoscopic diagnosis of the bleeding source and intensive care treatment. If endoscopy reveals a visible vessel or active bleeding, the pattern of blood loss is monitored by transfusion requirements (determined by frequent hematocrits), nasogastric aspiration, and central venous monitoring. During this surveillance time, the patient is treated with antacids or cimetidine to maintain acid and pepsin neutralization (gastric pH greater than 5). We favor early surgical intervention in the good risk patient if bleeding continues or recurs within the first 12-24 hours. If the patient has a potentially lethal disease, e.g., tumor or systemic illness, or if the patient is a poor surgical candidate, clot embolization of a discrete ulcer bleeding source is attempted by an experienced operator early after admission. Operation is then undertaken only if embolization fails to stop bleeding. The finding of erosive upper gastrointestinal disease suggests prolonged conservative management [10]. Vasoconstrictive therapy or operation is rarely needed. After bleeding has been arrested, medical treatment with antithrombotic agents may be required postoperatively. Better attention to pre- and postoperative care may do much to decrease the mortality of patients with a bleeding ulcer.

If the patient survives and stops bleeding, future treatment is dependent upon the previous history. If this admission represents the first bleeding episode in an otherwise uncomplicated patient with ulcer disease, we favor medical treatment with full-dose cimetidine or antacids until the ulcer heals. Cimetidine on a continuous basis is our initial treatment option in the patient with recurrent but nondisabling bleeding. Patients who need frequent hospitalizations for bleeding, despite cimetidine or who have complicated ulcers and hemorrhage, usually require surgical intervention.

REFERENCES

1. Allan R, Dykes P: A study of the factors influencing mortality rates from gastrointestinal hemorrhage. Q J Med 45:533, 1976
2. Arias IM, Zamcheck N, Thrower WB: Recurrence of hemorrhage from medically treated gastric ulcers. Arch Int Med 101:369, 1958
3. Bardhan KD, Saul DM, Edwards JL, et al: Double-blind comparison of cimetidine and placebo in the maintenance of healing of chronic duodenal ulceration. Gut 20:158, 1979
4. Boles RS Jr, Cassidy WJ, Jordan SM: Medical vs surgical management for the complication of hemorrhage in duodenal ulcer. Gastroenterology 32:52, 1957
5. Borland JL Sr, Hancock RW, Borland JL Jr: Recurrent upper gastrointestinal hemorrhage in peptic ulcer. Gastroenterology 52:631, 1967
6. Buckingham JM, ReMine WH: Results of emergency surgical management of hemorrhagic duodenal ulcer. Mayo Clin Proc 50:223, 1975
7. Cargill JM, Peden N, Saunders JH, et al: Very long-term treatment of peptic ulcer disease with cimetidine. Lancet 2:1113, November 25, 1978
8. Chinn AB, Littell AS, Badger GF, et al: Acute hemorrhage from peptic ulcer. A follow-up study of 310 patients. N Engl J Med 255:973, 1956
9. Chinn AB, Weckesser EC: Acute hemorrhage from peptic ulceration. An analysis of 322 patients. Ann Int Med 34:339, 1951
10. Cody HS, Wichern WA: Choice of operation for acute gastric mucosal hemorrhage. Report of 36 cases and review of the literature. Am J Surg 134:322, 1977
11. Czaja AJ, McAlhany JC, Pruitt BA Jr: Acute gastro duodenal disease after thermal injury. N Engl J Med 291:925, 1974
12. Donaldson RM, Handy J: Five year follow-up study of patients with bleeding duodenal ulcer with and without surgery. N Engl J Med 259:201, 1958
13. Dronfield MW, Ferguson R, McIllmurray MB, et al: Policies on mortality for bleeding peptic ulcer. Lancet 1:1126, May 26, 1977
14. Dronfield MW, Atkinson M, Langman MJS: Effects of different operation policies on mortality for bleeding peptic ulcer. Lancet 1:1126, May 26, 1979
15. Enquist IF, Karlson KE, Dennis C, et al: Statistically valid ten year comparative evaluation of three methods of management of massive gastro duodenal hemorrhage. Ann Surg 152:550, 1965

16. Farris JM, Smith GK: Appraisal of long term results of vagotomy and pyloroplasty in one hundred patients with bleeding duodenal ulcers. Ann Surg 166:630, 1967
17. Festen HPM, Lamers BH, Driessen MM, et al: Cimetidine in anastomotic ulceration after partial gastrectomy. Gastroenterology 76:83, 1979
18. Fordtran JS, Grossman MI: Third symposium on histamine H_2-receptor antagonists-clinical results with cimetidine. Gastroenterology 74:338, 1978
19. Fry J: Peptic ulcer. A profile. Br Med J 2:809, 1964
20. Gilbert DA, Silverstein DE, Tedesco FJ, et al: Prognosis of upper gastrointestinal bleeding preliminary results of the ASGE national bleeding survey. Gastroenterology 76:1138, 1979
21. Goligher JC, Pulvertaft CN, DeDombol FT: Five to eight year results of Leeds-York controlled trial of elective surgery for duodenal ulcer. Br Med J 2:781, 1968
22. Grace WJ, Mitty WF: Does subtotal gastrectomy in bleeding peptic ulcer prevent recurrence of bleeding? Am J Dig Dis 7:69, 1962
23. Griffith WJ, Neumann DA, Welsh JD: The visible vessel as an indicator of uncontrolled or recurrent gastrointestinal hemorrhage. N Engl J Med 300:1411, 1979
24. Hallenbeck GA: Elective surgery for treatment of hemorrhage from duodenal ulcer. Gastroenterology 59:784, 1970
25. Hallenbeck GA, Gleysteen JJ, Aldrette JS: Proximal gastric vagotomy. Effects of two operative techniques on clinical and gastric secretory results. Ann Surg 184:435, 1976
26. Hastings PR, Skillman JJ, Bushnell LS, et al: Antacid titration in the prevention of acute gastrointestinal bleeding. N Engl J Med 298:1041, 1978
27. Himal HS, Watson WW, Jones CW, et al: The management of upper gastrointestinal hemorrhage. A multi parametric computer analysis. Ann Surg 179:489, 1974
28. Horrocks JC, Dedombal FT: Clinical presentation of patients with "dyspepsia". Gut 19:19, 1978
29. Howard RJ, Murphy WR, Humphrey EW: A prospective randomized study of the elective surgical treatment for duodenal ulcer. Two to ten year follow-up study. Surgery 73:256, 1973
30. Janicki P, Alfidi RJ: Selective visceral angiography in the diagnosis and treatment of gastroduodenal hemorrhage. Surg Clin N Am 56:1365, 1976
31. Ivy AC, Grossman MI, Bachrach WH: Chapt 16, Peptic Ulcer. Philadelphia, Blakiston, 1950, p 557
32. Johansson C, Barany F: A retrospective study on the outcome of massive bleeding from peptic ulceration. Scand J Gastroenterol 8:113, 1973
33. Johnston D: Operative mortality and post-operative morbidity of highly selective vagotomy. Br Med J 4:545, 1975
34. Kiefhaber P, Moritz K, Schildberg FW: Endoskopische Nd-YAG laserko gulation blutender akuter und chronischer ulcera langenbecks. Arch Chir 347:567, 1978
35. Kozell PD, Meyer KA: Massively bleeding duodenal ulcers. General factors influencing incidence and mortality. Arch Surg 86:445, 1963

36. Krag E: Acute hemorrhage in peptic ulcer. A clinical radiographic and statistical follow-up study. Acta Med Scand 180:339, 1966
37. Linscheer WG, Fazio TL: Control of upper gastrointestinal hemorrhage by endoscopic spraying of clotting factors. Gastroenterology 77:642, 1979
38. Littman A: VA cooperative study on gastric ulcer. Gastroenterology 61:567, 1971
39. McAlhany JC, Czaja AJ, Pruitt BA: Antacid control of complications from acute gastro duodenal disease after burns. J Trauma 16:645, 1976
40. McEwen A, Johnston S, Needham CD, et al: Factors affecting the mortality in hemorrhage from benign peptic lesions of the stomach and duodenum. Br Med J 2:1056, 1968
41. McGregor DB, Savage LE, McVay CB: Massive gastrointestinal hemorrhage. A twenty-five year experience with vagotomy and drainage. Surgery 80:530, 1976
42. Moore FD, Peete WBJ, Richardson JE: The effects of definitive surgery on duodenal ulcer disease. A comparative study of surgical and nonsurgical management in nine hundred and ninety-seven cases. Ann Surg 132:652, 1950
43. Morris DW, Levine GM, Soloway RD, et al: Prospective randomized study of diagnosis and outcome in acute upper gastrointestinal bleeding. Endoscopy vs. conventional radiology. Am J Dig Dis 20:1103, 1975
44. Nielsen SD, Ambrupe E: Mortality following surgical treatment for massive gastroduodenal hemorrhage. Acta Chir Scand (Suppl) 396:29, 1969
45. Norbye E: Ulcer statistics from Drammen Hospital, 1936-1945. Acta Med Scand 143:50, 1962
46. Northfield TC: Factors predisposing to recurrent hemorrhage after acute gastrointestinal bleeding. Br Med J 1:26, 1971
47. Pickard RG, Sanderson I, Northfield TC: Controlled trial of cimetidine in acute upper gastrointestinal bleeding. Br Med J 1:661, March 10, 1979
48. Postlethwait RW: Five year follow-up results of operations for duodenal ulcer. Surg Gynecol Obstet 137:387, 1973
49. Price WE, Grizzle JE, Postlethwait RW: Results of operations for duodenal ulcer. Surg Gynecol Obstet 131:233, 1970
50. Regan RP, Malagelada JR: A reappraisal of clinical roentgenographic and endoscopic features of the Zollinger-Ellison syndrome. Mayo Clin Proc 53:19, 1978
51. Roberts WM: Gastroduodenal hemorrhage. Experience with two hundred sixty four consecutive cases. S Afr Med J 41:207, March 4, 1967
52. Schiller KFR, Truelove SC, Williams DW: Haematemesis and melaena with special reference to factors influencing the outcome. Br Med J 1:7, April 4, 1970
53. Serebro HA, Mendeloff AI: Late results of medical and surgical treatment of bleeding peptic ulcers. Lancet 2:505, September 3, 1966
54. Silverstein FE: A staunch approach to endoscopic therapy. Gastroenterology 77:797, 1979
55. Snyder EM, Stellar CA: Results from emergency surgery for massively bleeding duodenal ulcer. Am J Surg 115:170, 1968

56. Stolte JB: Gross bleeding from the digestive tract. 2. The frequency of manifest bleeding in peptic ulcer, with regard to the duration of the disease and the age of the diseased. Acta Med Scand 116:584, 1944
57. Twiford TW, Goldstein HM, Zornoza J: Transcatheter therapy of gastrointestinal arterial bleeding. Am J Dig Dis 23:1046, 1978
58. Walker CO: Complications of peptic ulcer disease and indications for surgery in Sleisenger and Fordtran (eds): Gastrointestinal Diseases (2nd ed). Philadelphia, Saunders, 1978, p 914
59. Wenckert A, Borg I, Lindblom P: Review of medically treated bleeding gastric or duodenal ulcers. Acta Chir Scand 120:66, 1978

Aaron S. Fink, M.D.
Richard G. Fiddian-Green, M.A., M.D., F.R.C.S.

Pathophysiological Considerations in the Management of Patients With Bleeding Ulcers

ABSTRACT

The overall mortality in patients with bleeding ulcers has not improved, despite improvements in medical care and reduction in surgical mortality, but it would be reduced if peptic ulcer disease could be prevented or effectively treated before the complication of bleeding appeared.

In patients who have had a gastrojejunostomy, jejunal ulcers are caused by an abnormal exposure to acid. The mortality from bleeding jejunal ulcers could be reduced by lessening the frequency with which gastrojejunostomies are constructed, and especially by reducing the frequency with which ulcerogenic operations are performed. Most duodenal and gastric ulcers appear not to be caused by an abnormal exposure to acid but by an impaired resistance to a normal exposure to acid. Medical treatment of ulcer disease might be more effective if, in addition to being directed towards reducing the exposure to acid, it were directed towards enhancing the ability of the mucosa to withstand exposure to acid.

Patients in whom the bleeding will not stop require early occlusion of their bleeding vessel for optimal results. These patients might be identified sooner by consideration of various factors associated with an increased risk of rebleeding. An improvement in the technique for monitoring the rate of blood loss might help to identify these patients sooner and with greater precision. The overall mortality from bleeding ulcers might be reduced if patients were referred for surgery earlier and with greater frequency.

Hemorrhage from peptic ulcer presents a major therapeutic challenge to both internists and surgeons. Fifteen to 20% of patients afflicted with peptic ulcers

---

Aaron S. Fink, M.D.: Chief Resident, Department of Surgery, University of Michigan Medical Center; Richard G. Fiddian-Green, M.A., M.D., F.R.C.S.: Associate Professor of Surgery, Director, Gastrointestinal Endocrine Laboratory, University of Michigan Medical Center, Ann Arbor, Michigan.

will have at least one hemorrhage if followed for fifteen to twenty-five years [53]. Twenty-five to 37% [42, 49] of patients with duodenal ulcers and 13% [43] of patients with gastric ulcers present with bleeding; further, one-quarter of all hospital admissions for duodenal ulcer disease are for bleeding [49].

The mortality in patients with bleeding ulcers is dependent on multiple factors but may be as high as 30%-50% in poor-risk patients [25, 34]. Both Chalmers et al [7] and Schiller et al [47] have shown that there has been no reduction in the mortality from bleeding ulcers during the past 15 years despite our improvements in medical care during this period. These findings indicate that new approaches are necessary if we are to reduce the mortality associated with bleeding ulcers.

In this chapter we shall discuss various pathophysiological factors that may contribute to the development and maintenance of bleeding ulcers with the object of identifying ways in which we might improve management of patients afflicted with this disease. These factors will be considered from four vantage points: the disease; the patient; the hemorrhage; and the ulcer.

THE DISEASE

Most ulcers develop as the result of an intensely investigated but poorly understood disease process. Acid seems to be essential for the development and maintenance of this disease process, for ulcers are invariably present in patients who secrete "abnormal" amounts of acid and rarely, if ever, present in individuals who are achlorhydric. Further, ulcers heal when their exposure to acid is abolished. The onset of bleeding does not appear to be associated with any alteration in the relationship between acid and ulcers [1].

Jejunal ulcers are found in individuals whose jejunal mucosa is abnormally exposed to acid. Under normal conditions, jejunal mucosa is not exposed to acid. Jejunal mucosa may be exposed to acid in patients who have a normal anatomy if they have the Zollinger-Ellison syndrome [15]. Jejunal mucosa is most often exposed to acid in patients who have a gastrojejunostomy (Figs. 1-7). Ulceration is especially common in patients with a gastrojejunostomy if their exposure to acid is increased, which occurs when alkaline secretions from the pancreas and liver are prevented from reaching the anastomosis by a Roux-en-y or jejuno-jejunal anastomosis [4, 38] or long afferent loop (Figs. 1-3). The exposure to acid is especially increased under these circumstances when acid secretion is increased by the autonomous release of gastrin from a retained antrum [37] (Fig. 4) or gastrinoma [15]. Jejunal ulcers will heal if their exposure to acid is abolished. Thus, jejunal ulcers seem to be caused by an abnormal exposure to acid.

It is generally agreed [2] that the majority of duodenal ulcers are found in individuals who are exposed to normal amounts of acid. Thus, in contrast to

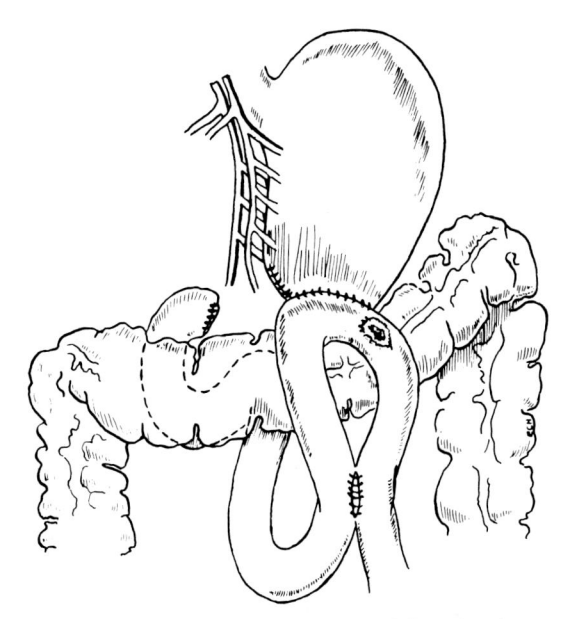

Fig. 1. Ulcerogenic operation caused by the diversion of alkaline secretions from the anastomosis without vagotomy. Treatment by vagotomy.

jejunal ulcers, the majority of duodenal ulcers are not caused by an abnormal exposure to acid. Since acid is the sine qua non for the development and maintenance of all duodenal ulcers, most of them must be caused by an impaired resistance to a normal exposure to acid.

The minority of duodenal ulcers are found in individuals who are exposed to abnormal amounts of acid. Indeed, the majority of individuals who are exposed to abnormal amounts of acid have duodenal ulcers [2]. Several studies, however, have raised the possibility that the abnormal exposure to acid found in the minority of patients with duodenal ulcers may be the result rather than the cause of their ulcer disease [17, 27, 52]. Furthermore, duodenal ulcers are found in those areas of the duodenum intermittently exposed to acid rather than in those areas continuously exposed to acid [46]. Indeed, duodenal bulb ulcers have been observed to heal in patients with normal anatomy who were exposed to abnormal amounts of acid; these ulcers were replaced by new ulcers at more distal sites as the disease progressed [22] and the abnormal exposure to acid increased (Table 1, p 102). Thus, a causal relationship between duodenal bulb ulcers and an abnormal exposure to acid has not been firmly established.

Most gastric ulcers are also found in individuals who are exposed to normal amounts of acid [3]. Since acid also appears to be the sine qua non for development and maintenance of gastric ulcers, it would seem that most gastric

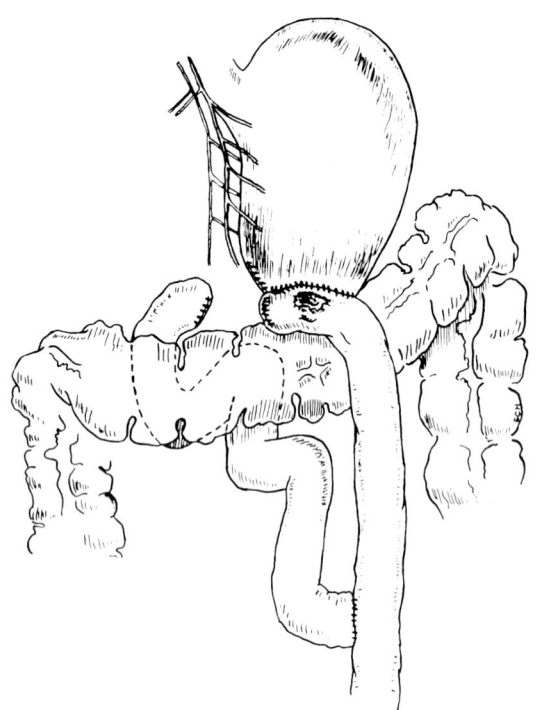

Fig. 2. Ulcerogenic operation caused by the diversion of alkaline secretions from the anastomosis without vagotomy. Treatment by vagotomy.

ulcers are also caused by an impaired resistance to a normal exposure to acid rather than by an abnormal exposure to acid.

The mucosal resistance to acid depends upon a number of factors (Fig. 10). The ability of acid to exert a negative feedback control on its own secretion and to stimulate the secretion of bicarbonate governs the intensity and duration of the exposure to acid. The permeability of mucosa to acid determines the rate at which acid can enter it. The mucosal blood flow aids in the removal of any acid that happens to enter the mucosa, while the respiratory and renal buffer systems are crucial to the disposal of any acid that has penetrated the mucosa. Finally, the remarkable ability of intestinal mucosa to repair itself [23] enables the patient to maintain a barrier between luminal acid and submucosal tissues.

Local differences in these protective mechanisms appear to be responsible for the gradient in mucosal resistance to acid that extends from the stomach distally [21, 31]. Thus, the relative impermeability of gastric mucosa [12] contributes to its remarkable ability to withstand a prolonged exposure to acid. The generation of an alkaline tide [32] by the secretion of acid enhances this ability. The generation of alkaline secretions from the pancreas, the liver,

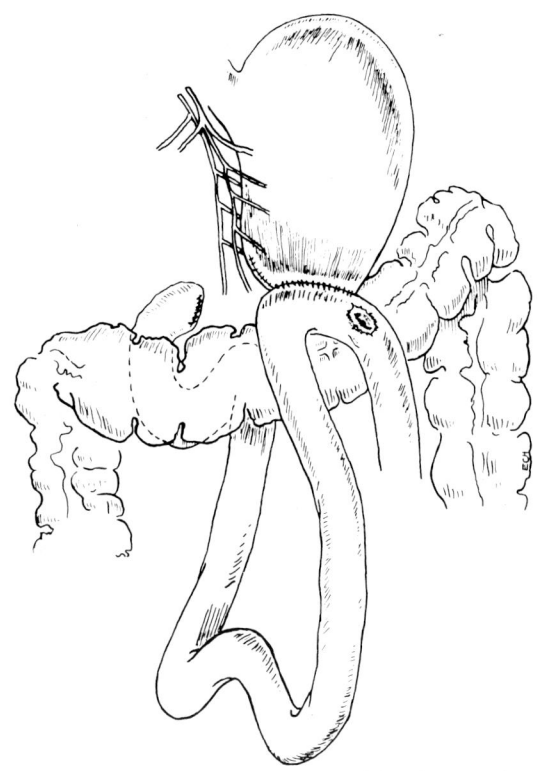

Fig. 3. Ulcerogenic operation caused by the creation of an inordinately long afferent limb. The afferent limb should be kept to a hand's breadth in length. Treatment by revision and vagotomy.

Brunner's glands, and from intestinal mucosa contributes to the ability of duodenal mucosa and, to a lesser degree, jejunal mucosa to withstand lesser exposure to acid [14, 18, 39, 40]. The metaplastic change within duodenal mucosa [44] and the hyperplasia of Brunner's glands that occur when the duodenum is exposed to abnormal amounts of acid may enhance the mucosal resistance to acid and contribute to the healing of ulcers in areas exposed to abnormal amounts of acid (Figs. 8 and 9).

An impairment of mucosal resistance to acid may be caused by a number of factors. Some of these factors impair the ability of mucosa at all sites to withstand an exposure to acid. The failure of acid to inhibit the secretion of gastrin increases the amount of acid to which the mucosa is exposed by increasing the parietal cell mass [6]; it also increases the intensity and duration of the exposure to acid within the exposed area. This occurs in patients with retained antra [37], with antral G cell hyperplasia [5, 10] and in patients with

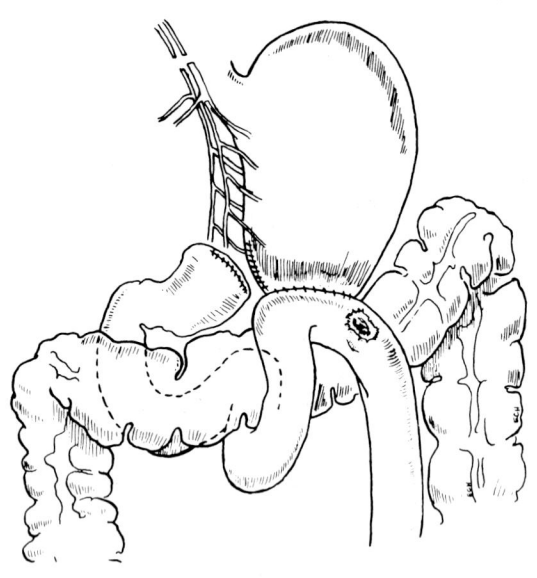

Fig. 4. Ulcerogenic operation created by retaining an antral stump isolated from the acid stream. Treatment by excision of the retained antral stump.

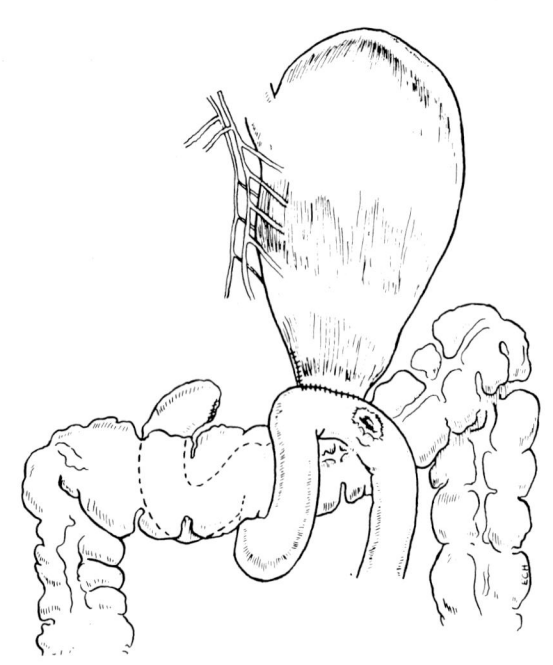

Fig. 5. Lesser ulcerogenic operation created by partial resection (30%) without vagotomy. Treatment by vagotomy.

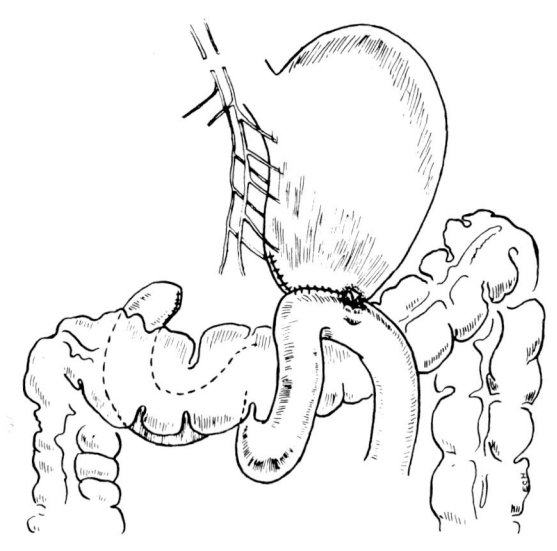

Fig. 6. "Stitch-ulcer" created by the use of non-absorbable sutures. Treatment by endoscopic removal.

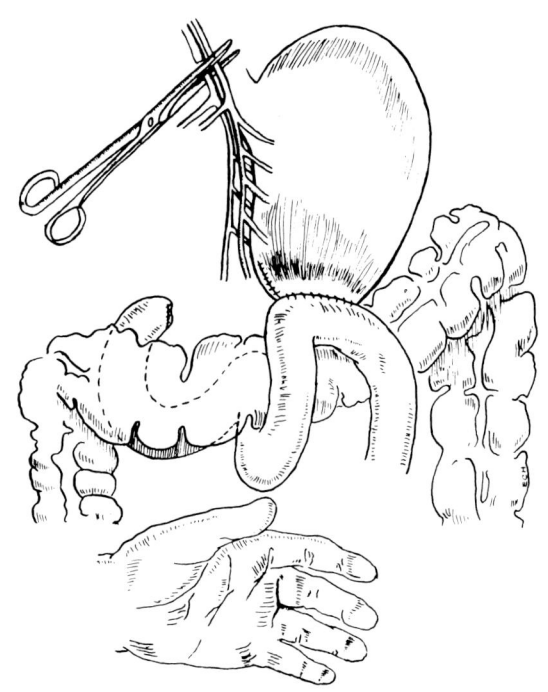

Fig. 7. "Ideal" Billroth II operation with 40% resection, vagotomy and short afferent loop (limited to a hand's breadth in length).

Table 1
Clinical Course and Concentration of Acid in Fasting Gastric Juice of Two Patients With Zollinger-Ellison Syndrome

			Location				Diagnosis	
Patient	Date	Antrum	DU Bulb	Post bulbar	Jejunal	UGI	Endos- copy	Lapa- rotomy
A	1957	Ulcer				+		
	1961		74 mEq/l Ulcer			+		
	1962		Ulcer			+		
	1963				135 mEq/l Ulcer			+
B	1974		Ulcer				+	
	1975		60 mEq/l Ulcer	60 mEq/l Ulcer			+	
	1976				120 mEq/l Ulcer		+	+

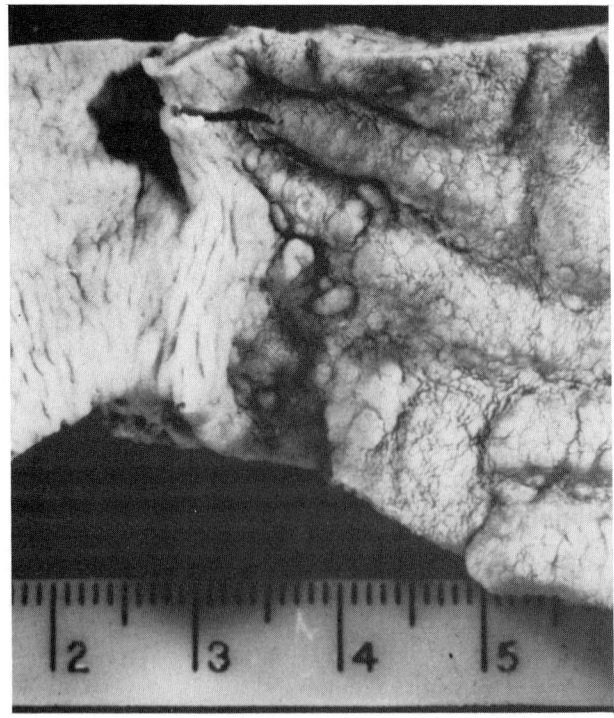

Fig. 8. Brunner's gland hyperplasia in the duodenum of a patient with the Zollinger-Ellison syndrome. [Courtesy Dr. Henry Appleman.]

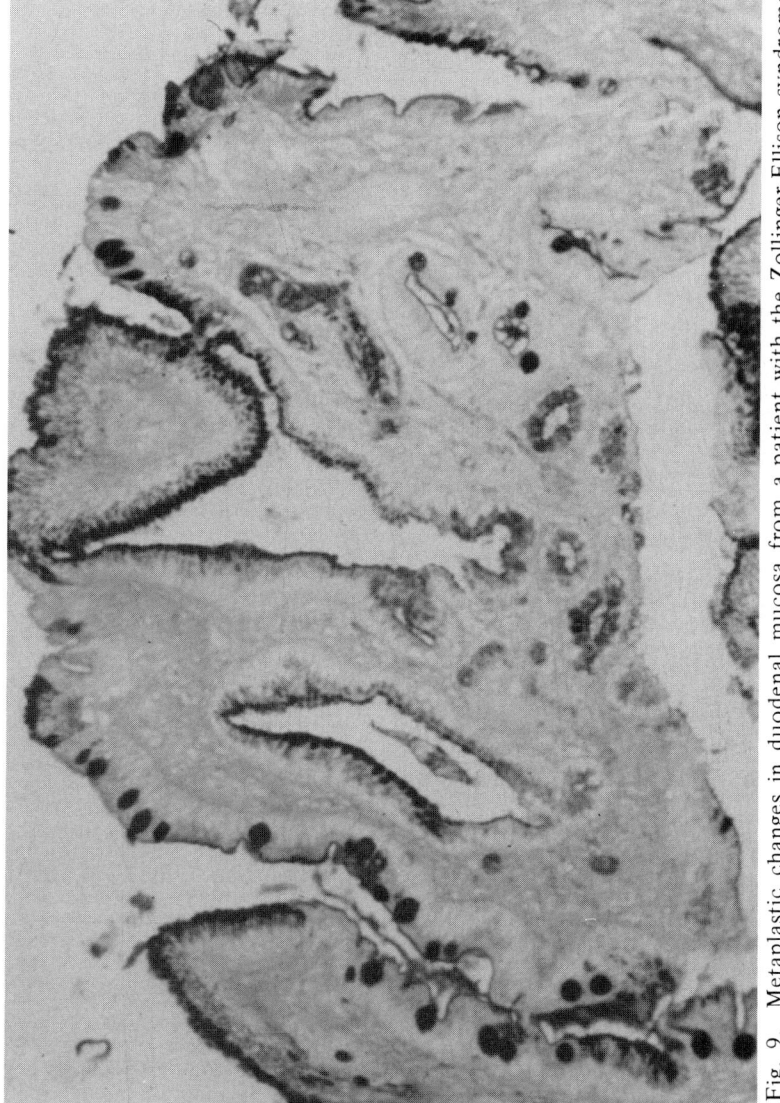

Fig. 9. Metaplastic changes in duodenal mucosa from a patient with the Zollinger-Ellison syndrome. [Courtesy Dr. Henry Appleman.]

gastrinomas [15], as has been alluded to above. Hypercalcemia may also contribute to the hypergastrinemia and to the increased exposure to acid in patients with the multiple endocrine adenoma syndrome [36, 51, 55]. It is of interest that luminal calcium has recently been observed to impair the ability of acid to inhibit the release of gastrin in vitro [19]. An impairment in mucosal blood flow, such as occurs in hemorrhagic shock, must hinder the removal of any acid that penetrates intestinal mucosa. Any deterioration in respiratory function or renal function further impedes the ability to buffer any acid that is removed from intestinal mucosa. Finally, sepsis, starvation, and steroids impair mucosal resistance at all sites by impairing the ability of mucosa to repair itself when breached.

Other factors impair the ability of mucosa in one specific area to withstand an exposure to acid. Gastric outlet obstruction may increase the intensity and duration of exposure to acid in the stomach by enhancing the release of gastrin [16], although this relationship has been questioned. Salicylates, urea and bile [12, 13] increase the permeability of gastric mucosa to acid. Bile may also increase the permeability of duodenal mucosa to acid [20]. Cimetidine will impair the production of the alkaline tide. Finally, as alluded to above, diversion of alkaline secretions from the pancreas and liver from a gastrojejunal anastomosis will also impair the ability of jejunal mucosa to withstand its "abnormal" exposure to acid (Figs. 1-3).

THE PATIENT

The patient threatened by gastrointestinal bleeding from a peptic ulcer relies upon a number of compensatory responses to maintain hemostasis and preserve life. These responses are most vividly demonstrated in the patient suffering from acute massive (>1500 ml or 25% of intravascular blood volume) [35] hemorrhage. The acute intravascular volume depletion causes a fall in cardiac output and diastolic blood pressure. The body responds with a massive release of catecholamines, which increase peripheral resistance and pulse rate in an attempt to maintain perfusion of vital organs. The ability to remove acid that enters intestinal mucosa is impaired by these compensatory mechanisms. If these responses do not compensate for the blood loss, shock ensues which, if untreated, culminates in acidosis, anoxia and cellular dysfunction. These events further impair the ability of intestinal mucosa to withstand an exposure to acid and thereby enhance the ulcerogenic process.

In addition to these cardiovascular responses, hormonal and hematological responses assist the patient in adjusting to the recent hemorrhage. Thus, increased secretion of ADH and aldosterone help reestablish intravascular volume at the expense of urinary output and extravascular volume. This, in turn, leads to a fall in hematocrit and a dilution in plasma proteins [35]. Further, after an initial leukocytosis and thrombocytosis in response to the stress of hemorrhage, the hematopoietic system is eventually stimulated to increase red blood cell production. These compensatory mechanisms are aided by the replacement of blood and of clotting factors lost *pari passu* with the hemorrhage. Restoration of mucosal blood flow restores the ability to remove acid from the mucosa, while restoration of renal blood flow restores the ability to dispose of acid removed from intestinal mucosa.

These compensatory responses are influenced by many factors. Certainly the patient's *age* influences the capacity to respond and, therefore, to withstand the life-threatening insult [35]. Numerous studies have emphasized the increased mortality associated with bleeding from peptic ulcers in patients over the age of 60 [25, 47, 54]. Associated illnesses, such as cardiovascular, pulmonary and renal disease, also limit the degree of compensatory response [35]; these illnesses have been shown to increase mortality significantly following surgical therapy for bleeding ulcers [50]. Such associated disease must also impair the ability to remove and dispose of any acid that may enter intestinal mucosa.

THE HEMORRHAGE

Several characteristics of the presenting hemorrhage have prognostic significance (Table 2). These characteristics all relate to the magnitude of the hemorrhage and the rate of bleeding. Schiller et al [47] reported that patients presenting with hematemesis, in lieu of melena, have a higher fatality rate. These patients are also more likely to experience recurrent hemorrhage [41], a pattern of bleeding which also predisposes to a lesser chance of surviving the hemorrhage [28]. These recurrent hemorrhages, according to Northfield [41], occur predominantly within 48 hours of the initial bleed. As expected, continuous bleeding is the least favorable pattern and is associated with a significant increase in the expected mortality rate [41]; therefore, the same association exists between mortality rate and duration of the bleed [9]. The severity of the hemorrhage, as reflected by the number of transfusions [26, 47], the presence of anemia [25] and of hypotension [47] also influences fatality

Table 2
Factors Associated With Increased Risk of Rebleeding

Factor	Ref.
Hematemesis	41
Admission HB < 9 g%	25
Hypotension	47
Spurting vessel	24

rate. These findings suggest that the risk of continued bleeding, or of recurrent bleeding, is a function of the rate of blood loss.

THE ULCER

Prognosis may also be influenced by the various attributes of the bleeding ulcer itself. Certainly, the ulcer's location is important; several studies have alluded to the poorer prognosis associated with hemorrhage from gastric ulcers as opposed to hemorrhage from duodenal ulcers [28, 53]. Further, other reports have emphasized the fact that postbulbar [45, 49] and giant posterior duodenal ulcers [33, 48] tend to bleed more frequently and more severely than the usual bulbar duodenal ulcers. This is probably related to the close proximity between post bulbar and giant posterior duodenal ulcers and the gastroduodenal artery.

The size of an ulcer crater is also of significance in assessing an ulcer and the likelihood of bleeding. This factor is underscored by the above-cited risks of giant (>2.5 cm) posterior duodenal ulcers. In addition, Wenckert et al [54] have indicated that an ulcer that is demonstrated on an upper gastrointestinal series is more likely to bleed than an ulcer that cannot be detected by this investigation; clearly, larger ulcers are more easily discerned by upper gastrointestinal series than smaller ulcers.

The chronicity of an ulcer influences the nature of an ulcer's hemorrhage. Key [30], in a classic study in 1950, demonstrated that the base of an acute ulcer is characterized by a haphazard, diffuse hypervascularity in the submucosa; these vessels, although increased in number, appear to be normal right into the ulcer crater. In contrast, the chronic ulcer base demonstrates a severe underlying hypovascularity due to widespread vascular occlusion (endarteritis obliterans) into the adjacent mucosa and replacement of normal tissue by fibrous tissue; the mucosal edges surrounding the chronic ulcer tend to be hypovascular. When massive ulcer hemorrhage occurs from a chronic ulcer, therefore, it is most likely to be due to erosion into a major artery. When massive ulcer hemorrhage occurs from an acute ulcer, on the other hand, it is most likely to occur from a multitude of hyperemic vessels. Thus, massive bleeding from a chronic ulcer occurs from ulcers located in the proximity of a select group of major vessels, whereas massive bleeding from an acute ulcer may occur from a multitude of different sites.

MANAGEMENT

It is distressing that despite our improvements in medical care and our reduction in operative mortality for patients with bleeding ulcers, the mortality for bleeding ulcers has not changed during the past 15 years [7, 47]. If we are to reduce the mortality for patients with bleeding ulcers, we must either improve the efficacy of our medical treatment or increase the proportion of patients being referred for operation.

Medical management of ulcer disease is, however, most likely to reduce the mortality from bleeding ulcers if it can be used to prevent bleeding or recurrent bleeding in patients with established ulcer disease, or in patients known to have an increased risk of developing an ulcer. This prophylactic approach appears to have had some success in patients with renal transplants [29].

Management of patients with bleeding ulcers should include a detailed history and physical examination and tests to establish a specific diagnosis. Risk factors associated with an increased risk of rebleeding and, hence of need for surgical intervention should also be noted. Potential precipitating factors, such as the ingestion of salicylates, and remediable chest or renal disease, should be identified and reversed. Ulcerogenic operations (Figs. 1-3), gastric stasis, and the presence of a gastrinoma should also be identified and dealt with appropriately. Ulcerogenic operations are best avoided by attention to correct surgical technique (Fig. 7).

Medical treatment of the ulcer disease in patients with bleeding ulcers is currently directed towards reducing the exposure to acid with antacids and cimetidine. Since many ulcers seem to be caused by an impaired resistance to acid, consideration should also be given to maintaining and improving the mucosal resistance to acid (Fig. 10).

If the ability of mucosa to withstand an exposure to acid is to be improved in patients in shock from bleeding ulcers, then resuscitative efforts should be directed towards restoring mucosal blood flow so as to facilitate the removal of any acid that may be entering the intestinal mucosa. This may be achieved by volume replacement, the avoidance of vasopressors, and by the optimization of cardiac function (Fig. 10). Resuscitative efforts should then be directed towards the buffering of any acid that is removed from intestinal mucosa. This may be achieved by the systemic administration of bicarbonate and by optimizing respiratory and renal functions. It is of interest that the systemic infusion of alkali prevents the development of ulcers induced by the intraluminal infusion of exogenous acid in dogs [8, 11]. The observation raises the possibility that systemic infusions of alkali may be of some therapeutic benefit in patients with bleeding ulcers. Simultaneous treatment of coexisting sepsis, the avoidance of steroids, and the maintenance of body nutrition should further enable the patient to repair the ulcer that has caused his bleed.

Fortunately, most ulcers stop bleeding with "medical treatment." Some ulcers will, however, not stop bleeding until the bleeding vessel is occluded. Surgical occlusion has been achieved by *embolization, photocoagulation* and *electrocoagulation* but may not be permanent. Medical occlusion by vasopressin is pathophysiologically unsound. Occlusion by the correct placement of a nonabsorbable suture is most effective and most permanent, especially when the bleeding is coming from a large vessel in the depths of a chronic ulcer.

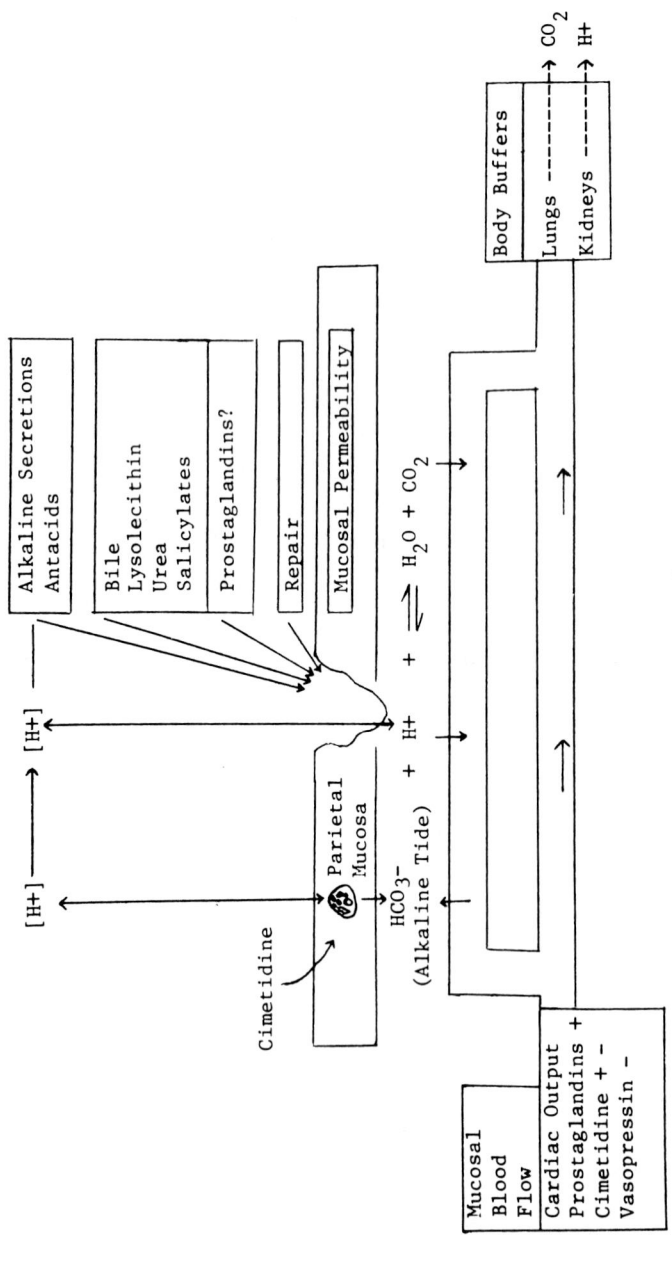

Fig. 10. Factors which may influence the ability of mucosa to withstand an exposure to acid.

Recognition that the overall mortality from bleeding ulcers has not improved despite advances in medical care and reduction in surgical mortality, should encourage the more frequent use of surgical occlusion. Furthermore, recognition that the operative mortality is greatly increased, if the decision to operate is delayed [9] and if intervention itself is delayed until after patients have received more than six units of blood, should encourage earlier surgical intervention. An appreciation of those factors associated with an increased risk of continued bleeding or rebleeding and, hence, of surgical intervention (Table 2) should aid in the timely selection of patients requiring surgical occlusion to arrest their hemorrhage. The development of better techniques for monitoring the rate of blood loss might help us to develop criteria for selecting with greater precision patients who will require occlusion to arrest their hemorrhage. Finally, the overall mortality from bleeding ulcers might be further reduced by exploiting our advances in medical care by managing patients in an ICU setting in collaboration with a skilled surgeon and a staff experienced in the management of hemorrhagic shock.

REFERENCES

1. Baron JH: Upper gastrointestinal bleeding. Clinical Tests of Gastric Secretion, New York, Oxford University Press, 1979, p 137
2. Baron JH: Duodenal ulcer. Clinical Tests of Gastric Secretion, New York, Oxford University Press, 1979, p 98
3. Baron JH: Gastric ulcer and carcinoma. Clinical Tests of Gastric Secretion, New York, Oxford University Press, 1979, p 86
4. Baugh CM, Bravo J, Dragstedt LR II, et al: The pathogenesis of the Exalto-Mann-Williamson ulcer II. Relation of the antrum to the hypersecretion of gastric juice in Mann-Williamson animals. Gastroenterology 39:330, 1960
5. Berson SA, Yalow RS: Progress in gastroenterology: radioimmunoassay in gastroenterology. Gastroenterology 62:1061, 1972
6. Card WI, Marks IN; The relationship between the acid output of the stomach following "maximal" histamine stimulation and the parietal cell mass. Clin Sci 19:147, 1960
7. Chalmers TC, Sebestzen CS, Lee S: Emergency surgical treatment of bleeding peptic ulcer: an analysis of the published data on 21,130 patients. Trans Amer Clin Climatol Assn 82:188, 1971
8. Cheung LY, Porterfield G: Protection of gastric mucosa against acute ulceration by intravenous infusion of sodium bicarbonate. Am J Surg 137:106, 1979
9. Cocks JR, Desmond AM, Swynnerton BF, et al: Partial gastrectomy for haemorrhage. Gut 13:331, 1972
10. Cowley DJ, Dymock IW, Boyes BE, et al: Zollinger-Ellison syndrome type I: clinical and pathological correlations in a case. Gut 14:25, 1973

11. Cummins GM, Grossman MI, Ivy AC: An experimental study of the acid factor in ulceration of the gastrointestinal tract in dogs. Gastroenterology 10:714, 1948
12. Davenport HW: Physiological structure of the gastric mucosa. In Code CW (ed): Handbook of Physiology, Section G, Vol II. Washington DC, American Physiological Society, 1967, p 759
13. Davenport HW: Destruction of the gastric mucosa barrier by detergents and urea. Gastroenterology 54:175, 1968
14. Dorricott NJ, Fiddian-Green RG, Silen W: Mechanisms of acid disposal in canine duodenum. Am J Physiol 228:269, 1975
15. Ellison EH, Wilson SD: Ulcerogenic tumor of the pancreas. Prog Clin Cancer 3:225, 1967
16. Feurle G, Ketterer H, Becker HD, et al: Circadian serum gastrin concentrations in control persons and in patients with ulcer disease. Scand J. Gastroenterol 7:177, 1972
17. Fiddian-Green RG, Bank S, Marks IN, et al: Maximum acid output and position of peptic ulcers. Lancet 2:1370, 1976
18. Fiddian-Green RG, Silen W: Mechanisms of acid and alkali disposal in rabbit duodenum. Am J Physiol 229:1641, 1975
19. Fiddian-Green RG, Pittenger G, Kothary P, et al: Luminal calcium reverses the ability of acid to inhibit the release of canine antral gastrin in vitro. (Abstr) Clin Res 27:632A, 1979
20. Fiddian-Green RG, Silen W: The influence of acid and bile on the viability of rabbit mucosa. (Abst) S Afr J Surg 12:69, 1974
21. Florey HW, Jennings MA, Jennings DA, et al: The reactions of the intestine of the pig to gastric juice. J Pathol Bacteriol 49:105, 1939
22. Friesen SR: A gastric factor in the pathogenesis of the Zollinger-Ellison syndrome. Ann Surg 168:483, 1968
23. Grant R, Grossman MI, Ivy AC: Histological changes in the gastric mucosa during digestion and their relationship to mucosal growth. Gastroenterology 25:218, 1953
24. Griffiths WJ, Neumann DA, Welsh JD: The visible vessel as an indicator of uncontrolled or recurrent gastrointestinal hemorrhage. N Engl J Med 300:1411, 1979
25. Himal HS, Watson WW, Jones CW: The management of upper gastrointestinal hemorrhage: a multiparametric computer analysis. Ann Surg 179:489, 1974
26. Himal HS, Perrault C, Mzabi R: Upper gastrointestinal hemorrhage: aggressive management decreases mortality. Surgery 84:448, 1978
27. Hobsley M, Whitfield PF, Faber RG, et al: Hypersecretion and length of history in duodenal ulceration. Lancet 2:101, 1975
28. Jones FA: Hematemesis and melena with special reference to causation and to the factors influencing the mortality from bleeding peptic ulcers. Gastroenterology 30:166, 1956
29. Jones RH, Rudge CJ, Bewick M, et al: Cimetidine: prophylaxis against upper gastrointestinal haemorrhage after renal transplantation. Br Med J 1:398, 1978

30. Key JA: Blood vessels of a gastric ulcer. Br Med J 2:1464, 1950
31. Kiriluk LB, Merendino KA: An experimental study of the buffering capacity of the contents of the upper small bowel. Surgery 35:532, 1954
32. Kivilaakso E, Silen W: Pathogenesis of experimental gastric mucosal injury. N Engl J Med 301:364, 1979
33. Klamer TW, Mahr MM: Giant duodenal ulcer: a dangerous variant of a common illness. Am J Surg 135:760, 1978
34. Kraus M, Mendeloff G, Condon RE: Prognosis of gastric ulcer: twenty-five year follow-up. Ann Surg 184:471, 1976
35. Law DH, Watts HD: Gastrointestinal bleeding. In Sleisenger MH and Fordtran JS (ed.): Gastrointestinal Disease, 2nd ed. Philadelphia, Saunders, 1978, p 217
36. McGuigan JE, Colwell JA, Franklin J: Effect of parathyroidectomy on hypercalcemic hypersecretory peptic ulcer disease. Gastroenterology 66:269, 1974
37. McKittrick LS, Moore FD, Warren R: Complications and mortality in subtotal gastrectomy for duodenal ulcer. Ann Surg 120:531, 1944
38. Menguy R, Mings H: Role of pancreatic and biliary juices in regulation of gastric secretion: pathogenesis of the Mann-Williamson ulcer. Surgery 50:662, 1961
39. Meyer JH, Way LW, Grossman MI: Pancreatic bicarbonate response to acidification of various lengths of proximal intestine in the dog. Am J Physiol 219:971, 1970
40. Meyer JH, Way LW, Grossman MI: Pancreatic bicarbonate response to various acids in the duodenum of the dog. Am J Physiol 219:964, 1970
41. Northfield TC: Factors predisposing to recurrent hemorrhage after acute gastrointestinal bleeding. Br Med J 1:26, 1971
42. Palmer ED: Complications of duodenal ulcer: some aspects of their natural history. Am J Dig Dis 6:68, 1961
43. Palmer ED: Gastrointestinal ulcer bleeding: pathologic and clinical features. In Palmer ED (ed): Upper Gastrointestinal Hemorrhage. Springfield, IL, Charles Thomas, 1970, p 101
44. Patrick WJA, Denham D, Forrest APM: Mucus change in the human duodenum: a light and electronic microscopic study and correlation with disease and gastric acid secretion. Gut 15:767, 1974
45. Pattison AC, Stellar CA: Surgical management of post bulbar duodenal ulcers. Am J Surg 111:313, 1966
46. Rhodes J, Prestwich CJ: Acidity at different sites in the proximal duodenum of normal subjects and patients with duodenal ulcer. Gut 7:509, 1966
47. Schiller KFR, Truelove SC, Williams DG: Haematemesis and melaena, with special reference to factors influencing the outcome. Br Med J 2:7, 1970
48. Snyder EN, Stellar CA: Results from emergency surgery for massively bleeding duodenal ulcer. Am J Surg 116:170, 1968
49. Spiro HD: Clinical Gastroenterology, New York, Macmillan, 1977, p 307
50. Stone AM, Stein T, McCarthy K, et al: Surgery for bleeding duodenal ulcer. Am J Surg 136:306, 1978

51. Stremple JF, Watson CG: Serum calcium, serum gastrin, and gastric acid secretion before and after parathyroidectomy for hyperparathyroidism. Surgery 75:841, 1974
52. Sircus N: Gastric secretion in peptic ulcer disease with special reference to body weight, duration of disease and stenosis. In Semb LS, Myren J (ed): The Physiology of Gastric Secretion. Baltimore, Williams and Wilkins, 1968, p 581
53. Walker CO: Complications of peptic ulcer disease and indications for surgery. In Sleisenger MH, Fordtran JS (ed): Gastrointestinal Disease. Philadelphia, W B Saunders Co, 1978, p 914
54. Wenckert A, Borg I, Lindblom P: Review of medically treated bleeding gastric or duodenal ulcers. Acta Chir Scand 120:66, 1960
55. Wilson SD, Singh RB, Kalkhoff RK, et al: Does hyperparathyroidism cause hypergastrinemia? Surgery 80:231, 1976

George Willeford, M.D.
Charles T. Richardson, M.D.

Medical Treatment of Bleeding Ulcers

ABSTRACT

Gastric and duodenal ulcers are the most common cause of hematemesis and melena. Medical therapy for bleeding ulcers has evolved, for the most part, from past experience and anecdote rather than controlled clinical trials.

Gastric lavage with either iced water or saline is usually instituted soon after a bleeding ulcer patient is admitted to the hospital. Lavage is continued until the stomach is clear of blood or clots. In addition to lavage, reduction in gastric acidity is an important part of therapy. We usually treat bleeding ulcer patients with 300 mg cimetidine (intravenously until lavage is complete and then orally) every four hours for 4-5 days and then reduce the dose to 300 mg four times daily. If desired, 30 ml of antacid, given every 30-60 min, may be substituted for cimetidine. In some patients both cimetidine and antacids may be required to effectively reduce gastric acidity.

Gastric and duodenal ulcers are the most common cause of hematesis and melena. Approximately 50% of hospital admissions for upper gastrointestinal (UGI) bleeding are the result of either bleeding gastric or duodenal ulcers or both [5, 16, 49, 50]. Despite new therapeutic modalities and use of intensive care units, the mortality from UGI bleeding has not changed over the past 30 years [1, 59]. Bleeding from ulcers may occur at any age but is most common in the fourth decade in women and fifth decade in men [7].

Medical therapy has been subjected to very few controlled clinical trials. Many decisions regarding therapy are based on past experience and anecdote rather than on objective data. In this chapter we will explore the historical

---

George Willeford, M.D.: Fellow in Gastroenterology, Veterans Administration Medical Center, and Department of Internal Medicine, University of Texas Health Science Center; Charles T. Richardson, M.D.: Chief, Gastroenterology, Veterans Administration Medical Center, Associate Professor of Internal Medicine, Department of Internal Medicine, University of Texas Health Science Center, Dallas, Texas.

development of current therapeutic regimens for treating actively bleeding ulcers. We will give our recommendations regarding therapy and, when available, the scientific basis for our approach.

INITIAL THERAPY

If facilities are available, all patients with UGI bleeding should be admitted to an intensive care unit. Optimal management can be achieved if both an internist and a surgeon participate in patient care. Following initial resuscitative measures, a sump type nasogastric tube (Fig. 1) should be placed through the nose into the stomach. The nasogastric tube (1) helps to localize the bleeding site to the UGI tract; (2) aids in clearing the stomach of blood and food (this is especially important if endoscopy is planned); (3) helps to gauge the rapidity of bleeding; and (4) allows medications to be administered to the confused or otherwise mentally compromised patient. Although aspiration of blood from the stomach suggests the source of bleeding is in the UGI tract, a negative NG aspirate does not exclude bleeding from a site above the ligament of Treitz. For example, bleeding from a duodenal ulcer can occur without reflux of blood into the stomach, thus resulting in a nasogastric aspirate negative for blood.

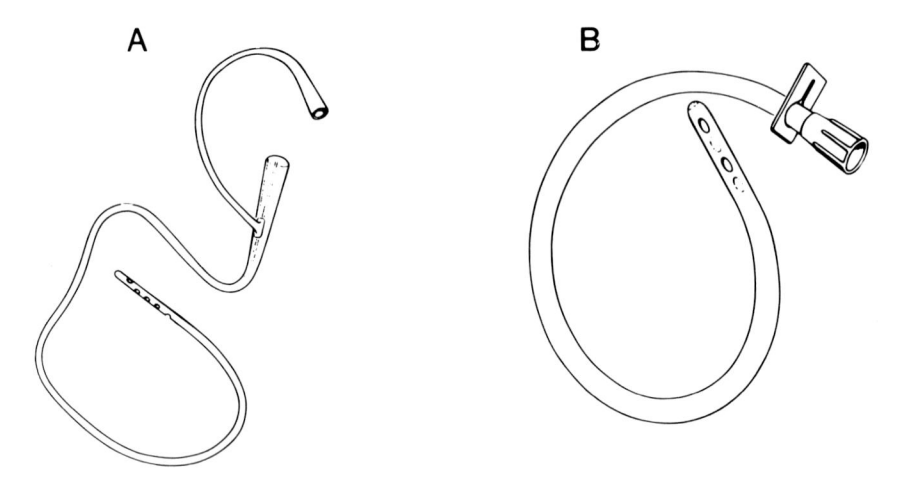

Fig. 1. (A) Sump type nasogastric tube. Length 48 inches, diameter 16 French (5.3 mm). (B) Oral gastric tube of Edlich or Ewald type. Length 36 inches, diameter 34 French (11.3 mm).

GASTRIC LAVAGE

Lavage, especially with cold solutions, is thought to be of value in treating UGI bleeding by lowering intragastric temperature, decreasing gastric blood flow, and removing blood clots from the stomach. To produce maximally effective lavage, the nasogastric tube should be removed and replaced with a large bore oral gastric tube of the Edlich or Ewald type (Fig. 1). When lavage is judged complete (the return from the stomach is either clear or only light pink in color and free of blood clots), the lavage tube is removed and replaced by a small diameter sump type nasogastric tube. If bright red blood continues to return despite vigorous lavage, then more invasive procedures (angiography, surgery) should be considered (see the chapters titled *Surgery for Massive Upper Gastrointestinal Hemorrhage, Rebleeding After Surgery for Bleeding Ulcers*, and *Therapeutic Angiography in Gastrointestinal Hemorrhage*).

The first in-depth study evaluating gastric cooling was performed by Wangensteen and co-workers [53]. Gastric juice was collected overnight from known duodenal ulcer patients. When gastric juice at room temperature was dripped into the esophagus of a cat, severe esophagitis resulted. However, when the experiment was repeated with cooled gastric juice, little or no esophagitis occurred. Experiments were then performed in 2 duodenal ulcer patients and several dogs. Local cooling using an intragastric balloon resulted in decreased gastric juice volume, hydrogen ion concentration, and pepsin concentration. Based on these results, 9 patients bleeding from duodenal ulcers and 1 patient bleeding from a gastric ulcer were treated by this technique [54]. All 10 patients stopped bleeding after an average cooling time of 15.7 hours. Because these studies were not controlled, it is not known how many patients would have stopped bleeding without gastric cooling in the same (or even shorter) period of time.

Direct gastric lavage of iced solutions through a large bore tube was later popularized because it was easier than perfusing cold solution through an intragastric balloon [48]. Once again, it must be emphasized that there have been no controlled studies evaluating this technique. However, based on the studies described above, gastric lavage with iced solutions has become an established part of the management of UGI bleeders.

Investigators have attempted to determine the physiologic effects of iced gastric lavage [56]. One study measured left gastric artery blood flow in dogs before and after cold saline lavage. Cooling of the dog stomach (Fig. 2, top) resulted in a progressive fall in gastric blood flow (Fig. 2, bottom). With rewarming, blood flow promptly returned to precooling levels. In addition, these authors evaluated the effect of gastric cooling on coagulation. They found that cooling resulted in prolongation of the bleeding time, clotting time and prothrombin time. These studies suggest that iced saline lavage may have undesirable as well as desirable effects.

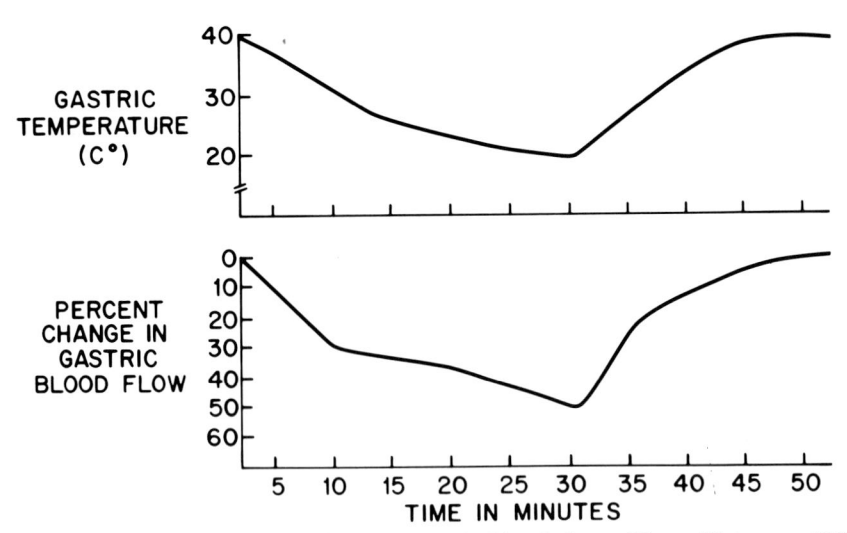

Fig. 2. Effect of gastric cooling on gastric blood flow. [From Waterman NG and Walker BA. The effect of gastric cooling on hemostasis. Surg Gynecol Obstet 137:80, 1973. Used with permission.]

Although most investigators recommend that saline be used for lavage, Bryant and colleagues [8] compared iced saline with iced water in lavaging the stomachs of dogs. No change occurred in serum osmolality, serum sodium or hematocrit when either water or saline was used. A slight fall in serum potassium occurred with either solution. These results suggest that tap water may be as good as saline for gastric lavage. In fact, water may be preferable due to lower costs and ease of supply. Monitoring of serum potassium may be necessary during and after lavage with either water or saline.

INTRAGASTRIC VASOCONSTRICTORS

In addition to iced solutions, some investigators have suggested that intragastric lavage with levarterenol (Levophed) may decrease UGI bleeding by reducing gastric blood flow [15, 29, 31]; but results depicted in Fig. 3 suggest that levarterenol has no significant advantage over cold saline [55]. Thus, because the addition of levarterenol to iced saline lavage produces no significant advantage over iced saline alone, we do not recommend the routine use of intragastric vasoconstrictors. If desired in certain circumstances (a final effort to stop bleeding before the patient is taken to surgery, for example), 8 mg of levarterenol should be mixed with 100-200 ml of lavage solution, infused into the stomach, and left for 20-30 minutes [29]. This may be repeated once or twice.

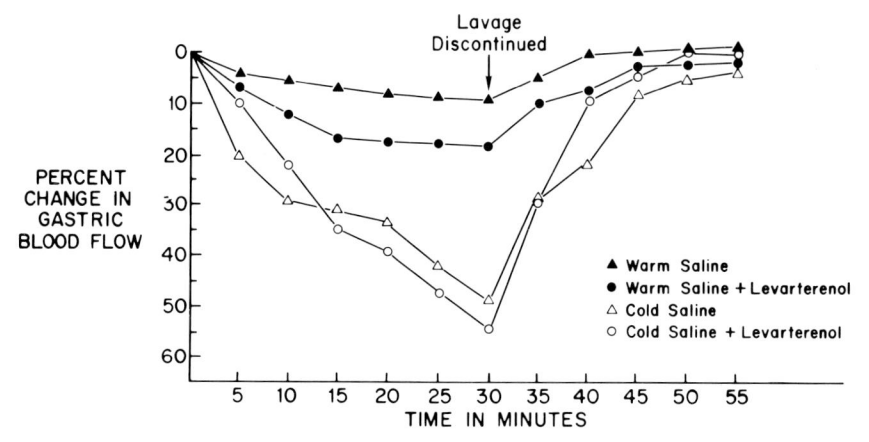

Fig. 3. Changes in gastric artery blood flow resulting from warm and cold saline lavage with and without levarterenol. [From Waterman WG and Walker JL. Effect of a topical adrenergic agent on gastric blood flow. Amer J Surg 127:241, 1974. Used with permission.]

INITIAL THERAPY SUMMARIZED

Our current routine is as follows: (1) a sump type nasogastric tube is placed through the nose into the stomach; (2) if clots or bright red blood are present and the aspirate does not clear with less than a liter of cold tap water lavage, the sump tube is removed and replaced with a large bore tube passed through the mouth into the stomach; (3) with the patient on his side and oral suction available, lavage is begun with iced tap water (saline is also acceptable); (4) lavage is continued until all clots are removed and the return is clear or light pink; (5) the large tube is removed and a smaller tube replaced through the nose; (6) the nasogastric tube is left in place for only the initial 8 to 12 hours of treatment, allowing time to initiate medical therapy and to insure that bleeding has ceased before the tube is removed. Attention should be paid to serum electrolytes, especially serum potassium, during and after lavage. There is evidence suggesting a marked fall in left gastric artery blood flow with iced lavage with or without levarterenol [55]. Therefore, caution should be exercised in lavaging anyone, especially the elderly, with possible mesenteric vascular compromise.

Although we and others currently recommend and use gastric lavage in treating bleeding patients, we recognize that gastric lavage may not be therapeutically helpful and in fact may be harmful. An accurate assessment will come only from good controlled clinical trials.

REDUCTION OF GASTRIC ACIDITY

Rationale

Currently, most pharmacologic methods used to treat or prevent peptic ulcers are aimed at reducing gastric acidity by either decreasing acid secretion (H_2-receptor antagonists and anticholinergic drugs) or neutralizing acid (antacids). There are several reasons to believe that if gastric acidity is reduced, ulcers may be prevented; or, if an ulcer is already present, there is an improved chance that it will heal. First, duodenal ulcers and, except in rare instances, gastric ulcers do not occur in the absence of gastric acid. Second, in a cat esophagus model, esophagitis, which was produced by dripping acid and pepsin on the esophagus, was prevented by increasing the pH of the bathing solution [21]. Third, antacid and cimetidine have been shown to heal gastric or duodenal ulcers in a large percentage of patients [6, 28, 40, 42], and cimetidine has been shown to be better than placebo in preventing ulcer recurrence [20, 24].

There is an additional reason to believe that reducing acidity may be beneficial in treating bleeding ulcers. In vitro studies have shown that clotting parameters become abnormal as gastric pH decreases [11, 22]. For example, when pH was reduced below 6.8, prothrombin time and activated partial thromboplastin time were progressively prolonged. As pH was reduced below 6.4, platelet aggregation was less than 50% of normal and clotting time was prolonged to twice normal [22]. When pepsin was added, platelet aggregation was further reduced. None of these abnormalities could be demonstrated when pH was maintained above 7.4. It should be remembered that these experiments were carried out in vitro, and whether the results apply to patients with bleeding ulcers is not known.

One of the most important questions in treating bleeding ulcer patients is to what extent intragastric pH should be increased. The studies using a cat esophagus model suggest that mucosal injury can be prevented if pH is maintained above 2.5 [21]; however, in vitro studies have shown that peptic activity which is maximum at 2.0 is not reduced markedly until pH is increased to 5.5 [43]. Further support for increasing pH can be gained from the studies mentioned above in which clotting abnormalities occurred when pH was below 6.8. Whether or not such pH elevations aid in the treatment of the bleeding ulcer patient is not known.

We have adopted the arbitrary policy that, at least during the first few days of treatment of the bleeding ulcer patient, gastric pH should be increased to, and maintained between, 5.5 and 7.0. In most patients this can be achieved with proper usage of available drugs. The remainder of this chapter will deal with methods used to increase gastric pH and thus reduce gastric acidity.

METHODS OF REDUCING GASTRIC ACIDITY

H_2-Receptor Antagonists

There are two receptors for histamine which have been labeled H_1 and H_2-receptors. The H_1-receptors are blocked by the classic antihistamines such as diphenhydramine hydrochloride (Benadryl). However, since H_1-receptors are not located on gastric acid secreting cells (parietal cells), these drugs have no inhibitory effect on acid secretion. Recently, analogs of histamine have been synthesized which block the effect of histamine on H_2-receptors located on the acid secreting cell. These compounds have been labeled histamine H_2-receptor antagonists. The structure of the currently available H_2-receptor antagonist, cimetidine (Tagamet), is shown in Figure 4 and is compared with the structure of histamine.

Cimetidine reduces basal and nocturnal acid secretion as well as acid secretion stimulated by histamine, pentagastrin, caffeine, bethanecol, 2-deoxyglucose, insulin, sham feeding, and food [9, 26, 32, 46]. Controlled clinical trials [6, 40] have shown that cimetidine is superior to placebo in healing duodenal ulcers. In addition, studies [20, 24] have shown that patients treated with cimetidine for 6 months or a year have a lower incidence of ulcer recurrence than patients treated with placebo. Results of studies [2, 12] evaluating the effect of cimetidine in the treatment of patients with gastric ulcers have been inconsistent. Thus, the role of cimetidine in the treatment of gastric ulcers remains unclear.

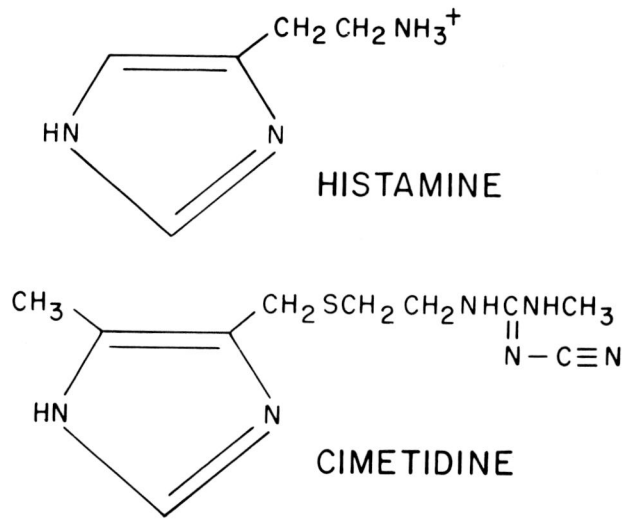

Fig. 4. Structure of histamine and cimetidine.

Two studies [17, 34] have suggested that cimetidine may be helpful in the treatment of UGI bleeding from superficial mucosal lesions. A recent study [27] in a small group of patients evaluated the effect of cimetidine in the prevention of rebleeding from endoscopically documented bleeding gastric or duodenal ulcers. Results suggested that cimetidine may be useful in preventing rebleeding from gastric ulcers but not duodenal ulcers.

Although there are no controlled clinical trials establishing that cimetidine is effective in treating actively bleeding ulcers, we recommend that it be used routinely since reducing gastric acidity is one of the goals of therapy and since, so far, the incidence of drug side effects has been low. Also, once the bleeding episode has subsided, cimetidine should be useful in aiding ulcer healing.

Cimetidine reduces acid secretion by increasing intragastric pH and also by reducing the volume of gastric juice secreted. However, even though the volume of gastric juice is low, preliminary data from our laboratory suggest that 300 mg cimetidine given every six hours (as routinely recommended in the patient who is not eating) will not always maintain pH in the 5.5 to 7 range throughout the six hour period. In addition, a recent study [41] has shown that if cimetidine is given three times daily with meals and again at bedtime, gastric juice pH is below 5.5 during much of the 24 hour period. Therefore, in treating a bleeding ulcer patient, we usually prescribe 300 mg cimetidine every four hours for 4-5 days and then reduce the dose to 300 mg four times daily, with meals and at bedtime. We monitor gastric pH for the first 6-8 hours after admission and add antacid to the regimen if cimetidine alone does not increase pH above 5.5.

Cimetidine may be given orally or intravenously. We give cimetidine intravenously as long as the patient is being lavaged; however, once lavage is complete and nasogastric suction is no longer needed, we prescribe cimetidine orally.

Care must be exercised when giving cimetidine to the bleeding patient with reduced glomerular filtration rate. This may be especially important in treating elderly patients in whom the use of cimetidine has been associated with reversible alterations in mental status [37]. Recommended dosage regimens for various degrees of renal insufficiency are shown in Table 1 [33]. Note that in patients with mild to severe renal insufficiency, the frequency of drug administration is decreased. In some patients, however, these dosage recommendations may not be sufficient to maintain an intragastric pH in the 5.5 to 7 range. Therefore, it is important to monitor intragastric pH and either alter the frequency of cimetidine administration accordingly or add antacid.

Anticholinergic Drugs

Anticholinergic drugs are thought to reduce acid secretion by blocking an acetylcholine receptor on or near the gastric parietal cell. When given orally, they reduce basal or nocturnal acid secretion by about 50% [4] and reduce food stimulated acid secretion by 25-30% [44]. This contrasts with cimetidine which

Table 1
Recommended Dosage Intervals for Cimetidine in Renal Disease Patient Bleeding From Gastric or Duodenal Ulcers

Degree of Renal Failure (Creatinine Clearance, ml/min)	Recommended Dose of Cimetidine
Normal (> 87)	300 mg q 4 hr
Mild (49.3 – 86.9)	300 mg q 6 hr
Moderate (19.1 – 34.1)	300 mg q 8 hr
Severe (0 – 19.1)	300 mg q 12 hr*

*Patients on dialysis should receive an extra 300 mg dose at the completion of dialysis. Degree of renal failure based on data from [33].

reduces basal acid secretion by approximately 90-95% [26] and food-stimulated secretion by 60-75% [46].

A number of controlled clinical trials have evaluated the effect of anticholinergic drugs on the healing of ulcers and the results have been conflicting. Therefore, because of lack of data supporting their use, anticholinergic drugs are not recommended as part of the routine therapy of bleeding gastric or duodenal ulcers. If, however, a patient has a hypersecretory state such as Zollinger-Ellison syndrome, anticholinergic drugs may be useful as an adjunct to cimetidine in reducing acid secretion. Studies suggest that anticholinergic drugs prolong the inhibitory effect of cimetidine on acid secretion in patients with Zollinger-Ellison syndrome [36, 45].

Antacids

Antacids increase intragastric pH by neutralizing gastric acid. Several studies [13, 25, 35, 51] suggest that antacids may be effective in preventing or treating bleeding from superficial gastric mucosal lesions, but there are no controlled clinical trials evaluating the use of antacids in the treatment of bleeding ulcers. However, investigators have demonstrated that antacids aid in the healing of nonbleeding gastric or duodenal ulcers [28, 42]. Recognizing these results and assuming that it is helpful to reduce gastric acidity, it seems reasonable to use antacids either alone or in combination with cimetidine in treating the bleeding ulcer patient.

Most antacids contain aluminum, magnesium or calcium salts but differ in neutralizing capacity and rate of reaction with gastric acid. The difference in potency (neutralizing capacity) can vary widely and should be taken into consideration when prescribing an antacid. Therefore, antacid dosage should be based on milliequivalents of neutralizing capacity rather than on the volume of a specific antacid. In vivo antacid potency can be judged by a relatively simple in vitro assay [18]. There are several good magnesium-aluminum hydroxide antacids, and detailed information is available to determine which antacids are the most effective [18]. We recommend an 80 mEq dose which, on the average, is equivalent to about 30 ml of most antacids. The dose may be reduced if one of the new, more potent antacids is prescribed.

It may not be sufficient just to neutralize gastric acid for a short period of time. Rather, sustained elevation of gastric pH may be required if antacids are to be of benefit in treating bleeding ulcer patients. It is difficult to achieve sustained elevations of gastric pH when antacids are given to a fasting patient. Under these circumstances the duration of antacid effect is brief (only 20-30 minutes) because gastric emptying is accelerated in the absence of food [23]. This fact is important when treating bleeding ulcer patients who may not eat for several days. Therefore, if antacids alone are used, it may be necessary to give a dose every 30 minutes to achieve adequate reduction of acidity. Doubling the antacid dose (for example, from 30 to 60 ml every hour) may not be as effective in raising pH over prolonged periods as shortening the dosage interval because the rate of gastric emptying is the major factor determining duration of action.

Thus, to be effective in increasing intragastric pH, antacid should be given at a dose and frequency to produce sustained neutralization of acid. This can best be established by monitoring pH every 15 to 30 minutes during the first several hours after admission and adjusting the dose of antacid to maintain pH above 5.5. In some patients a continuous drip of antacid per nasogastric tube may be necessary.

When the acute bleeding phase has passed, the patient may begin eating. When antacids are taken after food, the duration of action is prolonged because food delays gastric emptying allowing antacids to remain in the stomach for a longer time period. Once bleeding ulcer patients are eating, we recommend an 80 mEq dose (usually 30 ml) of antacid every hour during the day for a week and then the same dose one and three hours after each meal. A recent study [38] has shown that a bedtime dose of antacid is not as effective as cimetidine in reducing nocturnal acidity. Therefore, in patients treated with antacid during the day, a 300 mg dose of cimetidine should be given at night.

The major side effect of antacid is diarrhea. Diarrhea usually can be controlled by alternating a magnesium-aluminum hydroxide antacid with an antacid containing only aluminum hydroxide.

Milk Drip

Between 1933 and 1955 milk drips were popularized as a treatment for peptic ulcerations and therefore were applied to the therapy of UGI bleeding. In 1956 Dawson [14] reported a controlled, randomized trial of milk drips in the treatment of UGI bleeding and found no difference in the numbers of deaths, percent rebleeding or emergency operations between the patients treated with milk drips and those treated with placebo; pH was not measured and the volume of milk was chosen arbitrarily. A similar study in 1969 [50] likewise showed milk drips to be of no benefit in reducing transfusion requirements or emergency operation. Thus, there is no evidence to suggest that milk-drips are useful in treating actively bleeding ulcers or in preventing rebleeding.

Combination Therapy

In many patients cimetidine every four hours or antacid at frequent intervals should be sufficient to maintain gastric pH at 5.5 or above. However, in some patients both drugs may be necessary. The need for combination therapy in an individual patient can be determined by monitoring pH of the gastric aspirate at frequent intervals during the first few hours after admission.

NEW THERAPIES

H_2-Receptor Antagonists

Several new H_2-receptor antagonists have been developed. Preliminary studies suggest that these new compounds may be more potent than cimetidine, and at least one of these compounds may have a longer duration of effect. What role these new drugs will play in the management of bleeding ulcers remains to be seen.

Prostaglandins

Studies [10, 19] have shown that prostaglandins prevent stress ulcers in animals and may improve ulcer healing in man. These beneficial effects of prostaglandins may result from inhibition of gastric secretion [52, 58] or from a direct cytoprotective effect [47] of prostaglandins on gastric and perhaps duodenal mucosa. To date there have been no attempts to study the effect of prostaglandins in the actively bleeding ulcer patient. If prostaglandins do prove to be useful in the treatment of nonbleeding ulcers, then perhaps their use in the bleeding patient can be further explored.

Bismuth Compounds

Bismuth-peptide complex compounds have been shown to be effective in the treatment of gastric and duodenal ulcers [30, 39, 57]. In contrast to bismuth containing antacids, these bismuth compounds do not neutralize acid. The mechanism of action is uncertain and controversial but most likely includes (1) chelation with proteins produced by necrotic ulcer tissue which may protect during the healing phase of ulceration or (2) the binding by colloidal bismuth of pepsin [3].

Bismuth-peptide complex compounds are not marketed in the United States at present.

SUMMARY

The therapy of bleeding gastric and duodenal ulcers is based, for the most part, on anecdote and theory rather than on objective data. Admittedly without strong basis in fact, our recommendations for therapy of bleeding gastric and duodenal ulcers include:

1. Admit the bleeding patient to an intensive care unit, if possible, where care is best provided by an internist-surgeon team with a consulting gastroenterologist, if available.
2. Soon after admission, place a sump type nasogastric tube. Lavage with 1-2 liters of either cold or room temperature tap water (or saline) depending on individual preference. There is no evidence that the addition of levarterenol or other pressors to gastric lavage solutions is of therapeutic value. If lavage clears the stomach of blood, begin therapy as described below to increase intragastric pH.
3. If the nasogastric aspirate contains clots or does not clear easily, remove the small sump tube and replace it with a large bore tube (Edlich, Ewald) placed through the mouth into the stomach. Lavage with patient positioned on his side. Be sure oral suction is available to clear secretions and blood from the mouth. Continue lavage until the return from the stomach is free from clots or blood. Most large bore tubes do not have a sump mechanism; therefore allow gravity and intraabdominal pressure to drain the stomach. Do not withdraw with a syringe from a large bore tube without a sump attachment because suction may damage the gastric mucosa. When the gastric aspirate clears, remove the large tube, replace the nasogastric tube and proceed with medical therapy. If evidence of active bleeding continues despite lavage, consider more invasive therapeutic modalities (i.e., angiography, surgery).
4. Begin cimetidine intravenously. Once lavage is complete and if nasogastric suction is not needed give cimetidine orally. We suggest giving 300 mg every four hours initially. The frequency of dosage must be adjusted in patients with renal insufficiency. Thirty ml antacid every 30-60 min may be used as an alternate form of therapy.
5. Measure intragastric pH every 15-30 min during the first several hours that nasogastric tube is in place. If pH is not maintained above 5.5 with cimetidine alone or antacid alone, use the drug combination.
6. Remove the nasogastric tube within 8 to 12 hours if bleeding has stopped and medical therapy has been initiated.

7. Four to five days after bleeding has stopped change cimetidine dosage to 300 mg four times daily (with meals and at bedtime). If the patient has been treated initially with antacid rather than cimetidine, alter the antacid dose to 30 ml one and three hours after meals and give 300 mg cimetidine at bedtime.

REFERENCES

1. Allan P, Dykes P: A study of factors influencing mortality rates from gastrointestinal haemorrhage. Q J Med 180:533, 1976
2. Bader JP, Morin T, Mondor H, et al: Treatment of gastric ulcer by cimetidine. a multicentre trial. In Burland WL, Simkins MA (eds): Cimetidine. Proceedings of the Second International Symposium on Histamine H_2-receptor Antagonists. Amsterdam, Excerpta Medica, 1977. p 287
3. Banks S, Marks IN: Evaluation of new drugs for peptic ulcer. Clin Gastroenterol 2:379, 1973
4. Barman MC, Carson RK: The effect of glycopyrrolate on nocturnal gastric secretion in peptic ulcer patients. Am J Med Sci 246:325, 1963
5. Berkowitz D: Fatal gastrointestinal hemorrhage: diagnostic implications from a study of 200 cases. Am J Gastroenterol 40:372, 1963
6. Bodemar G, Norlander B, Walan A: Cimetidine in the treatment of active peptic ulcer disease. In Burland WL, Simkins, MA (eds): Cimetidine. Proceedings of the Second International Symposium on Histamine H_2-receptor Antagonists. Amsterdam, Excerpta Medica, 1977 p 224
7. Bogoch A: Hematemesis and melena. In Bockus HC, ed: Gastroenterology 3rd ed. Philadelphia, Saunders, 1974, p 770
8. Bryant LR, Mobin-Uddin K, Dillon ML, et al: Comparison of ice water with iced saline solution for gastric lavage in gastroduodenal hemorrhage. Am J Surg 124:570, 1972
9. Cano R, Isenberg JI, Grossman MI: Cimetidine inhibits caffeine-stimulated gastric acid secretion in man. Gastroenterology 70:1055, 1976
10. Carmichael HA, Nelson L, Russell RI, et al: The effect of the synthetic prostaglandin analog 15(R) 15 methyl-PGE_2 methyl ester on gastric mucosal hemorrhage induced in rats by taurocholic acid and hydrocholic acid. Am J Dig Dis 22:411, 1977
11. Chaimoff C, Creter D, Djaldehi M: The effect of pH on platelet and coagulation factor activities. Am J Surg 126:257, 1976
12. Ciclitira PJ, Machell RJ, Farthing MJ, et al: A controlled trial of cimetidine in the treatment of gastric ulcer. In Burland WL, Simkins MA (eds): Cimetidine. Proceedings of the Second International Symposium on Histamine H_2-receptor Antagonists. Amsterdam, Excerpta Medica, 1977 p 283
13. Curtis LE, Simonian S, Burk CA, et al: Evaluation of the effectiveness of controlled pH in management of massive upper gastrointestinal bleeding. Am J Surg 125:474, 1973

14. Dawson AM: Continuous intragastric milk drip in the treatment of upper gastrointestinal haemorrhage. Lancet 1:73, 1976
15. Douglass HO: Levarterenol irrigation. JAMA 230:1653, 1974
16. Dronfield MW, Langman MJS: Acute upper gastrointestinal bleeding. Br J Hosp Med 19:99, 1978
17. Dunn DH, Fischer RC, Siluis SE, et al: The treatment of hemorrhagic gastritis with cimetidine. Surg Gynecol Obstet 147:272, 1978
18. Fordtran JS, Morawski SG, Richardson CT: In vivo and in vitro evaluation of liquid antacids. N Engl J Med 288:923, 1973
19. Gibinski K, Rybicha J, Mikos E, et al: Double-blind clinical trial on gastroduodenal ulcer healing with prostaglandin E_2 analogues. Gut 18:636, 1977
20. Gillespie G, Gray GR, Smith IS, et al: Short term and maintenance treatment in severe duodenal ulceration. In Burland WL, Simkins MA (eds): Cimetidine. Proceedings of the Second International Symposium on Histamine H_2-receptor Antagonists. Amsterdam, Excerpta Medica, 1977 p 240
21. Goldberg HI, Dodds WJ, Gee S, et al: Role of acid and pepsin in acute experimental esophagitis. Gastroenterology 56:223, 1969
22. Green FW, Kaplan MM, Curtis LE, et al: Effect of acid and pepsin on blood coagulation and platelet aggregation. Gastroenterology 74:38, 1978
23. Grossman MI: Duration of action of antacids (Abstr). Clin Res 8:125, 1960
24. Hansky J, Korman MG: Long term cimetidine in duodenal ulcer disease. Am J Dig Dis 24:465, 1979
25. Hastings PR, Skillman JJ, Bushnell LS, et al: Antacid titration in the prevention of acute gastrointestinal bleeding: a controlled, randomized trial in 100 critically ill patients. N Engl J Med 298:1041, 1978
26. Henn RM, Isenberg JI, Maxwell J, et al: Inhibition of gastric acid secretion by cimetidine in patients with duodenal ulcer. N Engl J Med 293:371, 1975
27. Hoare AM, Bradby GUH, Hawkins CF: Cimetidine in bleeding peptic ulcer. Lancet 2:671, 1979
28. Hollander D, Harlan J: Antacids vs placebo in peptic ulcer therapy. JAMA 226:1181, 1973
29. Kiselow MC, Wagner M: Intragastric instillation of levarterenol. Arch Surg 107:387, 1973
30. Lanza FL: An endoscopic evaluation of gastric ulcer treated with a mixture containing bismuth ammonium citrate. Curr Ther Res 12:1, 1970
31. Leveen HH, Diaz C, Wynkoop BJ, et al: Control of gastrointestinal bleeding. Am J Surg 123:154, 1972
32. Longstreth GF, Malagelada J-R: Cimetidine suppression of nocturnal gastric secretion in active duodenal ulcer. N Engl J Med 294:801, 1976
33. Ma KW, Brown DC, Masler DS, et al: Effects of renal failure on blood levels of cimetidine. Gastroenterology 74:473, 1978
34. MacDougall BRD, Bailey FJ, Williams R: Histamine H_2-receptor antagonists in the prophylaxis and control of acute gastrointestinal haemorrhage in liver disease. In Burland WL, Simkins MA (eds): Cimetidine. Proceedings of the Second International Symposium on Histamine H_2-receptor Antagonists. Amsterdam, Excerpta Medica, 1977, p 329

35. McAlhany SC, Czaja AJ, Pruitt BA: Antacid control of complications from acute gastroduodenal disease after burns. J Trauma 16:645, 1976
36. McCarthy DM, Hyman PE: Cholinergic influence on gastric acid selection in the Zollinger-Ellison syndrome (Abstr). Gastroenterology 76:1198, 1979
37. McMillen MA, Ambis D, Siegel JH: Cimetidine and mental confusion. N Engl J Med 298:284, 1978
38. Milton-Thompson GJ, Wright B, Vincent D, et al: Comparison of 24 hour intragastric acidity in duodenal ulcer patients on high dose antacids or cimetidine (Abstr). Gastroenterology 76:1204, 1979
39. Moshal MG: A bismuth-peptide complex in the treatment of duodenal ulceration. S Afr Med J 49:1157, 1975
40. Northfield TC, Blackwood WS: Controlled clinical trial of cimetidine for duodenal ulcer. In Burland WL, Simkins MA (eds): Cimetidine. Proceedings of the Second International Symposium on Histamine H_2-receptor Antagonists. Amsterdam, Excerpta Medica, 1977, p 240
41. Peterson WL, Barnett C, Feldman M, et al: Reduction of twenty-four hour gastric acidity with combination drug therapy in patients with duodenal ulcer. Gastroenterology 77:1015, 1979
42. Peterson WL, Sturdevant RAL, Frankl HD, et al: Healing of duodenal ulcer with an antacid regimen. N Engl J Med 297:341, 1977
43. Piper DW, Fenton BH: pH stability and activity curves of pepsin with special reference to their clinical importance. Gut 6:506, 1965
44. Richardson CT, Bailey BA, Walsh JH, et al: The effect of an H_2-receptor antagonist on food stimulated acid secretion, serum gastrin, and gastric emptying in patients with duodenal ulcers. Comparison with an anticholinergic drug. J Clin Invest 55:536, 1975
45. Richardson CT, Walsh JH: The value of a histamine H_2-receptor antagonist in the management of patients with Zollinger-Ellison syndrome. N Engl J Med 294:133, 1976
46. Richardson CT, Walsh JH, Hicks MI: The effect of cimetidine, a new histamine H_2receptor antagonist, on meal-stimulated acid secretion, serum gastrin, and gastric emptying in patients with duodenal ulcer. Gastroenterology 71:19, 1976
47. Robert A, Nezamis J-E, Lancaster C, et al: Cytoprotection by prostaglandins in rats. Gastroenterology 77:433, 1979
48. Salmon PA: Local gastric hypothermia induced by direct perfusion of the gastric lumen: experimental basis and clinical application. Can Med Assoc J 97:944, 1967
49. Schiller KFR, Truelove SC, Williams DG: Hematemesis and melena with special reference to factors influencing the outcome. Br Med J 2:7, 1970
50. Scobie BA: Milk drip therapy for upper gastrointestinal bleeding. Med J Aust 1:1028, 1969
51. Simonian SJ, Curtis LE: Treatment of hemorrhagic gastritis by antacid. Ann Surg 184:429, 1976
52. Shultz RA, Nezamia J-E, Lancaster C: Gastric antisecretory and anti-ulcer properties of PGE_2 15-methyl PGE_2, and 16,16-Dimethyl PGE_2. Gastroenterology 70:359, 1976
53. Wangensteen OH, Root HD, Jenson CB, et al: Depression of gastric

secretion and digestion by gastric hypothermia: its clinical use in massive hematemesis. Surgery 44:265, 1958
54. Wangensteen OH, Root HD, Salmon PA, et al: Depressant action of local gastric hypothermia on gastric digestion. JAMA 169:1601, 1959
55. Waterman WG, Walker JL: Effect of a topical adrenergic agent on gastric blood flow. Am J Surg 127:241, 1974
56. Waterman NG, Walker BA: The effect of gastric cooling on hemostasis. Surg Gynecol Obstet 137:80, 1973
57. Weiss G, Serfontein WJ: The efficiency of bismuth-protein complex compound in the treatment of gastric and duodenal ulcers. S Afr Med J 45:462, 1970
58. Wilson DE, Phillips C, Levine RA: Inhibition of gastric secretion in man by prostaglandin A. Gastroenterology 61:201, 1971
59. Yajho RD, Norton LW, Eiseman B: Current management of upper gastrointestinal bleeding. Ann Surg 181:474, 1974

Philip E. Donahue, M.D.
Lloyd M. Nyhus, M.D., F.A.C.S.

Surgery for Massive Upper Gastrointestinal Hemorrhage

ABSTRACT

Massive upper gastrointestinal hemorrhage is a frequent occurrence in almost any hospital setting. Because the patients affected are often chronically ill, and because of the serious physiologic consequences of massive bleeding, the surgeon must be prepared to treat all of the associated problems which may arise.

There are well established "rules" which help decide when an operation is indicated. Once this point has been reached, a careful and thorough exploratory laparotomy can identify the source of bleeding, even if a preoperative diagnosis is not available.

The role of gastrointestinal endoscopy is still controversial; it is best viewed as a valuable adjunct in the aggressive evaluation of patients with bleeding, and an important part of a comprehensive treatment program. Endoscopic diagnosis must be combined with surgical judgment in treating the individual patient.

Operative therapy is tailored to the patient and to the bleeding lesion. There is a general tendency to avoid resection, or resect "less" when possible, to avoid the prohibitive mortality generally associated with massive resection.

By attention to the many details associated with gastrointestinal hemorrhage, the morbidity of a bleeding episode can be reduced. One must be aware of the high mortality in most series of patients with bleeding and do everything possible to prevent it.

The treatment of the bleeding patient is a continuing challenge to all clinicians. Although there is still considerable morbidity and mortality with major hemorrhage, major advances have been made in the care of such patients. For example, the ability to evaluate and compensate for circulatory deficits has

---

Philip E. Donahue, M.D.: Assistant Professor of Surgery, Department of Surgery, University of Illinois Hospital and Chief, General Surgery, West Side Veterans Administration Hospital, Chicago, Illinois; Lloyd M. Nyhus, M.D., F.A.C.S.: Warren H. Cole Professor and Head, Department of Surgery, University of Illinois at the Medical Center, Chicago, Illinois.

been markedly improved by the routine use of pulmonary artery pressure monitoring devices; impending or frank respiratory failure can now be treated by volume respirators and the utilization of positive airway pressure apparatus; cardiac arrhythmias are managed with transvenous pacing wires; acute renal failure can be treated successfully by temporary hemodialysis. Still, none of the modalities by itself has altered the fact that major hemorrhage has significant risk for mortality [31].

The most important aspect of the care of bleeding patients is selection of the optimal treatment for the underlying condition from which the bleeding episode has resulted. For example, a patient with recurrent bleeding from a duodenal ulcer requires a definitive operation to control the source of bleeding and reduce secretion of acid; on the other hand, a patient with massive trauma, hypotension, and bleeding from acute gastric mucosal lesions needs intravenous fluid therapy.

Given the complexity of comparing individual patients with bleeding ulcers, the problem of making all-inclusive statements about such patients sometimes seems futile. However, the clinician has a different problem. He or she has the task of determining which of many possible approaches should be undertaken in the care of an individual patient [9, 41]. All decisions must be firmly grounded in the known pathophysiology of the various conditions that result in gastrointestinal hemorrhage. Ideally, the practitioner should have extensive personal experience in the treatment of such patients. As in most areas of medicine, there is no substitute for mature judgment.

When reviewing the staggering number of publications concerned with this problem, we are always impressed by the diversity of opinion about all aspects of the natural history of bleeding ulcers. Several excellent studies have compared the efficacy of alternative approaches to both diagnosis and treatment of massive hemorrhage [1, 2]. Considerable disagreement still exists about approaches to management of these patients [10, 11, 13, 15, 17, 18, 26].

All studies agree that there is considerable mortality in large groups of patients with bleeding ulcers and that no single approach can guarantee a favorable result [6]. A major controversy continues to surround the efficacy of aggressive diagnosis in lowering the mortality of massive upper gastrointestinal hemorrhage. Several recent studies reached the conclusion that endoscopic diagnosis has not affected the mortality [10, 11, 15, 34]. This conclusion must be viewed in the context of the patients studied, since there is great variability in the severity of the hemorrhage and in the number of patients with bleeding esophageal varices or stress ulcers, lesions which have prohibitive mortality as a rule. Whether or not the study is limited to patients who have sustained truly massive hemorrhage is extremely important since the inclusion of many patients with melena alone, without hematemesis or hypotension, will underestimate the value of aggressive measures. Likewise, a great number of patients with stress gastritis or varices, a group with 50% mortality, can conceal the effectiveness of prompt diagnosis in lowering the mortality of bleeding duodenal and gastric ulcers.

The age and general medical condition of the patients are difficult to "control" in studies such as these, and it is a fact that most of the patients who die do so because of associated organ failure, although hemorrhage certainly serves as the precipitating event.

Given this reality, the operating surgeon must be aware of the risk factors in massive hemorrhage so that operation can be recommended at the optimal time for the patients under consideration [19].

The studies previously referred to do not determine another critical factor — to what extent endoscopic diagnosis has allowed the clinician to determine that surgical intervention is unavoidable, given the natural history of the lesion. Very large duodenal ulcers, large gastric ulcers, and chronic gastric ulcers are examples of lesions in which care is positively affected by endoscopic diagnosis. If one examines a cohort of such patients the benefits of prompt diagnosis become clear. Modern operative treatment should result in a surgical mortality of 10% or less [7, 18, 24] as opposed to a surgical mortality of 25-40% in some less favorable series.

Each of us wondered what the precise role of endoscopy should be in the overall management of patients with gastrointestinal bleeding when these devices were introduced; ten years' experience allows us to draw certain conclusions. We have been and are enthusiastic about the role of endoscopic diagnosis in bleeding patients because precise knowledge of the bleeding lesion allows more specific application of surgical therapy, shortens operative time, and helps us avoid operation in those patients who are best treated by nonoperative methods.

More reassuring studies have shown a convincing decrease in the mortality of massive bleeding when an aggressive diagnostic and therapeutic approach was used [18, 21]. These studies do not claim that endoscopic examination alone made the difference; on the contrary, endoscopic diagnosis is only a part of a complex diagnostic and therapeutic process [2, 28]. Identification of the bleeding point, adequate volume resuscitation, reference to the patient's age and previous medical history, and frequent assessment of the patient's response to therapy remain the vital factors. It is incorrect and misleading to contend that endoscopic examination in most medical centers is anything more than a diagnostic tool which aids in the selection of appropriate therapy. The advent of therapeutic endoscopy for managing hemorrhage by electrocautery or laser beams may force revision of the previous statement.

WHEN TO OPERATE

Surgeons are often faced with the question, "When do you recommend operation for bleeding ulcers?" The obvious answer — "when necessary, and at the appropriate time" — may seem too simple, but it is meant to suggest that individual factors have to be considered at all times [9].

Patients with massive hemorrhage are at grave risk, however, and frequently require operation in the course of their treatment; this is especially true of those whose bleeding episode is associated with frank shock on admission to the hospital [19, 32]. Two types of presentation of hemorrhage bear comment. Type I includes those patients who experience exsanguinating hemorrhage (≥50 ml/min) and who cannot tolerate any delay in definitive treatment. Type II includes all other types of hemorrhage. Patients with Type I hemorrhage cannot tolerate long delays for diagnostic efforts; likewise they are not candidates for endoscopic examination (except after intubation and resuscitation). Operative exploration in such instances must serve both a diagnostic and therapeutic function (see below). For example, the portacaval shunt performed for bleeding ulcer (mistakenly assumed to be a bleeding varix because varices are present) has small chance of success; the suggested diagnosis must be verified by direct inspection. Patients with type II hemorrhage, the large majority of individuals with massive hemorrhage, are those whose rate of bleeding slows or even stops during or possibly as a result of initial therapy. These patients are best managed by methodical and simultaneous diagnostic and therapeutic maneuvers [8].

MANAGEMENT OF TYPE II HEMORRHAGE

Many institutions are now organizing a team of physicians to manage all patients with gastrointestinal hemorrhage. The team, consisting of a general surgeon, a medical gastroenterologist and a primary physician, should be notified every time a patient enters the emergency room with a complaint resembling upper gastrointestinal hemorrhage [3]. The general steps in the management of a patient with upper gastrointestinal hemorrhage are: (1) confirmation of gastrointestinal hemorrhage, (2) adequate resuscitation, (3) evacuation of stomach of blood clots and detritus, (4) early endoscopy, (5) adequate angiography, if indicated, (6) conservative measures to control bleeding, (7) possible radiologic control of bleeding, and (8) operation, if necessary.

Barium meal is not included as part of the evaluation of upper gastrointestinal hemorrhage: it is accurate only 50% of the time and in all instances obscures both endoscopic and angiographic findings.

The patient is usually admitted to the emergency room with a chief complaint of having vomited blood. As the physicians are being notified, the nurses prepare the patient for examination and obtain vital signs. If the patient is in a state of shock, the situation is urgent, and immediate steps are taken to correct hypotension. After presence of hemorrhage has been confirmed, early resuscitation is carried out by rapid colloid or crystalloid infusion through large-bore intravenous portals. Prior history of known ulcer disease, alcoholism, or of having taken any medications such as aspirin are especially pertinent. A nasogastric tube is passed; "coffee grounds" or blood-flecked material is not a great cause for alarm since the patient is not bleeding as rapidly as someone with emesis of large amounts of frank blood. The nasogastric tube is removed and an Ewald tube inserted.

There are multiple variations in the tube which may be used, but an Ewald tube is best suited for removal of blood and clots from the stomach. The Ewald tube is vigorously irrigated with one-half iced water and one-half iced saline solution (which need not be sterile) until the returns begin to lighten. If, after 30 minutes or so of irrigation, it becomes evident that the stomach cannot be cleared of blood, preparations are begun for immediate operation. In more than 75% of instances, however, the treatment just described will stop gastrointestinal hemorrhage. Lest the description of the success of lavage seem too enthusiastic, mention is made of the invariable presence of 700-1000 ml of clot in the stomachs of patients requiring surgical exploration. No tube can empty the stomach of clots if the rate of hemorrhage is too rapid.

When the Ewald returns are pink, the stomach has been evacuated as completely as possible, and the gastrointestinal panendoscope can be inserted. Inspection at this point has been shown to be 90% accurate in diagnosing the source of bleeding. If the hemorrhage continues to be rapid, endoscopic examination should not be attempted because it may result in pulmonary aspiration. The course of action at this point is dictated by the patient's history and medical condition, endoscopic findings, angiographic facilities (and immediate availability of a radiologist), and other technical factors. Individualization of treatment is mandatory [8].

The patient who has had severe trauma or is having a stormy postoperative course (e.g., sepsis, fistula) is likely to have stress ulceration. Hemorrhage in this situation would mandate endoscopy followed by selective angiogram to establish the sites of bleeding. Attempts to control bleeding with selective infusion of vasopressin or by neutralization of intragastric acidity should be made.

At times the surgeon will be pressured to operate blindly upon a patient with ongoing hemorrhage and to have endoscopic examination performed only after the patient has been intubated in the operating suite. Though there are instances in which this may be necessary, an aggressive approach to the therapy of patients with massive hemorrhage will minimize the number of occasions for this approach.

Indications for Operation

The goal of conservative management of massive gastrointestinal hemorrhage is sometimes overly optimistic. We propose the indications for surgical treatment in Table 1 — they have passed the test of time, and their efficacy has been proved. Since mortality associated with massive upper gastrointestinal hemor-

Table 1
Absolute and Relative Indications for Operation

Absolute indications

    1500 ml whole blood replacement during any 24-hour period, after initial stabilization

    Continuous bleeding for more than 48 hours (24 hours in patients older than 50 years of age)

    Recurrent bleeding during vigorous medical therapy

    Coincident bleeding and perforation

    Lesions which invariably continue bleeding (such as aortoduodenal fistula)

Relative indications

    Age greater than 50 years

    Serious medical problem, especially heart disease

    Severe pain persisting during hemorrhage

    Shortage of available blood because of

        Rare blood type

        Preformed antibodies that make cross-match difficult

        Patient's refusal to accept transfusion

    Endoscopic demonstration of actively bleeding arterial lesion

rhage is related to the timing of operation, patients with less than optimal resuscitation should not be operated upon, just as patients should not be permitted to continue bleeding day after day until moribund. Likewise, patients with serious systemic disease can not be allowed to continue bleeding without risking multisystem failure; in general such patients are operated upon sooner than "healthy" persons.

PREPARATION FOR OPERATION – THE TRANSOPERATIVE APPROACH

Physiological Considerations

Physiological preparation is the mainstay of modern surgical treatment, and massive hemorrhage provides a dramatic opportunity to maintain cardiopulmonary stability [12]. Cardiac monitoring techniques should include routine use of pulmonary artery catheters when possible, especially in patients older than 60 years of age, the group of patients who have the greatest mortality during bleeding episodes [5, 35, 38].

Pulmonary care must be directed toward minimizing the chances for aspiration of gastric contents, for alveolar hypoventilation or frank respiratory failure, and for pneumonia or atelectasis, postoperatively. Frequent monitoring of respiratory rate and arterial and central venous oxygen tensions allows early recognition of respiratory failure or cardiac insufficiency. Early intubation and institution of positive airway pressure continue to be the most beneficial means of protecting pulmonary function. New devices for achieving positive airway pressure by mask alone without intubation are not without risk in this type of patient, and are not recommended.

Patients who are brought to the operating room in optimal condition will have had adequate volume replacement as determined by blood pressure, pulse and urine output. At times, judicious volume replacement is not accompanied by satisfactory return to normal of these measurements; the usual reason is that resuscitation is lagging behind the rate of bleeding. These patients need two prompt changes in therapy as a rule; the first is an increase in the rate of fluid therapy, and the second is prompt surgical exploration. Such patients probably have unrecognized Type I hemorrhage, and procrastination or indecision can be a fatal mistake.

A practice which is recommended for all bleeding patients is the maintenance of a structured flow diagram which records the dynamic aspects of transfusion therapy and the patient's response (Table 2). Such a hemorrhage sheet can greatly simplify the tabulation of all significant aspects of the hemorrhage and serves as a valuable teaching device for residents, medical students and paramedical personnel.

A note of caution regarding the use of prophylactic antibiotics is in order for patients with massive bleeding. Such patients, even if they secrete adequate amounts of acid in the basal state, will have considerable contamination of their normally sterile gastric contents by swallowed bacteria which thrive because the blood in the stomach neutralizes any effect of endogenous acid. Effective antibiotic therapy is best directed against a wide spectrum of aerobic and anaerobic bacteria. Gram-positive bacteria, including Clostridia, may be present in large numbers and are the major pathogens. Beta lactam antibiotics (either the first generation cephalosporins or later modifications) should be given to any patient operated upon, preferably several hours before the operation. This policy implies that any patient who continues to bleed should have an antibiotic given during the first several hours of admission to the hospital. We also recommend Gram stain and culture of gastric contents whenever the stomach is entered.

At the conclusion of the operative procedure the skin and subcutaneous tissues are best left open to eliminate the possibility of subcutaneous wound infection. All of these considerations are especially applicable to patients with gastric ulcer.

Table 2
Massive Hemorrhage – Critical Management of a Case

	Day 1 (Admission)	Day 1 – $\bar{p}$ Initial Rx	Day 2
Pulse (postural ∆)	100 (130)	100 (115)	80 (80)
Blood pressure (postural ∆)	100/70 (80/0)	111/80 (100/79)	110/80 (110/80)
CVP pressure (cm H$_2$O)	2	8	8
PAD/PCW pressure (mm Hg)	2/0	8/4	10/4
Cardiac output	5 l/min	5 l/min	5 l/min
Hct	36	38	40
Intravenous therapy			
Crystalloid (cc)	2000	2000	
Colloid (g Alb)	25	–	
Whole blood	–		
Packed cells (units)	2	2	
Fresh frozen plasma	–		
PT/PTT	17.0/36.0	10.5/37.0	
Platelet count	250,000		
Urine output/hr; SG	30 (1.026)	50 (1.015)	50 (1.010)
Bloody bowel motion	1 black	2 tarry	1 tarry/brown
Color of gastric lavage	Bright red	Coffee grounds	Clear

Age, sex, duration of bleeding: 66 years; male; 4 days.
Significant medical history: Starr-Edwards aortic value, 1974.
Medications: Coumadin 5 mg/day.
Endoscopy (E)/Arteriography (A): E – normal esophagus; normal duodenal bulb; possible GU.

Psychological Preparation

The surgeon should be aware of the intense strain which massive hemorrhage places on the individual and his family members. The important quality of assurance depends much upon what the surgeon says, how he says it, and his style of management [20]. The surgeon should be firm and understanding, sharing his or her knowledge with the family so that they know the rationale of the treatment plan. The family should know that the surgeon is familiar with all of the conditions that cause bleeding, and that he or she will not spare any effort to correct the condition.

If surgeons do not develop this awareness and ability, then less knowledgeable individuals will fill the void, and a further step toward committee medicine will have been taken. We firmly believe that the surgeon is the logical individual to set the tone for all of the events surrounding the bleeding episode, and that the results of the surgeon's efforts — successful or not — will be most acceptable if the surgeon accepts personal responsibility for supervising all aspects of the patient's care.

PLAN OF OPERATION

The patient is brought to the operating room, prepared and draped while awake, and intubated. Although intubation while conscious sometimes seems a terrifying experience for the patient it is less dangerous than a "crash" induction complicated by difficulty intubating the patient or by aspiration of gastric contents. The proper psychological support by the operating room staff during this period is vital; the patient will always remember who held his or her hand or gave him or her an encouraging look when the situation was critical.

A midline incision is desirable, allowing maximal exposure in minimal time with little bleeding; the incision must be adequate for proper exposure. Mechanical retractors can provide excellent, tireless exposure. This is especially important if the number of surgical assistants is limited.

Intraoperative Endoscopy

If for any reason endoscopic examination was impossible preoperatively, it is sometimes advantageous to consider such an examination at this time [23]. The operating surgeon will want to know what the esophagus looks like. Are these varices? Are they bleeding? Is there gross esophagitis or a bleeding lesion at the gastroesophageal junction? All of these critical questions are best answered by direct visual examination. Surgeon-endoscopists can accomplish this examination in a few minutes without the attendant risks of aspiration or hypotension which might occur if endoscopic examination were performed under less optimal conditions.

Examination of the Abdominal Organs

Examination of the abdominal mass often provides rapid identification of the source of bleeding [14]. The condition of the liver and the presence of gastric or esophageal varices can be established quickly, though it is important to recognize that simultaneous ulcer or gastritis may be the source of bleeding in 50% of the patients with concomitant varices [40]. That is precisely why at some point in the diagnostic process the source of bleeding should be specifically identified in any patient with bleeding varices.

Next, inspection of the gastroesophageal junction, the body and lesser curvature of the stomach, and the duodenum is performed. If subserosal ecchymosis surrounds the gastroesophageal junction, a Mallory-Weiss tear at the gastroesophageal junction should be suspected; such a sign can be expected in 25% to 50% of patients with such lesions.

The lesser curvature of the stomach may have a contiguous inflammatory process from a chronic gastric ulcer or a marginal ulcer. Inflammatory reaction and petechial hemorrhage are characteristic in the vicinity of any active ulcer in either the duodenum or stomach.

Following this, digital palpation of the stomach and duodenum, including manual indentation of the anterior wall of these tissues may allow discovery of an ulcer crater on the posterior wall [14]. The induration of chronic pancreatitis should not be mistaken for an ulcer; the hardened pancreas can mimic the presence of an ulcer. The pyloric ring stretched over a swollen pancreas or retrogastric lymph nodes is another source of error.

If none of these investigations reveals the source of bleeding, the next step is a carefully planned gastrotomy. Planning is crucial in this step; the patient should not undergo gastrectomy as a hasty maneuver.

The first opening should be made along the anterior surface of the stomach in a way that allows either closure of the opening after inspection of the mucosa, distal gastrectomy (antrectomy) with tubularization of the gastric remnant, or partial gastrectomy in the manner of Pauchet [29, 30].

No External Evidence of Bleeding Site

The gastrotomy is performed after isolation of the stomach by laparotomy pads to minimize contamination of the abdomen. Generous use of electrocautery helps minimize bleeding from the edematous mucosa, and Babcock clamps placed upon mucosal arterioles can control this source of additional bleeding. Manual extraction of the clot is then performed.

Inspection of the mucosa sometimes shows numerous small acute ulcers. Even if several of these ulcers are found, it is important to determine whether there is an active source of bleeding within the stomach. This is done by first irrigating residual blood from both the proximal and distal stomach segments, placing moist laparotomy pads in each portion of the stomach, and removing these pads in sequential fashion from each portion of the stomach. The gastroesophageal junction should be checked carefully; the nasogastric tube will provide rapid identification of the gastroesophageal junction, and narrow metal retractors placing upward traction on the anterior gastric wall will allow complete evaluation of this critical area. Any bleeding superficial ulcers are oversewn with silk sutures. Then, thought is given to more definitive treatment of the condition (see below).

If no bleeding sites are found it is sometimes helpful for the surgeon to palpate the gastric tissues between his or her fingers; a small ulcer will sometimes be hidden between folds of mucosa and can be found in this way. Any bleeding chronic gastric ulcer is treated initially in the same manner as the bleeding duodenal ulcer (see below).

If no lesion is found in the stomach, an incision should be made that traverses the pylorus. This incision is made with the possibility of subsequent pyloroplasty in mind. Our choice, therefore, is an incision approximately one centimeter from the greater curvature side of the stomach and duodenum, since we favor the Finney pyloroplasty. The alternate incision midway between greater and lesser curvatures is satisfactory as well, but is not preferred because of difficulty in calibrating the subsequent "ostomy" precisely. With serious early dumping or alkaline reflux gastritis as the complication of too generous openings, the surgeon must be cognizant of the physical size of the connection he or she creates. If a duodenal or pyloric channel ulcer is found it should be carefully examined for the presence of an arterial wall in its base. We perform suture ligation of arteries proximally and distally with 2-0 silk sutures, then pass a "u" stitch beneath the center of the artery to obliterate any anastomosing vessels which might join the posterior wall. A note of caution is sounded regarding ulcers overlying the portal triad; the lumen of the common duct should not be compromised and operative cholangiography should be performed if there is any question of a hemostatic suture impinging upon this structure.

The preceding approach localizes the bleeding in most instances. The surgeon should beware if no bleeding lesion has been found! Such a circumstance requires rapid assessment of other potential sources of hemorrhage, including prosthetic-enteric fistula, pancreato-enteric fistula and hemobilia. If no source of bleeding is found we recommend that the abdomen be closed without any definitive procedure being performed. Just as blind gastrectomy is a historical footnote in the treatment of bleeding [36], so also is the vagotomy and pyloroplasty performed without specific indications.

SPECIFIC SURGICAL THERAPY

With the source of bleeding controlled, the next step is the performance of the definitive surgical procedure best suited to the bleeding lesion. A few minutes spent in evaluation of the next move are not only well spent but allow the anesthesiologist to correct any circulatory volume deficits.

Chronic Gastric Ulcer

The position of the ulcer determines several specific aspects of the operation. Most chronic gastric ulcers are situated on the lesser curvature of the stomach near the incisura; these are excised with ease by the Schoemaker modification of distal gastric resection. This technique utilizes a 40% resection with care taken to include the tongue-like projection of antrum along the lesser curvature. Typically, the greater curvature is freed from the gastroepiploic vessels along its distal margin up to the point at which resection will be performed. The gastroduodenal junction is mobilized and a Kocher maneuver elevates the duodenum to assure that the subsequent gastroduodenostomy can be performed without tension.

Then, the right gastric artery is identified and ligated. Look for a convex, pulsatile elevation along the cephalad border of the pylorus to identify this vessel. After division of the duodenum, the limits of gastric resection can be determined. Next, the left gastric artery is divided between clamps. Preliminary spreading maneuvers in this edematous tissue should be avoided; instead, the surgeon should place his or her left hand within the lesser sac with fingers beneath the stomach and the thumb anteriorly. When the surgeon compresses the stomach and withdraws the left hand the lesser curvature will be apparent, and clamps can be applied. Double ligation of the proximal left gastric artery is prudent [25].

A Payr clamp is then applied perpendicularly to the greater curvature of the stomach, encompassing 4.5 to 5.0 cm of stomach, the exact size required for subsequent anastomosis. A second Payr clamp or stapling device is inserted from the tip of the first clamp toward the gastroesophageal junction. The only difference in the approach to the bleeding patient is preliminary ligation of the left gastric artery, either through a gastrotomy as described or along the lesser curvature if bleeding is not massive.

The high gastric ulcer cannot be encompassed by clamps and is managed best by the Pauchet type of resection. This technique used in the early 1900's differs from the two clamp techniques just described in that instead of application of the second clamp, a free-cut is made along the anterior surface of the stomach, saving enough of the anterior wall to allow tubularization of the gastric remnant and avoid subtotal gastrectomy [37]. The resulting suture line will rotate to the posterior wall of the stomach as shown. The subsequent anastomosis should be neither too large nor too small; a 15-20 mm opening is perfectly adequate. We prefer the Billroth I anastomosis, but will on rare occasions perform a gastrojejunostomy if some physical factor, such as fatty liver, prohibits Billroth I anastomosis without tension.

An alternative treatment for a high-lying gastric ulcer is the distal resection without removal of the ulcer. Kelling and Madlener proposed this operation at the turn of the century, and it is reported to be efficacious. If this distal resection is used, the ulcer bed must be suture-ligated to control bleeding, and frozen section of the margin should be performed to exclude cancer.

No specific recommendation for lesser procedures can be made at this time. Although encouraging preliminary results of selective gastric vagotomy and pyloroplasty or highly selective vagotomy alone have been reported, their use must be categorized as experimental. In the patient at extremely poor risk, truncal vagotomy and pyloroplasty with wedge resection of the ulcer can be performed with the realization that recurrence of the ulcer is more likely.

Finally, any gastric ulcer seen in conjunction with a scarred pyloroduodenal area must be viewed as a combined ulcer, and vagotomy must be added to the gastric resection.

Chronic Duodenal Ulcer

The operative treatment of bleeding duodenal ulcer must include a procedure to arrest hypersecretion of acid. In our clinic vagotomy is recommended for all such situations. The technique of vagotomy must include a careful search for main and accessory vagal branches. We subscribe to the original technique (which has not received sufficient emphasis in the past) which results in a circumferential area of esophagus completely bared of adventitial-neural tissues [27].

The single most valuable maneuver in performing this type of vagotomy is the identification of the potential space at the anterior wall of the esophagus where the hepatogastric ligament joins the esophagogastric junction. When this landmark is used, subsequent baring of the esophagus is performed easily. In patients who have recurrent bleeding duodenal ulcers after previous vagotomy, this plane is often intact and inviolate. A complete vagotomy then can be performed with surprising ease. Likewise, the posterior trunk is often found intact in instances of recurrent bleeding, and care must be taken to guarantee that it is not left intact. Missed vagal nerves and incomplete vagotomy are the cause of most recurrent ulcers.

In general, resection is not recommended for the initial treatment of bleeding duodenal ulcers. Complete vagotomy with adequate pyloroplasty is safe, effective, and has less associated morbidity than gastric resection [16, 39]. However, there are instances in which resection must be performed: for example, large ulcers which virtually destroy the pyloroduodenal junction. Likewise, recurrent ulcers in the aftermath of complete vagotomy (as determined by repeat exploration) or primary ulcers in which control of the bleeding artery results in irreparable damage to the pyloroduodenal segment require distal gastric resection. The common causes of recurrent duodenal ulcer are:

incomplete vagotomy, inadequate gastric resection, retained antrum not in continuity with gastric secretions (Billroth II), too long afferent limbs, ulcerogenic tumor of the pancreas, ingestion of irritating drugs, and unphysiologic operations, such as truncan vagotomy without drainage, gastroenterostomy without vagotomy, and gastroileostomy.

In this setting, a 25% gastrectomy is adequate, and Billroth I reconstruction preferred. If a Billroth II operation is performed (a rare necessity), biopsies of the duodenal margin should be performed to preclude a margin of retained antral tissue.

The danger zone in any resection for duodenal ulcer is the distal segment containing the ulcer. The surgeon should beware of the large ulcer penetrating the head of the pancreas or portal triad. The base of such an ulcer should never be resected.

The Strauss maneuver, named for the late Alfred Strauss of Chicago, is eminently suited to the safe treatment of these penetrating ulcers. The base of the ulcer remains in situ and is excluded from the mainstream. Damage to contiguous structures, risk of pancreatitis, or needless hemorrhage is thus avoided. The surgeon should perform this maneuver from the left side of the table, elevating the pyloroduodenum with the left hand, incising the posterior mucosal layer alone under direct vision.

Stress Ulcers — Acute Gastric Mucosal Lesions

Surgical treatment is a last resort for such lesions, and the procedure of choice is debatable [4, 22, 32]. There is little question that total gastrectomy or near total gastrectomy will stop the hemorrhage. However, the associated mortality risk is so great that routine use of the procedure cannot be recommended. Alternatives such as vagotomy and pyloroplasty with oversewing of bleeding lesions are as effective in general as any procedure and must be considered. A more recent innovation which is also less risky than massive resection is ligation of all major arteries to the stomach [33]. While not as attractive in terms of definitive treatment as some other operations, the minimal morbidity does much to recommend the procedure.

The surgeon who manages a patient with gastrointestinal hemorrhage must be aware of all the options for treatment of a given lesion. It is impossible to state a priori which procedure must be employed when operation is necessary. The patient's age, the presence of additional organ pathology, and the previous experience of the surgeon must all be considered.

In all probability, massive upper gastrointestinal hemorrhage will continue to occur in all age groups; the surgeon can have a positive effect on the morbidity of massive hemorrhage by operating at just the right time and by performing an operation tailored to the specific patient.

Careful consideration must be given to cardiac, respiratory, and renal physiology in order to avoid multisystem failure. Furthermore, infectious complications must be anticipated and prevented where possible.

By attention to all of the possible systemic complications in patients with gastrointestinal hemorrhage we can provide optimal treatment for this critical problem.

REFERENCES

1. Allen HM, Block MA, Schuman BM: Gastroduodenal endoscopy. Arch Surg 106:450, 1973
2. Blackstone MO, Kirsner JB: Establishing the site of gastrointestinal bleeding. JAMA 241:599, 1979
3. Bombeck CT, Donahue PE, Nyhus LM: Complications of gastric and duodenal ulcer. In RM Zollinger (ed): General Surgery, Current Principles in Practice. Huntingdon Station, Physicians Programs Inc, 1979
4. Bryant LR, Griffen WO: Vagotomy and pyloroplasty, an inadequate operation for stress ulcers? Arch Surg 93:161, 1966
5. Chang FC, Drake JE, Farha G: Massive upper gastrointestinal hemorrhage in the elderly. Am J Surg 134:721, 1977
6. Ching E, ReMine WH: Surgical management of emergency complications of duodenal ulcer. Surg Clin N Am 51:851, 1971
7. Cocks JR, Desmond AM, Swynnerton BF, et al: Partial gastrectomy for hemorrhage. Gut 13:331, 1972
8. Donahue PE, Nyhus LM: Massive upper gastrointestinal hemorrhage. In Nyhus LM, Wastell C, (eds): Surgery of the Stomach and Duodenum, 3rd ed. Boston, Little, Brown, 1977
9. Donahue PE, Marrie AJ, Krystosek RJ, et al: Role of vagotomy in duodenal ulcer. Postgrad Med 62:156, 1977
10. Dronfield MW, Atkinson M, Langman MJS: Effect of different operation policies on mortality from bleeding peptic ulcer. Lancet 1:1126, 1979
11. Dronfield MW, McIllmurray MB, Ferguson R, et al: A prospective, randomized study of endoscopy and radiology in acute upper gastrointestinal bleeding. Lancet 1:1167, 1977
12. Eisenberg MM: Physiologic approach to the surgical management of duodenal ulcer. Curr Prob Surg 14:1, 1977
13. Enquist IF, Karlson KE, Dennis C: Statistically valid ten year comparative evaluation of three methods of management of massive gastroduodenal hemorrhage. Ann Surg 162:550, 1965
14. Freeark RJ, Norcross WJ, Baker RJ: Exploratory gastrotomy in management of massive upper gastrointestinal hemorrhage. Arch Surg 94:684, 1967
15. Graham DY: The value of endoscopy in the management of acute gastrointestinal bleeding: a prospective controlled randomized study. Gastroenterology 74:1125, 1978

16. Hallenbeck GA: Elective surgery for treatment of hemorrhage from duodenal ulcer. Gastroenterology 59:784, 1970
17. Hellers G, Ihre T: Impact of change to early diagnosis and surgery in major upper gastrointestinal bleeding. Lancet 2:1250, 1975
18. Himal HS, Perrault C, Mzabi R: Upper gastrointestinal hemorrhage: aggressive management decreases the mortality. Surgery 84:448, 1978
19. Kelly HG, Grant GN, Elliot DW: Massive gastroduodenal hemorrhage. Arch Surg 87:6, 1963
20. Kessel N: Reassurance. Lancet 1:1128, 1979
21. Kim V, Rudick J, Aufses AH Jr: Surgical management of acute upper gastrointestinal bleeding. Arch Surg 113:1444, 1978
22. Lindkaer-Jensen S, Nielsen OV, Pagel V, et al: Acute hemorrhagic gastritis-diagnosis and treatment. Acta Chir Scand 142:246, 1976
23. Lucas CE, Sugawa C: Diagnostic endoscopy during laparotomy for acute hemorrhage from the upper part of the gastrointestinal tract. Surg Gynecol Obstet 286:285, 1972
24. McGregor DB, Savage LE, McVay CB: Massive gastrointestinal hemorrhage: a twenty-five year experience with vagotomy and drainage. Surgery 80:530, 1976
25. Michels NA: Blood supply and anatomy of the upper abdominal organs. Philadelphia, J.B. Lippincott, 1955
26. Morris DW, Levine GM, Soloway RD, et al: A prospective randomized study of diagnosis and outcome in acute upper gastrointestinal bleeding: endoscopy versus conventional radiography. Am J Dig Dis 20:1103, 1975
27. Nyhus LM, Donahue PE, Krystosek RJ, et al: Complete vagotomy, the evolution of an effective technique. Arch Surg (in press)
28. Palmer ED: The vigorous diagnostic approach to upper gastrointestinal hemorrhage. JAMA 207:1477, 1969
29. Pauchet V: Practical Surgery Illustrated, Vol 5. London, Ernest Benn LTD, 1925, p 85
30. Pauchet V: La Pratique Chirurgicale Illustrée (fasc VII). Paris, Gaston Doin & C, 1927, p 145
31. Postlethwait RW: Retrospective study of operations for peptic ulcer. Surg Gynecol Obstet 149:703, 1979
32. Read RC, Huebl HC, Thal AP: Randomized study of massive bleeding from peptic ulceration. Ann Surg 162:561, 1965
33. Richardson JD, Aust JB: Gastric devascularization: a useful salvage procedure for massive hemorrhagic gastritis. Ann Surg 185:649, 1977
34. Sandlow LJ, Becker GH, Spellberg MA, et al: A prospective randomized study of the management of upper gastrointestinal hemorrhage. Am J Gastroenterol 61:282, 1974
35. Snyder EN, Stellar CA: Results from emergency surgery for massively bleeding duodenal ulcer. Am J Surg 116:170, 1968
36. Stewart JD, Schaer SM, Potter WH, et al: Management of massively bleeding peptic ulcer. Ann Surg 128:791, 1948
37. Tanner NC: Non-malignant affections of the upper stomach. Ann Roy Coll Surg Eng 10:45, 1952

38. Thorne FL, Nyhus LM: Treatment of massive upper gastrointestinal hemorrhage. Am Surg 31:413, 1965
39. Vogel TT: Critical issues in gastroduodenal hemorrhage: the role of vagotomy and pyloroplasty. Ann Surg 176:144, 1972
40. Waldram R, Davis M, Nunnerly H, et al: Emergency endoscopy after gastrointestinal hemorrhage in 50 patients with portal hypertension. Br Med J 4:94, 1974
41. Yajko RD, Norton LW, Eiseman B: Current management of upper gastrointestinal bleeding. Ann Surg 181:474, 1975

Terence Kennedy, M.S. (Lond),
F.R.C.S. England, F.R.C.S.I.

Rebleeding After Surgery for Bleeding Ulcers

ABSTRACT

Rebleeding after surgery for bleeding ulcers is rare when the primary operation has been properly conducted and special attention has been paid to the meticulous technique of suturing of the bleeding ulcer. The causes for recurrent bleeding include reactionary or secondary hemorrhage, incorrect diagnosis, and multiple bleeding sites. The appearance of new ulcers, and the development of a bleeding diathesis, are rare causes of rebleeding. The identification of the primary source of bleeding may be difficult and requires particular care. Preoperative endoscopic diagnosis is very useful but in cases of doubt palpation by the surgeon's finger may prove surprisingly accurate.

When hemorrhage recurs within hours or days of an emergency operation for bleeding ulcer, it is a disappointment to the surgeon and more importantly a potent cause of death. Rebleeding months or years later usually indicates recurrent ulceration at the same site or elsewhere; it is in fact no more than a restatement of the original problem and will not be considered in this chapter. The principal causes will now be discussed, not necessarily in their order of importance or frequency.

REACTIONARY AND SECONDARY HEMORRHAGE

After any gastric operation there is some risk of bleeding from suture lines. Because of the great vascularity of the stomach this risk is much higher than

---

Terence Kennedy, M.S. (Lond), F.R.C.S. England, F.R.C.S.I.: Consultant Surgeon, Royal Victoria Hospital, Belfast, Honorary Lecturer in Gastrointestinal Surgery, The Queens University, Belfast, Northern Ireland.

with anastomoses elsewhere in the gastrointestinal tract. Minor bleeding, discovered only by aspiration of small amounts of blood from a nasogastric tube, is quite common after any gastric operation. All that is generally required is careful observation until the bleeding stops, usually within an hour or two. More persistent bleeding may require transfusion, but it is very seldom sufficiently severe to cause alarm. It is difficult to assess the precise incidence of suture line hemorrhage but reoperation is probably required less than 1% of the time in operations performed by an experienced surgeon.

Attempts have been made to control bleeding of this kind by lavage with iced saline or instillation of dilute solutions of adrenalin (epinephrine). There is no good evidence that these maneuvers are of any benefit.

Accurate differential diagnosis of suture line bleeds during the first few hours is virtually impossible. Endoscopy is probably contraindicated because of the fear that inflation might damage a suture line. It is perhaps not very important since the decision to reoperate depends upon the quantity and rate of blood loss. At reoperation the suture lines should be opened up and resutured.

True secondary hemorrhage seven or more days after operation may occur as the result of sepsis. A small leak from an anastomosis may lead to the formation of a perigastric abscess. If this is in the vicinity of a major vessel, perhaps the stump of the left gastric artery after a gastrectomy, an infective arteritis is caused and this may lead to severe hemorrhage. This form of bleeding is probably very rare; I have seen it only once.

INCORRECT DIAGNOSIS

At the primary operation for bleeding, it is not always easy to determine the source of hemorrhage precisely. One often encounters, for example, a patient with an obvious chronic duodenal ulcer and a small relatively acute gastric ulcer which is easily overlooked. The latter may be the source of bleeding yet the surgeon may suture the duodenal ulcer neglecting the gastric ulcer.

This error is quite common, perhaps more so since it has become popular to treat bleeding ulcers by suture and vagotomy rather than gastrectomy. If such a patient requires reoperation a very careful search of the whole stomach and duodenum must be made. When searching for a bleeding point in the stomach, if preoperative endoscopy has not localized the lesion, there are various options open to the surgeon. The stomach may be widely opened and the mucosa inspected directly, but in the fundus rugosity may conceal the lesion. Alternatively a proctoscope or cytoscope may be inserted and the mucosa inspected after suitable inflation. Perhaps the most effective technique is to palpate the mucosa through a small gastrotomy. When there is a small acute ulcer it is often possible to feel the bleeding point, a small projecting vessel, which feels like a tiny grease nipple. In my experience palpation is a very accurate and useful method of locating a bleeding point within the stomach.

MULTIPLE BLEEDING SITES

Gastric ulcers induced by drugs like phenylbutazone and salicylates are often multiple. In these cases it is easy to suture one bleeding ulcer and overlook another which continues to bleed. In acute erosive gastritis there may be many bleeding points scattered throughout the stomach. Generally, it is possible to avoid emergency operation, but where it is essential the surgeon faces a difficult problem. The only certain way of preventing further bleeding is by total gastrectomy. Subtotal gastrectomy has been advocated and a less radical alternative is vagotomy with suture of individual bleeding points. There is considerable dispute about the relative merits of these alternatives. Vagotomy, gastrotomy and suture of bleeding points is strongly favored by Donahue and Nyhus [2]. It is a simpler procedure with less primary mortality than total or near total gastrectomy but there is a very real risk of further bleeding which inevitably is associated with a very high mortality. Menguy [6] takes the opposite view and advocates near-total gastrectomy, suggesting that when the risk of rebleeding is high the extent of gastric resection should be nearer to total. When erosive gastritis or stress ulceration is associated with rebleeding after operation, the situation is indeed grave. Where anything less than total gastrectomy has been performed the rebleeding rate is high. Kirtley and his colleagues from Nashville [5] reported rebleeding in 4 patients after vagotomy and suture of bleeding points. Two of these had multiple acute bleeding ulcers and were treated by subtotal gastrectomy. One bled again and died.

My own view is that operation should be avoided if at all possible in these cases. When it is essential, I favor gastrotomy and suture of bleeding points with associated vagotomy and drainage. Should there be further severe bleeding it is probably advisable to proceed to total gastrectomy, the high risk notwithstanding.

Gastric hypothermia has been used for erosive gastritis with some success [4] but the technique is not simple. It seems likely that control by endoscopic diathermy or laser may well become the treatment of choice in the future.

It is to be hoped that the need to operate in these very difficult cases will be diminished or even abolished by the routine use of cimetidine or other H_2-receptor blockers in stress situations. In many centers stress ulceration has already become much less common following the routine use of alkalis after burns and major trauma.

NEW ULCERS

In the Zollinger-Ellison syndrome new stomal ulcers may form within a few days of operation, and these ulcers have a marked tendency to bleed.

Hypergastrinaemia is, however, a rare condition and careful exploration of the pancreas at the primary operation with increasing use of routine gastrin assays make it less likely that gastrinomas will be missed. More of these interesting lesions are now diagnosed before the first surgical intervention. This is probably the most important cause of rebleeding.

INADEQUATE PRIMARY OPERATION

Where bleeding is due to an established chronic ulcer there is disagreement whether suture of the ulcer with vagotomy and drainage is as effective as partial gastrectomy. When dealing with a bleeding gastric ulcer, Billroth I partial gastrectomy with complete removal of the ulcer is the operation of choice. If the ulcer is large and deep, eroding the pancreas, it is not unusual for the left gastric or splenic artery to be breached. Complete excision here is obviously impossible but the bleeding vessel can be sutured and excluded from the gastrointestinal lumen. Gastrotomy and suture of a gastric ulcer with vagotomy and drainage or with proximal gastric vagotomy without drainage has been widely advocated. There are two disadvantages: first, the possibility that suture will not control the bleeding completely and second the risk that the ulcer may be malignant. This risk demands that the ulcer must be completely excised and the operation may then be completed by vagotomy and drainage. Although gastric cancer is not a common cause of severe acute bleeding, peptic ulceration of a malignant mucosa may cause difficulty in diagnosis. These patients tend to bleed profusely but have a good prognosis after resection.

When bleeding is due to a chronic duodenal ulcer it is virtually always a deep posterior wall ulcer which has eroded the gastroduodenal artery. There is no other vessel near the duodenal wall sufficiently large to cause bleeding extensive enough to require emergency operation.

For bleeding duodenal ulcer the operation of choice used to be, and in many clinics still is, a Billroth II gastrectomy with occlusion of the duodenal stump. This was thought to give better control of the bleeding point and a lower incidence of re-bleeding than the lesser procedure of combined vagotomy, pyloroplasty and suture of the ulcer. Conversely it has been argued that the bigger operation, gastrectomy, is more dangerous and will carry a higher mortality. There is no controlled trial to answer this dispute but published evidence favours the lesser procedure, vagotomy and suture. Alexander-Williams [1] reviewed the literature and found a mortality of 15% after gastrectomy compared with 8% after vagotomy and pyloroplasty. The incidence of rebleeding after the two operations was precisely the same, 13.5%. This may seem surprising but it must be remembered that simple closure of the duodenum proximal to an ulcer does not immediately control the gastroduodenal artery. If the duodenal wall is rolled up and turned into the crater as a tampon "en escargot" as described by Gordon-Taylor [3], bleeding may be well controlled. With simple closure bleeding may persist even though the food and acid stream is diverted. I have seen bleeding recur from a duodenal ulcer as late as three weeks after a Billroth II operation when one would have expected the original ulcer to have healed completely.

The key to the prevention of recurrent bleeding is the proper suturing of the bleeding vessel whether the operation is completed as a gastrectomy or a vagotomy and pyloroplasty. Two terms are commonly used — oversewing the ulcer and underrunning the bleeding point — and herein lies the difficulty. If the ulcer is oversewn (Fig. 1A) sutures are simply passed through the edges of the ulcer drawing them together. The mucosal edges thus cover the ulcer and the bleeding point and to a certain extent they may have a tamponade effect. This however is not adequate to control massive bleeding from the gastroduodenal artery, particularly in an elderly or hypertensive patient.

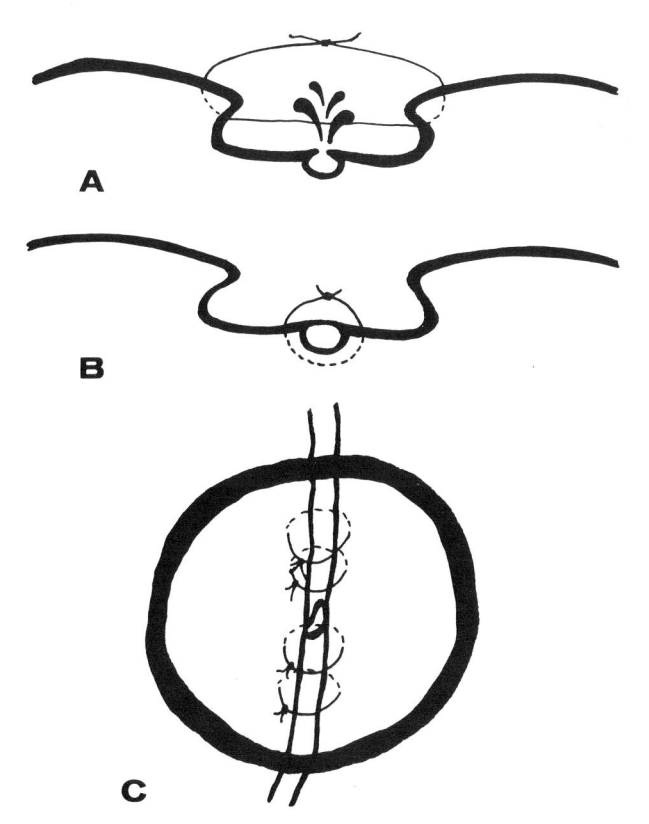

Fig. 1. (A) Oversewing; (B) underrunning; (C) sutures placed above and below the bleeding point.

The term underrunning is explicit (Fig. 1B). Here nonabsorbable sutures are passed through the fibrous tissue at the base of the ulcer and around the bleeding vessel. It is good practice to place two sutures around the vessel above the bleeding point and also two sutures below it (Fig. 1C). Often, at the time of operation, the bleeding point is temporarily occluded by clot. After suture of the vessel the surgeon should brush the ulcer base briskly with a gauze pledget to remove this clot; if bleeding follows it is obvious that the suturing is inadequate. After underrunning, oversewing is probably worthwhile as it may expedite ulcer healing.

There are two objections to the described technique. First, the use of nonabsorbable sutures could theoretically cause further ulceration, but this risk is very small. I use linen and oversew, and have never seen this complication. Secondly there is a fear that the common bile duct may be caught up in the suture and occluded. The bile duct in fact runs vertically some 1.5-2.0 cm to the right of the gastroduodenal artery. It is only with a very large bite that the common duct is at risk. I have never seen it occluded. It is vital to remember that the surgeon's objective is to save life by stopping the bleeding. Should obstructive jaundice follow it can be treated later.

When bleeding does recur, if the operation has been properly done, it may well come from another site. Yajko and his colleagues [7] experienced rebleeding in 14 of 130 patients treated surgically. Of these, 8 required further operation and in 7 a new bleeding source was found. Many authors have reported a high mortality when bleeding persists or recurs. When a second operation is required gastrectomy is probably advisable, provided that suture line bleeding has been excluded. Before deciding just how much stomach is to be resected it is advisable to inspect the fundal mucosa carefully, by endoscopy and gastrotomy, to exclude erosions or acute ulcers in the area to be retained.

BLEEDING DIATHESIS

Occasionally, after any form of gastric surgery postoperative bleeding occurs as a result of a coagulopathy. This risk is particularly high in patients where operation has been delayed until they have had many liters of blood transfused in the course of a few days. After massive hemorrhage and transfusion there will be a deficiency of functioning platelets and other clotting factors. Transfusion of fresh blood is indicated and often this is all that is required. If, however, bleeding continues after fresh blood transfusion, the problem may be more complex with other deficiencies, perhaps fibrinolysis or diffuse intravascular coagulation. Patients with associated liver disease are particularly liable to have severe clotting factor deficiencies. It is probably wise to seek the advice of an expert hematologist before giving Tranexamic acid or other drugs.

CONCLUSION

Rebleeding is rare when the primary operation has been properly conducted and special attention has been paid to the meticulous technique of suturing of a bleeding ulcer. The identification of the precise source of bleeding may be difficult and requires particular care. Preoperative endoscopy is very useful but in cases of doubt palpation of the mucosa by the surgeon's finger may prove surprisingly accurate.

With erosive gastritis there may be very real problems, but in general these patients should be treated medically. We do not yet know the precise value of cimetidine in these cases, though we may hope for considerable benefit.

REFERENCES

1. Alexander-Williams J: Emergency surgery: bleeding and perforation. In Williams JA, Cox AG (eds): After Vagotomy, London, Butterworth, p 337, 1969
2. Donahue PE, Nyhus LM: Massive upper gastrointestinal hemorrhage. In Nyhus LM, Wastell C (eds): Surgery of Stomach and Duodenum, 3rd Ed. Boston, Little Brown, 1977
3. Gordon-Taylor G: The problem of bleeding peptic ulcer. Br J Surg 33:336, 1946
4. Himal HS, Watson WW, Jones CW, et al: The management of bleeding acute gastric erosions; the role of gastric hypothermia. Br J Surg 62:221, 1975
5. Kirtley JA, Scott HW, Sawyers JL. The surgical management of stress ulcers. Ann Surg 169:801, 1969
6. Menguy R: Surgery of peptic ulcer. Philadelphia, Saunders, p 277
7. Yajko RD, Norton LW, Eiseman B: Current management of upper gastrointestinal bleeding. Ann Surg 181:474, 1975

W. P. Ritchie, Jr., M.D., Ph.D

Pathophysiology of Erosive Gastritis and Stress Ulceration

ABSTRACT

Acute erosive gastritis is probably the commonest cause of massive upper gastrointestinal hemorrhage. Bleeding from this source is most often related to salicylate or ethanol abuse, less frequently to acute posttraumatic hemorrhagic gastritis (stess ulcer). The pathogenetic common denominator appears to be an impairment of the so called gastric mucosal barrier, the ability of mammalian mucosa to maintain a high intraluminal pH gradient, which results in excessive back diffusion of acid into the mucosa itself. It is likely that both salicylates and ethanol produce damage by direct contact toxicity. The pathophysiology of stress ulcer is more complex and may involve the concomitant presence of secreted acid, reflux of upper intestinal content (of the bile acids, in particular), and concomitant gastric mucosal ischemia, in combination. The evidence to support this contention is persuasive, and includes the fact that, experimentally, increasing mucosal blood flow and neutralizing bile acids both protect the gastric mucosa from acute lesion formation. A consistent theme in all experimental models is that ulcerogenesis does not occur in the absence of intraluminal acid, a finding of significant clinical importance. Whether or not acute mucosal damage ensues may depend ultimately on whether or not the interstitial mucosal pH falls to levels inconsistent with cell survival. Recent research initiatives indicate that both H_2 receptor blocking agents and the prostaglandins may have real therapeutic potential when given prophylactically, although their precise mechanisms of action are unclear.

'As indicated elsewhere in this volume, the endoscope has become an indispensable tool in the evaluation of the patient with massive upper-gastrointestinal hemorrhage. An important consequence of its widespread employment

---

W. P. Ritchie, Jr., M.D., Ph.D.: Professor of Surgery, University of Virginia School of Medicine, Charlottesville, Virginia.
Established Investigator, American Heart Association, 1974-1979; supported by Contracts DAMD 17-74-C4014 and AM17591.

has been the realization that superficial erosive disease of the gastric mucosa may be responsible for as many as 30-40% of all bleeding episodes originating proximal to the ligament of Treitz [21]. Clinically, the vast majority of these are the result of the excessive use of either salicylate-containing compounds or of alcohol. While bleeding on this basis is usually easily managed, the sheer magnitude of the problem demands respect and attention. A much smaller fraction develops following profound and prolonged physiologic stress. Although a relatively infrequent occurrence, the difficulties encountered in arresting bleeding from this source and the considerable mortality associated with it justify the many research initiatives undertaken to elucidate its pathophysiology.

The present paper attempts to provide an overview of our current understanding of the pathophysiology of both the drug-related and the stress-related acute hemorrhagic gastropathies. In many respects, attempts to distinguish between the two on a pathogenetic basis are artificial. Nevertheless, their clinical behavior is sufficiently different to warrant making distinctions, whenever applicable. Where pathophysiologic features appear to be shared, appropriate notation will be made. The ensuing discussion will focus primarily on stress ulcer disease because it poses a much greater threat to patient survival.

MAGNITUDE OF THE CLINICAL PROBLEM

As indicated, superficial erosive disease of the gastric mucosa is most commonly associated with salicylate and ethanol abuse. Because our citizenry expends in excess of $30 billion on alcoholic beverages and consumes 12,000 tons of salicylate annually, the magnitude of the clinical problem is great [1, 27]. Although the numbers of patients with clinically significant hemorrhage from stess ulcer disease is much smaller, certain populations are predictably at risk: those hospitalized in intensive care units (5% may bleed from this source), those sustaining severe trauma (30%), and those with greater than 35% body burns (50%) [10, 29, 48]. Specific risk factors are detailed elsewhere. Despite scanty documentation, a strong impression exists that the incidence of stress ulcer has declined dramatically over the past several years. The factors responsible most likely relate to a combination of several developments: improved methods of ventilatory support for the severely traumatized or septic individual, a greater appreciation of the importance of maintaining adequate nutrition in the critically ill, and an enhanced appreciation of the possibility that stress ulcer can develop in susceptible patients, prompting greater vigilance with respect to methods of prophylaxis.

Both drug induced erosions and stress ulcers share certain unique clinical features which serve to distinguish them from other variants of the acid-peptic diathesis. The lesions responsible are invariably multiple in number; they are acute in onset; the mucosal disease is limited, in large part, to the proximal acid-peptic secreting area of the stomach; and, there is no evidence of hypersecretion of gastric acid in those patients who bleed. These distinctive features provide clues to the pathogenesis of the lesions under consideration.

CONCEPT OF THE GASTRIC MUCOSAL BARRIER

The mammalian parietal cell elaborates hydrochloric acid in concentrations which approach 160 mM at the cannulicular level. Pure parietal secretion is modified only slightly as it traverses the gastric pit. Thus, the concentration of hydrogen ion (H^+) in gastric content is still enormous relative to the gastric mucosa and blood. Yet, under ordinary circumstances, passive diffusion of H^+ in the direction of this large concentration gradient is minimal. This capacity of the gastric mucosa to maintain a high intraluminal pH gradient has been termed the gastric mucosal barrier [49]. Under certain circumstances, a variety of agents, when applied topically, damage this barrier by increasing the physical permeability of the mucosa. Not surprisingly, these agents include salicylic acid, acetylsalicylic acid, gall bladder bile, and the bile acids [11].

The precise anatomic locus of the barrier remains unclear. It was formerly thought that the tight junctions (desmosomes) which exist between adjacent surface epithelial cells were responsible for the relative impermeability of the gastric mucosa to cations. However, it is unlikely that this is the case since many compounds damage the barrier without disrupting these anatomic structures [13]. Current evidence suggests that the surface epithelial cells themselves may be the key factors responsible for the restricted permeability of undiseased gastric mucosa [19]. In the absence of an agreed-upon morphologic description, a definition of the "barrier" has evolved which is based on the consequences of damage to it. These include (1) increased luminal loss (back diffusion) of H^+; (2) increased luminal appearance of sodium ion (Na^+) and pepsin; (3) increased bidirectional movement of probing molecules, indicative of a physical increase in the permeability of the gastric mucosa [2]; (4) increased electrical conductance of the mucosa [14]; (5) alterations in gastric mucosal nutrient blood flow; and (6) liberation of histamine into gastric juice and into gastric venous effluent [22].

Although the exact pathophysiologic mechanism by which damage to the barrier results in injury to individual mucosal cells is unclear, the uniform electronmicrographic demonstration of striking intracellular edema indicates that disturbances of normal osmotic and pH equilibria may be involved. Martin [32] has suggested that, following the topical application of weakly acidic drugs (e.g., the salicylates and the bile acids) to the gastric mucosa, appreciable quantities of the drug anion accumulate intracellularly because, while applied as a salt, the acid becomes protonated and therefore lipid soluble in the relatively acid environment of the stomach. Once within the alkaline environment of the cell, however, the acid redissociates to an extent dictated by its pKa. Only the undissociated faction of the acid is available for removal from the cell by nonionic diffusion. For weak acids, with a pKa close to the normal intracellular pH, only small quantities of anion and H^+ accumulate intracellularly because relatively large amounts of the drug are undissociated and therefore removable. For stronger acids, the rate of anion and H^+ accumulation is greater since only a small fraction of the acid exists in undissociated form. Under these circumstances, progressive accumulation of anion might disturb the normal extracellular:intracellular osmotic equilibrium. Intraluminal acid could compound the injury by secondarily diffusing into the cell. If sufficient H^+ accumulates to overwhelm intracellular buffer systems, acid hydrolysis of intracellular protein would occur, aggravating the already existing osmotic imbalance. In addition, intracellular acidosis might also severely interfere with cell metabolism. If the insult is sufficiently severe or prolonged, cell lysis and death would eventuate.

A HYPOTHESIS CONCERNING STRESS ULCER

The Hypothesis

Considerable current interest centers on the hypothesis that the combination of intraluminal acid, reflux of upper intestinal content(of the bile acids in particular), and concomitant gastric mucosal ischemia is responsible for acute ulcerogenesis in the "stressed" patient. Guilbert et al [17] reported that dogs subjected to several hours of hemorrhagic shock developed typical erosive lesions in the proximal stomach following resuscitation, a circumstance which could be prevented if the pylorus was occluded during the period of hypotension. Hamza and DenBesten [18] demonstrated acute ulcerogenesis in shocked pylorus-occluded dogs when the intact stomach was exposed to endogenous acid and a 15 mM concentration of bile acids. Similarly, Mercereau and Hinchey [35] produced acute mucosal damage in ex vivo chambered rat mucosa using a combination of topically applied acid, a short period of shock, and a topical solution of crude bovine bile acids.

Our own laboratory has examined the hypothesis in dogs using chambered vascularized ex vivo wedges of proximal gastric wall [39, 41]. Mucosal ischemia was induced by infusing low doses of vasopressin directly into the blood supply of the wedge. It was found that extensive acute superficial mucosal necrosis with massive underlying interstitial hemorrhage occurred only in the simultaneous presence of topical acid, topical bile acid, and mucosal ischemia. None of these factors alone or in combination with only one other was capable of producing significant mucosal injury. Thus, lesion formation was not a function of bile acid induced excessive back diffusion of H^+ or of gastric mucosal ischemia, per se. Of considerable interest was the observation, subsequently confirmed by others, that blood flow increased significantly to nonischemic mucosa upon exposure to topical bile acids at low pH. Both acetylsalicylic acid and ethanol have been reported to induce comparable responses when applied to unmodified canine gastric mucosa [7]. This phenomenon probably represents an important compensatory mechanism by which the mucosa attempts to countervail the acute fall in interstitial pH which occurs during excessive H^+ back diffusion. When this mechanism is blunted, as in the model described, acute ulceration is the result.

Testing the Hypothesis

If this hypothesis is valid, it must be susceptible to testing using Koch's postulates; that is, if lesion formation is a function of excessive back diffusion of H^+ and concomitant gastric mucosal ischemia in combination, then vitiating either of these factors ought to ameliorate the severity of ulcer formation. In addition, to test the hypothesis in this manner, we studied three groups of animals. A control group was exposed to topical acid, topical bile acid, and mucosal ischemia. Both experimental groups were similarly treated except that, in one, wedge specific isoproterenol was infused and, in the other, the bile acid binding resin, cholestyramine, was applied topically. It was found that, despite H^+ back diffusion comparable to the control group, intraarterial isoproterenol significantly protected against lesion formation by increasing mucosal blood flow. Further, despite a reduction in mucosal blood flow comparable to the control group, topical cholestyramine significantly protected against lesion formation by preventing excessive back diffusion of H^+. Others have reported similar observations in different models [36, 50].

Factors Influencing Severity of Lesion Formation

A major difficulty in translating the hypothesis to the clinical situation is that many experimental studies have utilized concentrations of bile acids which are clearly inappropriate (10-40 mM). Black et al [3] studied bile acid reflux in patients with type I benign gastric ulcer, a disease in which pyloric incompetence has been convincingly demonstrated. Mean intragastric bile acid concentration in the fasting state was only 0.7 ± 0.2 mM. In a similar patient population, Rhodes et al [38] demonstrated a fasting intragastric bile acid concentration of 1.0 ± 0.5 mM. Our own laboratory has demonstrated comparable levels (mean concentration 1.9 ± 0.2 mM) in the intragastric content of postoperative patients. Using the model described, a study was designed to assess the ulcerogenic potential of differing bile acid concentrations over a range one might expect to encounter clinically (1-5 mM) [43]. The concentration of H^+ in contact with the mucosa was held constant. It was found that, in nonischemic mucosa, bile acids produce no ulcers, a significant concentration dependent increase in H^+ back diffusion, and a nonconcentration dependent increase in mucosal blood flow. In ischemic mucosa, in the face of a constant reduction in mucosal blood flow, lesions were produced at all concentrations of bile acids employed, the severity of which was bile acid concentration dependent. These data indicate that acute mucosal damage can occur in the presence of physiological bile acid concentrations, i.e., those routinely found in the gastric content of postoperative patients.

A second factor modulating the severity of lesion formation is the concentration of H^+ in contact with the mucosa. In a recent communication [40] we reported that, in nonischemic mucosa exposed to a constant concentration of bile acid, back diffusion of H^+ increased as a linear function of the concentration of H^+ in contact with the mucosa. No lesions were observed as mucosal blood flow also increased. Under the same circumstances in ischemic mucosa, H^+ back diffusion also increased with increasing concentration of intraluminal H^+ but, because no concomitant increase in mucosal blood flow was observed, acute mucosal damage was produced. Lesion severity was directly related to the concentration of H^+ in contact with the mucosa because this factor alone determined the degree of back diffusion induced. These findings may be applicable to the clinical setting, as suggested by recent reports demonstrating the efficacy of both prophylactic antacids and cimetidine in preventing stress ulcer disease [20, 30, 33].

Towards an Explanation

Any unifying concept which attempts to explain these seemingly disparate observations must account for the facts that lesion formation is absent in the absence of intraluminal acid, and that the severity of lesion formation is a linear function of the absolute magnitude of H^+ back diffusion, however it is produced. One thesis which has received considerable current scrutiny is that the acute ulcerogenesis which results under these circumstances is a consequence of inadequate tissue buffering of back diffused H^+, i.e., mucosal acidosis. The recent development of techniques designed to determine intramucosal pH directly has permitted a direct assessment of this possibility. Kivilaakso et al [25] have demonstrated a significant linear relationship between net H^+ flux and intramucosal pH in rabbit fundic mucosa exposed to intraluminal acid during hemorrhagic shock. With increasing back diffusion of H^+, the intramucosal pH fell to levels far below those found in systemic arterial blood and, concomitantly, severe mucosal damage was apparent. Conversely, under the same conditions, the pH of fundic mucosa exposed to intraluminal buffer fell to a much lesser extent, approximating the decrease in systemic arterial pH observed. Minimal mucosal damage was encountered. In the dog, fundic intramucosal pH was found to decline only slightly during shock in the presence of intraluminal buffer, decreased to a greater extent when challenged with a high intraluminal H^+ concentration, and was profoundly depressed when 10 mM bile acid was added to the acidic bathing solution. Only in this last circumstance was severe and extensive ulceration noted.

A recent study from our own laboratory complements these observations by demonstrating a strong association between bile acid-ischemia induced lesion formation and gastric venous acidosis, as manifested by low gastric venous pH, a decrease in gastric venous bicarbonate concentration, and an increase in gastric venous base deficit [42]. These alterations were highly significant when compared to gastric venous blood from appropriate controls, simultaneous derangements in all three parameters occurring only in those animals with severe mucosal damage. Since gastric venous acidosis was absent in the absence of an imposed topical acid load, it seems likely that back diffused H^+ was ultimately responsible. Data also exist to indicate that the relationship of mucosal acidosis to ulcerogenesis is one of cause and effect. The most direct evidence in this regard is contained in the recent report of Cheung and Porterfield [8] who showed that the systemic administration of alkali in large amounts vitiated the acute mucosal damage induced by topical acid and bile acid during shock. Taken together, these data indicate strongly that the acute gastric mucosal damage associated with excessive back diffusion of H^+ is indeed a consequence of uncompensated tissue acidosis.

Clinical Applicability of the Model

Despite the fact that, grossly and microscopically, the lesions produced in the model outlined bear a close resemblance to those observed in humans following severe trauma, the relevance of the model to the human circumstance cannot be stated with certainty. Evidence does exist to suggest that some degree of gastric mucosal ischemia is present in patients who develop stress ulcer: the gastroscopic evolution of the earliest detectable clinical lesions is compatible with an ischemic origin and sustained hypotension is a frequent antecedent event in patients who hemorrhage [58]. On the other hand, whether or not an inverse relationship exists between the ability of the human stomach to maintain a pH gradient and the development of stress ulcer is unclear. Skillman et al [48] noted that, when compared to healthy controls, 50% of critically ill patients demonstrated significantly greater than normal rates of back diffusion of an instilled H^+ load from the intact stomach. Conversely, McAlhany et al [34] using the flux of lithium to assess the barrier, were unable to demonstrate an association between lesion formation and increased mucosal permeability to this particular cation. In assessing these data, it must be recalled that the validity of the lithium technique has been questioned [46] and that the absolute magnitude of H^+ back diffusion is not as important a factor in experimental stress ulcer disease as is the capacity of the mucosa to dispose of it.

The final hypothetical factor involved is reflux of upper intestinal content. Although no direct assessment of this factor has been made in man, Kivilaakso et al [25] have shown experimentally that reflux precedes acute lesion formation in the intact stomach of animals subjected to hemorrhagic shock. As indicated, we have demonstrated that acute mucosal damage can occur in the presence of bile acid concentrations which are routinely found in the gastric content of postoperative patients. Finally, recent clinical reports, more in the nature of testimony than of evidence, suggest that reflux may be more common in intensive care unit patients than in appropriate controls, and that cholestyramine may have some benefit as prophylaxis against hemorrhage in these individuals [47].

RECENT EXPERIMENTAL DEVELOPMENTS

When administered prophylactically, H_2-receptor blocking agents have been shown to protect certain categories of susceptible patients from developing stress ulcer disease [20, 30, 33]. It is not surprising, therefore, that this class of agents, both alone in combination with H_1-receptor blockers, has been subjected to considerable scrutiny in an effort to demonstrate whether or not they possess a cytoprotective capacity. Cytoprotection refers to the ability of an agent to protect mucosal cells from morphologic or physiologic injury, independent of its antisecretory properties.

In support of the view that H_2 receptor blockers may be cytoprotective are the reports of Kauffman and Grossman [23] who demonstrated a reduction in lesion formation in rat antra exposed to topical acid and intravenous acetylsalicylic acid following pretreatment with intravenous cimetidine, and of Shirazi et al [45] who noted that a large dose of topical metiamide afforded protection to the intact stomach of the shocked dog exposed to topical acid and bile acid. In contrast, Carmichael [4] et al were unable to demonstrate significant cytoprotection in the intact stomach of the rat pretreated with topical metiamide and exposed to topical acid and topical acetylsalicylic acid.

The effects of H_2-receptor blockade on mucosal blood flow have also been assessed. Again no consensus is apparent. Delaney et al [12] found no significant alterations in microsphere measured flow in the intact resting stomach of the dog pretreated with antisecretory doses of cimetidine. On the other hand, Levine et al [26] reported that, when cimetidine was administered to bled piglets, fundic and antral mucosal blood flow were maintained at near normal — i.e., non-shock — levels. These latter observations are difficult to interpret in view of the known vasodilator properties of histamine in general and in view of the documented vasoconstriction observed during simultaneous H_1 and H_2-receptor blockade in the splanchnic circulation of the dog.

An alternative approach has been to examine the effects of the H_2-receptor blockers on the "gastric mucosal barrier" per se, independent of their capacity to influence blood flow or ulcer formation. The evidence clearly indicates that pretreatment with antisecretory doses of the H_2 antagonists alone does not alter the permeability characteristics of the gastric mucosa. On the other hand, Rees et al [37] reported that pretreatment with H_2 and H_1-receptor blocking agents together significantly attenuated the alterations in net cation flux observed when canine mucosa was exposed to topical bile acids. However, these observations could not be reproduced in the laboratories of at least two independent investigators. At the present time, I feel that it is unlikely that histamine receptor blocking agents are cytoprotective and that their clinical benefit is entirely related to their antisecretory properties.

A second class of compounds, the prostaglandins, is also undergoing extensive investigation because of their potential as therapeutic agents in all types of acid-peptic disease. The potent antisecretory properties of many of the prostaglandins (A, E, and I) have been amply documented, both in the intact stomach of man, dog, and rat, and, in an indirect fashion, in the isolated parietal cell as well. The precise mechanisms involved are unclear. Prostaglandins have also been shown to possess remarkable antiulcer properties. For example, in the rat, topical pretreatment with prostaglandin E_2 significantly ameliorates the acute gastric mucosal damage observed when acetylsalicylic acid, a potent inhibitor of prostaglandin synthetase, is given either intravenously or topically in the presence of exogenous acid. While studies of the effects of prostaglandins on bile acid-induced acute mucosal damage have been few, their general thrust has been similar [44].

In some models, protection from ulceration is undoubtedly secondary to prostaglandin-induced inhibition of gastric acid production. In others, however, the antiulcer properties of prostaglandins are evident even in the face of an exogenous acid load, are possessed by prostaglandins which do not inhibit acid secretion, and are apparent at doses of other prostaglandins which are totally without antisecretory effect. Thus, they are truly cytoprotective.

The possibility that decreased gastric mucosal permeability is involved in prostaglandin-mediated cytoprotection has received considerable attention. Unfortunately no consensus is apparent at the present time. For example, Cheung et al [6] have shown that topical PG E_2, in antisecretory doses, produces a small net luminal loss of H^+ and a marked net luminal gain of Na^+ in canine mucosa exposed to acid alone. On the other hand, under almost the same circumstances, Kenyon [24] observed no change in net H^+ flux, although a significant increase in net luminal gain of Na^+ was apparent. One possible explanation for these discrepancies, and for the apparent cytoprotection conferred by prostaglandins, is offered by the recent demonstration that prostaglandin E_2 stimulates a marked active secretion of alkali by both fundic and antral amphibian mucosa in-vitro [15]. Such a circumstance might account for the apparent increase in net H^+ loss (neutralization by alkali) was well as the large net Na^+ gain (coupled sodium and alkali flux) noted above.

The influence of prostaglandins on gastric mucosal blood flow has also been studied. While it is clear that the A type prostaglandins, given either intravenously or intraarterially, are potent vasodilators in the canine stomach, no such consensus exists for the E types. It has been reported that prostaglandin

E_2, when given either intravenously or topically, decreased gastric mucosal blood flow in the dog during histamine stimulation [5]. In contrast, an increase in gastric mucosal blood flow has been reported in nonsecreting canine mucosa during the intravenous administration of both E and A type prostaglandins [31].

To summarize: it seems likely that prostaglandins are cytoprotective against a wide variety of agents which damage the barrier, including acetylsalicylic acid and the bile acids. However, the manner in which this effect is produced remains unclear. Specifically, no consensus exists concerning the influence of prostaglandins on gastric mucosal permeability or blood flow in either the resting or secreting state.

REFERENCES

1. Beaver WT, Kantor TG, Levy G: On guard for aspirin's harmful effects. Patient Care 13:48, 1979
2. Birkett D, Silen W: Alteration of the physical pathways through the gastric mucosa by sodium taurocholate. Gastroenterology 67:1131, 1974
3. Black RB, Roberts G, Rhodes J: The effect of healing on bile reflux in gastric ulcer. Gut 12:552, 1971
4. Carmichael HA, Nelson LM, Russell RI: Cimetidine and prostaglandin: evidence for different modes of action on the rat gastric mucosa. Gastroenterology 74:1229, 1978
5. Cheung LY, Lowry SF: Effects of intra-arterial infusion of prostaglandin E_1 on gastric secretion and blood flow. Surgery 83:699, 1978
6. Cheung LY, Lowry SF, Perry J, et al: Topical effects of 16, 16 dimethyl prostaglandin E_2 on gastric acid secretion and mucosal permeability to hydrogen ions in dogs. Gut 19:775, 1978
7. Cheung LY, Moody FG, Reese RS: Effect of aspirin, bile, salt, and ethanol on canine gastric mucosal blood flow. Surgery 77:786, 1975
8. Cheung LY, Porterfield G: Protection of gastric mucosa against acute ulceration by intravenous infusion of sodium bicarbonate. Am J Surg 137:106, 1979
9. Collan Y, Kivilaakso E, Kalima TV, et al: Ultrastructural changes in the gastric mucosa following hemorrhagic shock in pigs. Circ Shock 4:13, 1977
10. Czaja AJ, McAlhany JC, Pruitt BA Jr: Acute gastroduodenal disease after thermal injury. N Engl J Med 291:925, 1974
11. Davenport HW: Destruction of the gastric mucosal barrier by detergents and urea. Gastroenterology 54:175, 1968
12. Delaney JP, Michel HM, Bond J: Cimetidine and gastric blood flow. Surgery 84:190, 1978
13. Eastwood GL, Kirchner JP: Changes in the fine structure of mouse gastric epithelium produced by ethanol and urea. Gastroenterology 67:71, 1974
14. Fromm D, Schwartz JH, Quijano R: Effects of salicylate and bile salt on ion transport by isolated gastric mucosa of the rabbit. Am J Physiol 230:319, 1976

15. Garner A, Heylings JR: Stimulation of alkaline secretion in amphibian-isolated gastric mucosa by 16, 16 dimethyl PGE_2 and $PGF_2\alpha$. Gastroenterology 76:497, 1979
16. Gordon MJ, Skillman JJ, Zervas NT, et al: Divergent nature of gastric mucosal permeability and gastric acid secretion in sick patients with general surgical and neurosurgical disease. Ann Surg 178:285, 1973
17. Guilbert J, Bounous G, Gurd FN: Role of intestinal chyme in the pathogenesis of gastric ulceration following experimental hemorrhagic shock. J Trauma 9:723, 1969
18. Hamza K, DenBesten L: Bile salts producing stress ulcers during experimental shock. Clin Res 19:393, 1971
19. Harding RK, Morris GP: Cell loss from normal and stressed gastric mucosae of the rat. Gastroenterology 72:857, 1977
20. Hastings PR, Skillman JJ, Bushnell LS, et al: Antacid titration in the prevention of acute gastrointestinal bleeding. N Engl J Med 298:1041, 1978
21. Himal HS, Watson WW, Jones CW, et al: The management of upper gastrointestinal hemorrhage. Ann Surg 179:489, 1974
22. Johnson LR, Overholt BF: Release of histamine in the gastric venous blood following injury by acetic or salicylic acid. Gastroenterology 52:505, 1967
23. Kauffman GL Jr, Grossman MI: Prostaglandin and cimetidine inhibit the formation of ulcers produced by parenteral salicylates. Gastroenterology 75:1099, 1978
24. Kenyon GS, Ansell IF, Carter DC: Methylated analogues of prostaglandin E_2 and the gastric mucosal barrier. Prostaglandins 15:779, 1978
25. Kivilaakso E, Fromm D, Silen W: Relationship between ulceration and intramural pH of gastric mucosa during hemorrhagic shock. Surgery 84:70, 1978
26. Levine B, Schwesinger W, Sirinek K, et al: Cimetidine prevents reduction in gastric mucosal blood flow during shock. Surgery 84:113, 1978
27. The Liquor Handbook. New York, Gavis-Jobson Associates, 1976
28. Lucas CE, Sugawa C, Friend W, et al: Therapeutic implications of disturbed gastric physiology in patients with stress ulceration. Am J Surg 123:25, 1972
29. Lucas CE, Sugawa C, Riddle J, et al: Natural history and surgical dilemma of "stress" gastric bleeding. Arch Surg 102:266, 1971
30. MacDougall BRD, Bailey RJ, Williams R: H_2 receptor antagonists and antacids in the prevention of acute gastrointestinal hemorrhage in fulminant hepatic failure. Lancet 1:617, 1977
31. Main IHM, Whittle BJR: The effects of E and A prostaglandins on gastric mucosal blood flow and acid secretion in the rat. Br J Pharmacol 49:428, 1973
32. Martin BK: Accumulation of drug anions in gastric mucosal cells. Nature 198:896, 1963
33. McAlhany JC, Czaja AJ, Pruitt BA Jr: Antacid control of complications from acute gastroduodenal disease after burns. J Trauma 16:645, 1976
34. McAlhany JC, Czaja AJ, Villarreal Y, et al: The gastric mucosal barrier in

thermally injured patients: Correlation with gastroduodenal endoscopy. Surg Forum 25:414, 1974
35. Mercereau WA, Hinchey EJ: Prevention of bile reflux induced acute gastric ulceration in the rat by cholestyramine. Ann Surg 179:883, 1974
36. Norton L, Matthews D, Avrum L, et al: Pharmacological protection against swine stress ulcer. Gastroenterology 66:503, 1974
37. Rees WDW, Rhodes J, Wheeler MH, et al: The role of histamine receptors in the pathophysiology of gastric mucosal damage. Gastroenterology 72:67, 1977
38. Rhodes J, Barnardo DE, Phillips SF, et al: Increased reflux of bile into the stomach. Gastroenterology 57:241, 1969
39. Ritchie WP Jr: Acute gastric mucosal damage induced by bile salts, acid and ischemia. Gastroenterology 68:699, 1975
40. Ritchie WP Jr, Cherry KJ Jr: Influence of [H^+] on bile acid-induced acute gastric mucosal ulcerogenesis. Ann Surg 189:637, 1979
41. Ritchie WP Jr, Cherry KJ, Gibb A: Influence of methylprednisolone sodium succinate on bile acid-induced acute gastric mucosal damage. Surgery 84:283, 1978
42. Ritchie WP Jr, McRae DB Jr, Felger TS: Arterial-venous acid-base balance during acute gastric mucosal ulcerogenesis. Am J Surg 139:22, 1980
43. Ritchie WP Jr, Shearburn EW III: Acute gastric mucosal ulcerogenesis is bile salt concentration dependent. Surgery 80:98, 1976
44. Robert A, Nezamis JE, Lancaster C, et al: Gastric cytoprotective property of prostaglandins. Gastroenterology 72:1121, 1978
45. Safaie-Shirazi S, Foster LV, Hardy BM: The effect of metiamide, an H_2 receptor antagonist, in the prevention of experimental stress ulcers. Gastroenterology 71:421, 1976
46. Saik RP, Brown D: Lithium: Not a sensitive indicator of hydrogen ion diffusion. J Surg Res 25:163, 1978
47. Schumpelick V, Rauchenberger B: Duodenogastric reflux and stress ulcer. Deutsch Med Wochshr 101:1647, 1976
48. Skillman JJ, Gould S, Chung RSK, et al: The gastric mucosal barrier: clinical and experimental studies in critically ill and normal man and in the rabbit. Ann Surg 172:564, 1970
49. Teorell T: Electrolyte diffusion in relation to the acidity regulation of the gastric juice. Gastroenterology 9:425, 1947
50. Zike WL, Safaie-Shirazi S, DenBesten L: The role of cholestyramine in the prevention of stress ulcers. J Surg Res 17:315, 1974

Charles E. Lucas, M.D.

Prevention and Treatment of Acute Gastric Erosions and Stress Ulcerations

ABSTRACT

An effort to prevent the development of acute erosive gastritis and stress ulceration can be made by preventing the development of iatrogenic sepsis, treating established sepsis, providing nutritional support, applying gastric decompression, and neutralizing the secretion of acid. The secretion of acid is most effectively neutralized by the intraluminal administration of Maalox whenever the pH of the gastric contents falls below 4.5. Some studies suggest that cimetidine may be of benefit in both the prophylaxis and treatment of this disease. However, three patients with acute gastric ulcers, treated at the Detroit General Hospital, perforated their ulcers while on cimetidine.

It is important to maintain the ability of blood to clot by the administration of platelets, fresh blood, and fresh plasma when necessary. Once bleeding occurs, gastric lavage and the replacement of blood loss form the basis of treatment. Vasopressin may be of transient benefit. Endoscopic electrocoagulation may be of more permanent benefit. If surgical intervention becomes necessary, vagotomy is advised in all patients both for its apparent effect on gastric mucosal blood flow and for its effect on acid secretion. Vagotomy and pyloroplasty is advised for acute erosive gastritis alone when the cause of the lesions has been controlled. Vagotomy and distal gastrectomy is advised for deeper stress ulcers especially when the cause has not been controlled. Total gastrectomy is advised for the failure of previous operations, for patients with very high secretion of acid, and for patients with Zollinger-Ellison syndrome.

Acute erosive gastritis and stress ulceration are catch-all terms which incorporate many different acute gastric mucosal lesions resulting from a wide

---

Charles E. Lucas, M.D.: Professor of Surgery, Wayne State University, and Chief, Emergency Surgical Service, Detroit General Hospital, Detroit, Michigan.

diversity of insults (Table 1). Accordingly, the histologic and pathologic features of these entities also vary. For simplicity, but not necessarily for accuracy, the term acute erosive gastritis will refer to superficial gastric erosions of multiple shapes (round, oval, irregular), measuring 2-15 mm in diameter, and extending, in depth, into the muscularis mucosa; stress ulceration is used to define those lesions which extend past the muscularis mucosa into the gastric muscle layer or beyond but lack the chronic inflammatory reaction with indurated and thickened borders typically seen with chronic peptic ulcers. Rokitansky in 1846 noted "decubiti of the gastric mucosa" at necropsy in patients who had died of pneumonia; these changes were attributed to postmortem autolysis. The advent of fiberoptic gastroscopy provided the means for appreciating the true significance of these lesions which may contribute to death [10, 19]. Since these lesions result from many different and diverse insults, reasonable prevention and therapy must be tailored to the specific insult. Physician exposure to acute

Table 1
Stresses Leading to Acute Erosive Gastritis and Stress Ulceration

Antiinflammatory drugs (mucosal barrier breakers)
   Aspirin
   Butazolamide
   Steroids
Hypovolemia and low perfusion (mucosal ischemia)
   Trauma with shock
   Nontrauma hemorrhage and shock
Anephric states (decreased gastrin degradation)
   Acute renal failure
   Nephrectomy for transplant
Sepsis (causes direct cellular insult)
   Complicating prior injury
   Peritonitis from hollow viscus soilage
   Interstitial pneumonitis and abscesses
Alcohol ingestion (full thickness gastric wall insult)
   Delirium tremens increases insult
Miscellaneous
   Postcardiopulmonary bypass
   Postpneumonectomy
   Postgastric surgery (bile reflux)
Laennec's cirrhosis
   Makes all above insults worse

erosive gastritis and stress ulceration varies with type of practice. Acute erosive gastritis in patients seen by a community internist is likely to be caused by aspirin; in patients at alcoholic rehabilitation centers it is likely due to alcohol. Abstinence, in both instances, eliminates the problem. Acute erosive gastritis and stress ulceration in the burn patient, septic patient, shock patient, uremic patient, or other critically ill patient, however, require a carefully coordinated regimen of therapy in conjunction with treatment of the underlying insult.

Since therapy varies with underlying insult, accurate diagnosis is essential. The diagnosis in most instances is based on a history of drug or alcohol exposure and concurrent associated illnesses. When the history is questionable or unreliable, the endoscopic picture may be helpful. The topography of acute erosive gastritis varies according to insult [17]. Shock, sepsis, and burns tend to produce proximal gastritis involving primarily the parietal cell mass area or fundic mucosa during the early phases and both the fundic and antral mucosa in the later phases; the fundic mucosa is much more involved, however, in both the early and late phases (Table 2) [10, 17]. In contrast acute erosive gastritis due to alcoholic insult involves much more of the antral mucosal area, whereas, aspirin-induced gastritis tends to involve both equally but is more likely to be associated with deeper stress ulceration (Fig. 1).

Table 2
Topography of Acute Erosive Gastritis and Stress Ulceration After Trauma, Shock, and Sepsis

LOCATION	Percent AEG Lesions		Percent SU Lesions	
Within 48 hours				
Fundic mucosa	98		0	
Proximal zone		89		
Junctional zone		9		
Antral mucosa	2		0	
Over 48 hours				
Fundic mucosa	88		4	
Proximal zone		65		3
Junctional zone		23		1
Antral mucosa*	8		0	

*In contrast, most benign gastric ulcers develop in antral mucosa.
AEG, acute erosive gastritis; SU, stress ulceration.

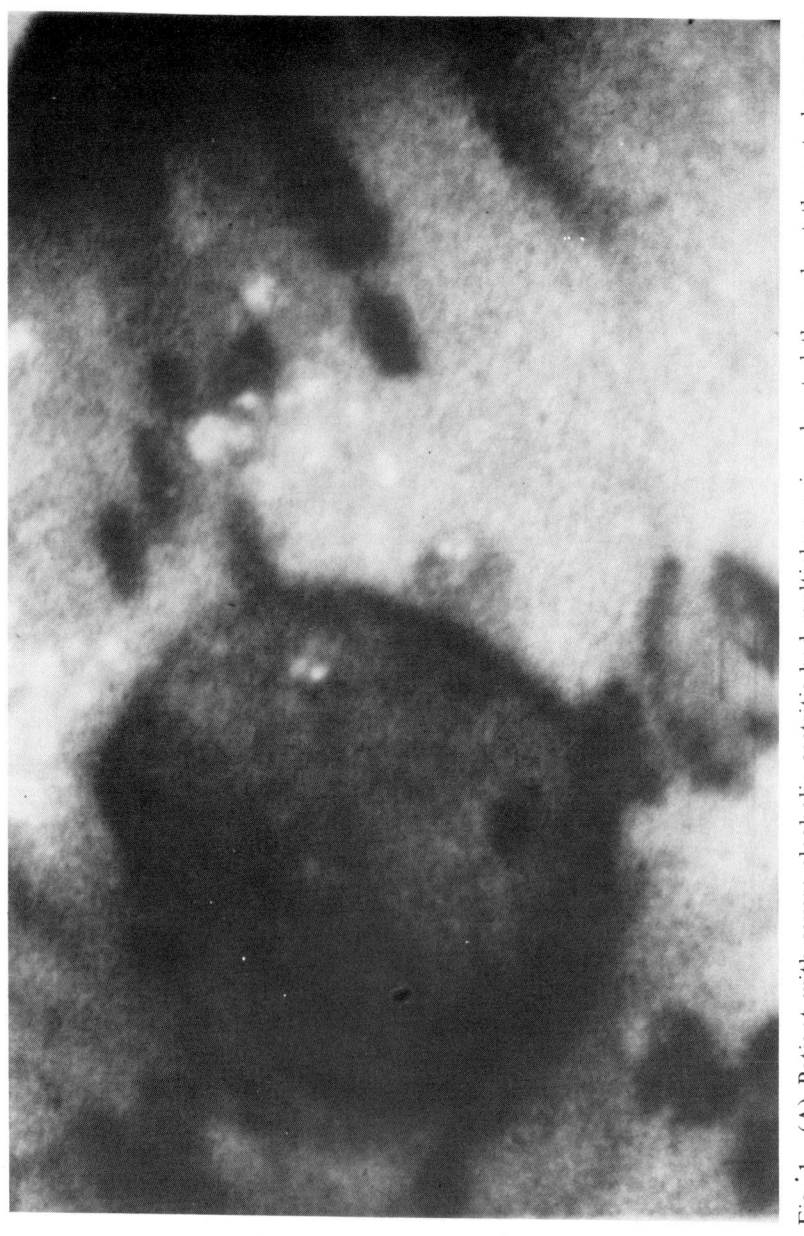

Fig. 1. (A) Patient with severe alcoholic gastritis had multiple erosions located throughout the antral mucosa. (B) Sparing of the fundic mucosa. This sequence is never seen with acute erosive gastritis due to sepsis, trauma, or burns.

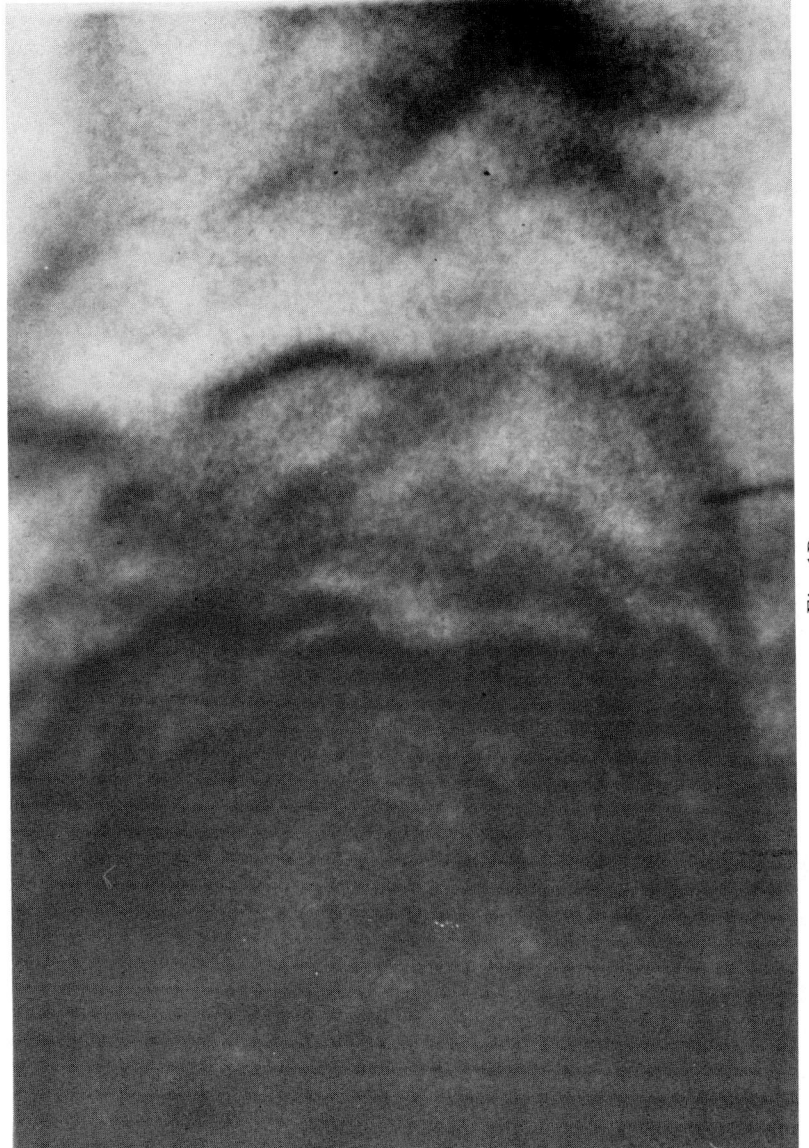

Fig. 1B

APPROACH TO THE ACTIVELY BLEEDING PATIENT

Regardless of etiology, the initial approach to the actively bleeding patient is consistent. Vital signs are stabilized with appropriate blood and salt solution replacement while vigorous nasogastric irrigation is maintained through a Levin tube or a larger Ewald tube. This latter tube facilitates clot removal. Frequently the patient vomits during gastric intubation or irrigation; this vomiting is fortuitous as it often completely evacuates the stomach of blood and clot, making subsequent irrigation and suction more effective in contracting the stomach and stopping active bleeding. When intragastric clots are retained, the gastric irrigation cannot be aspirated because the tube becomes occluded. When vomiting occurs at this time, aspiration must be avoided by either the conscious patient's normal gag response, appropriate suctioning, or proper positioning of the patient who has impaired sensorium. Since hypovolemic shock is one of the factors which leads to decreased gastric blood flow, especially to the fundic mucosa, early and effective plasma volume restoration helps minimize the hypoxic insult to the proximal stomach [1, 5]. This area of the proximal stomach is more susceptible to the later development of acute erosive gastritis and significant bleeding in traumatized hypotensive patients [9]. Once vital signs have been properly restored continued saline irrigation of the stomach helps keep the stomach empty so that contraction persists and thereby decreases the surface area of the open vessels within the erosions. When active bleeding continues despite judicious use of saline lavage, the addition of various vasopressor agents such as levarterenol to the lavage fluid may stop the bleeding. Unfortunately, the addition of a vasopressor agent in patients who are unresponsive to saline lavage has been uniformly unsuccessful in my own hands. The decision regarding immediate diagnostic and therapeutic regimens varies according to the early success in controlling bleeding.

When active hemorrhage is temporarily controlled by gastric lavage, diagnostic endoscopy can be performed immediately or deferred until the next morning depending upon the availability of the endoscopist and the patient's overall status. Early endoscopy within 24 hours of active bleeding maximizes the probability that an experienced endoscopist will be able to document the source of bleeding [19]. This allows for rational therapy and rational prophylaxis against rebleeding while in hospital. Early endoscopy, however, should not be done in patients who are no longer bleeding but are quite restless due to sepsis, alcohol withdrawal, or hypoxia.

Failure to stop bleeding with saline lavage or other modalities increases the urgency for emergency endoscopy that day in order to better plan therapy; this can be performed in either the emergency room or the regular endoscopy unit when the patient is stable and cooperative. When an actively bleeding patient is unstable or uncooperative, endoscopy, in this setting, is dangerous and leads to vomiting with aspiration, cardiovascular compromise, and extensive damage to the fiberoptic endoscope. When the unstable, actively bleeding patient appears to be a reasonable operative risk as judged by his general condition and the suspected cause of bleeding, emergency endoscopy is performed under general anesthesia during laparotomy [8]. When the patient's general condition is such that operative control of the underlying bleeding lesion would carry unacceptable risk and the emergency endoscopy would be unsafe because of possible vomiting and aspiration, the patient is maintained on nasogastric suction, gastric lavage, and general supportive care even though the actual source of bleeding is suspected but not actually confirmed. This is particularly true in patients with severe liver failure and suspected esophageal varices which, if treated operatively, would lead to almost certain hepatocellular failure and death.

PROPHYLAXIS

During the late 1960s acute erosive gastritis in severely injured and septic patients was the most common cause of transfusions in many trauma centers throughout North America. This was also true on the emergency surgical service at Detroit General Hospital where at least 2 new patients every week required transfusions for acute erosive gastritis due to sepsis or trauma or both. Ten years later severe acute erosive gastritis requiring multiple transfusions is rarely seen in injured or septic patients. The gastritis which does develop seldom requires operative intervention. The dramatic fall in morbidity and mortality from AEG in comparably injured and septic patients has prompted a careful retrospective and ongoing review of therapeutic regimens in order to identify the responsible factors. Based upon this analysis several factors can be cited (Table 3) [7].

Preventing Iatrogenic Sepsis

The most important factor leading to the decrease in severe acute erosive gastritis and stress ulceration is the overall reduction in iatrogenic septic complications related to phlebitis and airway sepsis. During the 1960s central venous pressure monitoring was usually accomplished through a long intravenous catheter or intravenous extension tube inserted through a peripheral basilic vein cutdown. This technique was considered to be relatively free of the hazards of phlebitis so commonly seen in association with peripheral intracaths. Such catheters were routinely left in place for a week. In retrospect, these catheters were not immune to the lethal hazards of phlebitis but were simply deep enough in the tissues so that venous sepsis was camouflaged. This sequence has been circumvented by the subclavian catheter which is now used for central venous pressure monitoring and is changed every 72 hours. Furthermore, pulmonary artery catheters are also changed within 60 hours of insertion. Airway sepsis has been dramatically reduced by decreasing the tidal volumes and eliminating positive end-expiratory pressure (PEEP) in critically ill and septic patients.

Table 3
Prophylaxis for Acute Erosive Gastritis and Stress Ulceration

---
Prevention of iatrogenic sepsis
  Airway sepsis — use lower tidal volume without PEEP
  Phlebitis — change all catheters within three days
  Avoid pasteurized plasma expanders — albumin

Nutritional support
  Provide total parenteral nutrition when sepsis controlled off antibiotics

Gastric decompression
  Remove ongoing acid secretion through patent tube

Neutralization of acid secretion
  Add Maalox for pH below 5
  Prevent tube blockage by Maalox

Acid inhibition by parietal cell blockade
  Cimetidine not as good as antacid

Maintain optimal coagulation profile
  Supplement with platelets, fresh blood, fresh plasma

Miscellaneous factors
  Vitamin A — probably not beneficial
  Steroids — probably not beneficial
  Intraarterial vasodilators — probably not beneficial
  Maintenance of reasonable arterial oxygen content
  Proper antibiotics coverage and drainage of abscess

Formerly, high tidal volumes (12-18 ml/kg bodyweight) and PEEP were often employed; currently lower tidal volumes (8-12 ml/kg) without PEEP are used for comparable septic patients. Airway sepsis has also been reduced by the elimination of supplemental albumin from all resuscitative regimens for shock and sepsis. The reduction in systemic and pulmonary sepsis resulting from the above changes has reduced the problems related to acute erosive gastritis and stress ulceration suggesting that the underlying sepsis was the major factor in causing so many of these lesions in the past.

Nutritional Support

Increased catabolism causing a negative nitrogen balance is well documented in the acutely ill patient. Hypoproteinemia and hypoalbuminemia accompany this catabolic state. Since acute erosive gastritis is associated with gastric mucosal edema, malnutrition and hypoalbuminemia have been incriminated as the causative factors leading to it. Total parenteral nutrition or enteral tube feedings have been proposed as effective prophylactics against the development of acute erosive gastritis in high risk patients [2]. More likely the hypoalbuminemia and mucosal edema in patients with acute erosive gastritis reflect the homeostatic response to the underlying insult rather than the gastritis being the result of hypoalbuminemia. Attempts to prevent the onset of acute erosive gastritis by early total parenteral nutrition in our septic patients has led to opportunistic superinfection and worse problems with bleeding from the gastritis. Nutritional support is best deferred until the acute shock or septic insult has been resolved.

Gastric Decompression

The etiologic role of the Levin tube in the development of acute erosive gastritis continues to be debated. Carrasquillia and co-workers [3] implicated the nasogastric tube in the evolution of AEG in dogs and suggested that suction disrupts the mucosa leading to significant bleeding from the proximal (fundic) mucosa in septic and injured patients; this sequence purportedly could be circumvented by using a tube gastrostomy placed through the antrum at the time of surgery for multiply injured patients who are at risk to develop AEG. This latter thesis was tested in 13 high risk patients with severe multiple organ injury who had antral gastrostomy performed at the initial operation for repair of multiple injuries. Ten of these 13 patients required transfusions for gastritis and 2 patients required vagotomy and subtotal gastrectomy [7]. The AEG in these latter two patients was located primarily in the fundic mucosa well away from the antral tube gastrostomy. Likely, the acute erosive gastritis in these patients is caused by those factors which produced the same lesion in Rokitansky's patients back in 1846 well before the invention of nasogastric tubes. Although nasogastric tubes may lead to superficial erosive gastritis, significant bleeding is avoided by continued gastric decompression and careful monitoring of tube patency. This regimen removes intraluminal acid and reduces the problems of adynamic ileus and abdominal distention. Currently, all critically ill patients should be maintained on continuous nasogastric suction until the acute episode has subsided and all sepsis has been eliminated.

PHARMACOLOGIC INTERVENTION FOR STRESS BLEEDING

Control of Acids

Most workers now agree that acute erosive gastritis and stress ulceration are caused, to some degree, by hydrochloric acid [5, 10, 15]. The acid factor is related to the amount of acid secreted, the amount which diffuses back from the lumen across the mucosa into the gastric wall, and the percentage of back-diffused acid which is neutralized by dynamic mucosal perfusion or the "alkaline tide" in the fundic area. Septic, trauma, and burn patients probably have both an increase in acid secretion and acid back diffusion [2]; erosive gastritis due to alcohol, bile, or antiinflammatory drugs is likely related to an increase in back diffusion caused by a physiological breakdown in the gastric mucosa barrier [4]. The end result in each instance is increased intramural acid with cellular destruction. Control of the acid problem is recognized as an essential of prophylaxis (Table 3). Much controversy exists however about the most effective modality for acid control.

This problem was studied prospectively at Detroit General Hospital in a group of 54 septic patients being treated in the surgical intensive care unit. The patients were allocated into three separate treatment groups which included: (1) continuous gastric suction interposed with hourly instillation of Maalox (30 ml) for 15 minutes whenever the intraluminal pH fell below 4.5; (2) hourly instillation of 30 ml milk and 30 ml Maalox which is allowed to remain intraluminally for 15 minutes prior to resumption of nasogastric suction for 45 minutes; (3) a repeated sequence of intraluminal drip of 150 ml of an antacid cocktail (milk, Maalox, and procaine) for 30 minutes, clamping of the nasogastric tube for 30 minutes followed by repeat nasogastric suction for another 30 minutes. The 54 patients were evenly divided between the three treatment groups, each treatment group having different problems (Table 4). All three groups had problems with maintaining nasogastric tube patency after the instillation of antacid. Patients in group II (routine milk and Maalox hourly) had moderate problems with metabolic alkalosis; patients in group three (sequence of drip, clamp, and suction) had severe problems with metabolic alkalosis,

Table 4
Prospective Study of Prophylactic Antacid Regimens

Antacid Regimen*	Number of Patients	Control of Bleeding	Problems With Alkalosis	Problems With Diarrhea	Problems With Ileus
Suction plus hourly Maalox (30 ml) for pH below 4.5	18	Same	Minimal	None	None
Suction plus hourly milk (30 ml) and Maalox (30 ml) for 15 minutes	16	Same	Moderate	Minimal	None
Repeated sequence of antacid cocktail (milk, Maalox, Procaine) infusion, occlusion of tube, and suction for 30 minute intervals	20	Same	Severe	Severe	Moderate

*The use of nasogastric suction alone was shown to be associated with excessive bleeding from acute erosive gastritis in very high risk patients.

abdominal distention, diarrhea, and occasionally aspiration. Although the differences in the number of transfusions required for the 3 groups of patients were not significant, the patients having selective instillation of antacid for confirmed low gastric pH did best. Currently, the regimen of intermittent antacid instillation for confirmed hyperacidity is used for all patients; it has been modified so that only 15 ml Maalox is instilled when the gastric pH is below 5 after which the suction is immediately reattached to preclude plugging of the nasogastric tube by Maalox.

Acid Inhibition

A more exciting trend toward acid control has evolved recently, namely, histamine receptor site blockade by such drugs as cimetidine [12]. Both experimental and clinical studies confirm the effectiveness of these drugs in reducing acid secretion. Although our own anecdotal experience does not support the prophylactic value of cimetidine in preventing rebleeding in patients with intermittent bleeding from acute erosive gastritis, prospective randomized studies in man and animals indicate its protective efficacy is similar to Maalox [12]. Ability to control gastric pH is better with Maalox than cimetidine [6]. Further studies on cimetidine are needed to better define its effect on gastric mucosal blood flow and neutralization of back-diffused acid and gastric mucosal regeneration.

Three patients were seen recently in our institution, actively bleeding from a high-lying gastric ulcer. All 3 were placed on cimetidine and all 3 developed perforation of gastric ulcers. The question as to whether this sequence is coincidental or related to cimetidine therapy can only be answered after further studies are made.

Another potentially useful group of drugs for effecting acid blockade are the prostaglandins [14]. Some prostaglandins not only decrease acid secretion, by a cryptic mechanism but also increase gastric mucosal blood flow thereby allowing for more efficient neutralization of that acid which is back diffused. Other reports suggest that the protective effects of prostaglandins are independent of acid secretion, back diffusion, and intramural neutralization but are more likely related to direct cytoprotection which can be provided by oral administration. Further evaluation of the prostaglandins as prophylactics against acute erosive gastritis is needed.

Coagulation Supplementation

Patients in shock, with active bleeding from nongastric sites, or severe sepsis develop specific defects in their coagulation profile. Hypotension leads to a reduction in fibrinogen and platelets which are consumed within small vessels; active hemorrhage and replacement with bank blood leads to thrombocytopenia, hypofibrinogenemia, and a reduction in factors 5, 7, and 8; septic patients develop thrombocytopenia and impaired platelet adhesiveness and aggregability [7, 9]. Careful monitoring of the prothrombin time, partial thromboplastin time, platelet count, and fibrinogen level will help document these changes before they lead to significant hemorrhage from associated erosive gastritis. Judicial use of fresh whole blood, fresh frozen plasma, and platelet concentrate is most rewarding. Heparin therapy, formerly advocated in actively bleeding patients with thrombocytopenia, hypofibrinogenemia, and increased fibrin split products, is contraindicated in patients with acute erosive gastritis; it only makes the bleeding worse [7]. Heparin is now reserved for only those patients with thrombocytopenia, hypofibrinogenemia, and no fibrin split products indicating consumption without concomitant lysis. I have never seen this combination in a patient with acute erosive gastritis.

Miscellaneous Factors

Different prophylactic regimens designed to help maintain mitochondrial integrity, restore the mucosal mucin barrier, or increase gastric mucosal blood flow have been advocated. Although steroids have been incriminated as a causative agent in the development of acute erosive gastritis, they have also been recommended in its treatment because of their purported ability to prevent gastric mucosal cellular disruption by helping to stabilize lysosome membranes [2]. More likely steroids are neither helpful nor harmful during the acute phase and should be used only if there is some other medical indication in the

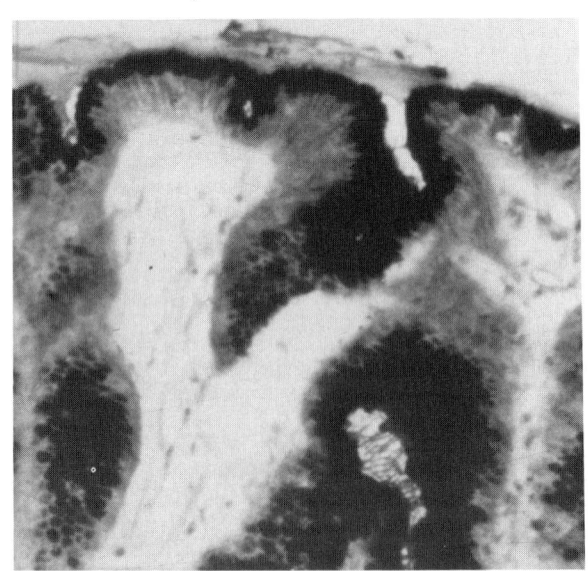

Fig. 2. Severe erosive gastritis producing bleeding requiring operative intervention. Immediately adjacent to bleeding erosions the mucosa is edematous but still contains a superficial and intracellular mucin layer (black staining).

acutely ill patient. Vitamin A has been proposed as a prophylactic against the development of acute erosive gastritis on the basis of its action on gastric mucosal regeneration and mucin secretion [9]. Although several animal models are known to develop a uniform reduction in both surface and intracellular mucin, histologic studies in patients undergoing gastrectomy for acute erosive gastritis show only focal ulceration interspersed with nonerosive edematous mucosa which has normal intracellular and surface mucin (Fig. 2). Furthermore, quantitative studies on gastric mucin secretion in Vietnam combat casualties and our own civilian casualties demonstrated an increased secretion of mucopolysaccharides including sialic acid, hexosamine, and total hexoses [10, 16].

Apparently the most important factor in acid back diffusion is not the mucin barrier but rather the integrity of the outer cellular membrane, tight junctions and terminal bars (Fig. 3). This membrane in turn is maintained by

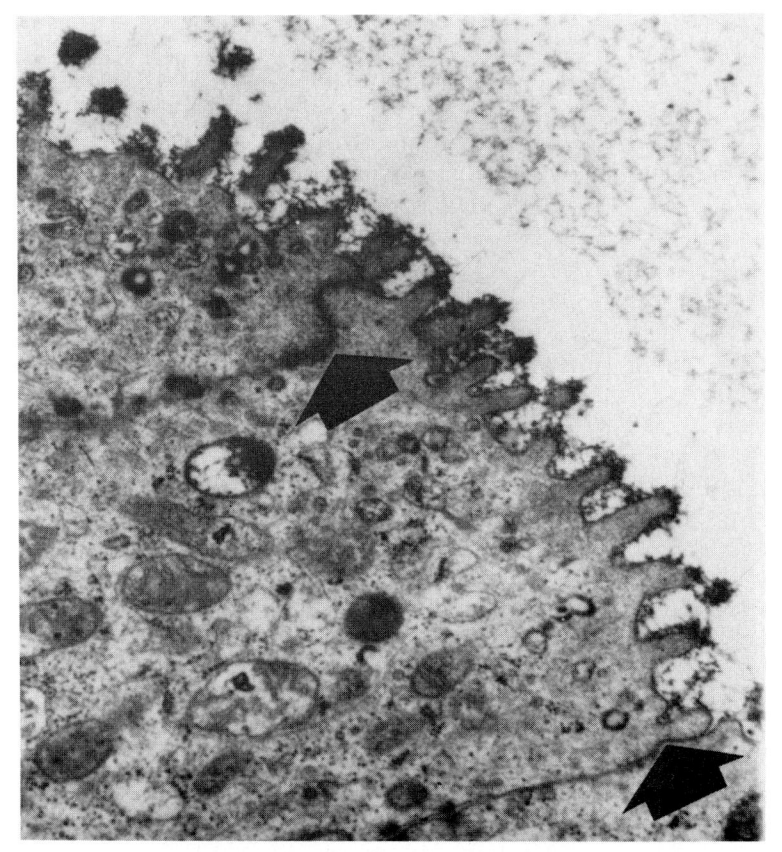

Fig. 3. Gastric mucosa immediately adjacent to bleeding erosions at the time of gastrectomy shows an intact mucosal surface with tight junctions or terminal bars (arrows).

ongoing gastric mucosal perfusion. Ritchie and co-workers suggested that augmentation of this gastric mucosal perfusion by selective intraarterial infusion of a vasodilator such as isoproterenol will help protect this surface membrane and also facilitate neutralization of back diffused acid [13]. Although mucosal hypoxia is an important etiologic factor during a hypotensive episode, the added gastric mucosal blood flow brought about by intraarterial vasodilator infusion in a stable patient is unlikely to result in an increased unloading of oxygen from the hemoglobin molecule. Such regimens of mucosal perfusion augmentation however have theoretical merit and deserve further study.

Finally, the absolute or total gastric mucosal blood flow appears to be even less crucial in septic patients who develop acute erosive gastritis. Both in vivo and intrachamber studies indicate that bacterial sepsis in animals produces a hyperdynamic state similar to that seen in humans, with increased cardiac

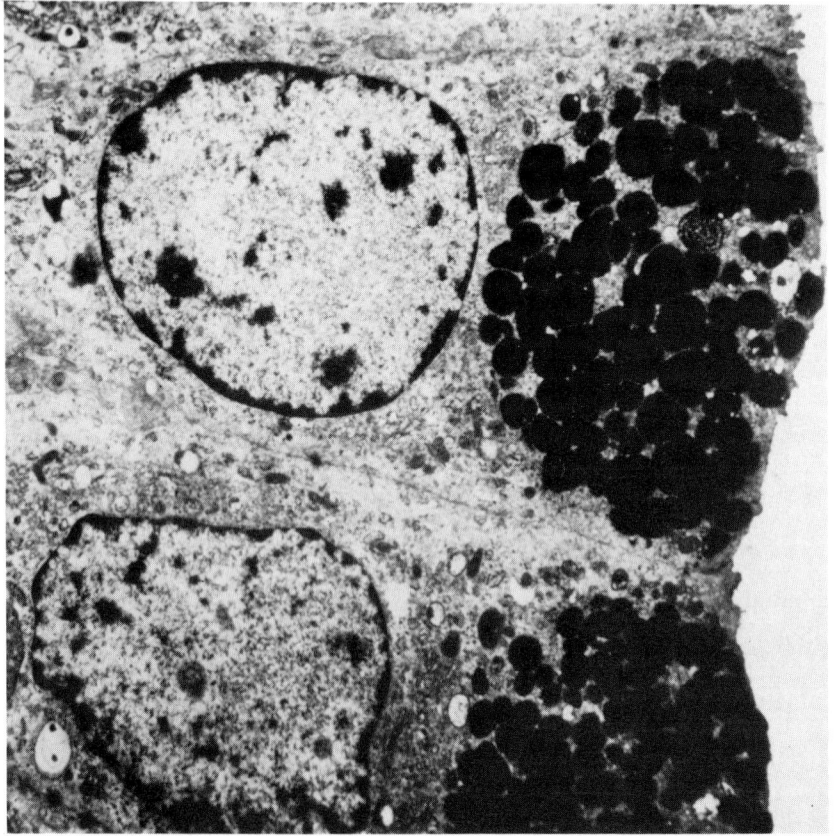

Fig. 4. Transmission electronmicrograph showing intact mucosal cells with normal apical mucin granules immediately adjacent to bleeding erosions which required gastrectomy.

output, decreased total peripheral resistance, and increased gastric mucosal blood flow during the period that acute erosive gastritis is evolving [11]. The development of AEG during sepsis may be related to a direct cellular insult produced by a circulating toxic byproduct of sepsis, thus, explaining the pattern of focal erosions interspersed with intact mucin covered mucosa (Fig. 4).

NONOPERATIVE THERAPY FOR ACTIVE BLEEDING

Local Agents

The initial regimen for active bleeding from acute erosive gastritis and stress ulceration includes vigorous gastric lavage with saline until the gastric aspirate is clear. The addition of cold (iced saline) to the lavage may provide a temporary cooling effect on the gastric mucosa and thereby cause vasoconstriction. Goodale has had good results in controlling active bleeding with the gastric cooling balloon using a technique similar to that popularized for duodenal ulcer disease [9]. This technique requires special expertise which has not yet been achieved or mastered in our hands. Supplemental cimetidine, vitamin A, steroids, and prostaglandins do not appear to be helpful during the active bleeding phase (Table 5).

The Endoscopic Hemostat

Endoscopy not only provides a means for instituting rational therapy based upon accurate diagnosis but also provides a means for obtaining hemostasis when

Table 5
Nonoperative Therapeutic Measures for Bleeding

Gastric lavage
   Saline (iced or room temperature)
   Added vasopressor to lavage

Gastric hypothermia — balloon cooling
   Results vary with expertise

Endoscopic hemostat
   Tedious but effective in expert hands

Intraarterial infusion of vasopressin
   Rebleeding likely

Coagulation replacement
   Very helpful

Blood replacement
   Volume varies with insult

the above regimens fail. Sugawa perfected the technique of electrocoagulation in animals and then applied this technique to critically ill, actively bleeding patients being treated on the emergency surgical service [18]. Endoscopic electrocoagulation of acute erosive gastritis is reasonably safe although several applications of current to multiple bleeding sites is often necessary and makes the whole process quite tedious. During this time the endoscopic assistant must monitor the patient closely and guard against vomiting and aspiration.

Intraarterial Infusion

Although selected intraarterial vasopressin infusion through the celiac axis, gastroduodenal artery, or left gastric artery in patients with peptic ulcer disease has received many plaudits, this technique has not received great acclaim for control of bleeding from acute erosive gastritis and stress ulceration. Some of the poor results obtained with this modality may be due to inadequate facilities or lack of expertise on the part of physician and hospital teams treating large numbers of patients with erosive gastritis. Our own limited experience with this technique as a hemostat has been unsuccessful. Although bleeding may be temporarily slowed, rebleeding is predictable [7].

Blood Replacement

The appropriate volume of blood replacement as part of a nonoperative regimen varies according to the underlying etiology. Alcoholic gastritis in general is a self-limiting process. Bleeding is often brisk during the first 24 hours, slows the second 24 hours, and ceases by the third day. The added factor of delirium tremens may extend the bleeding phase for 24-48 more hours. During the actively bleeding phase, the gastric mucosa and the remaining gastric wall are edematous, friable, and easily injured during operative manipulation. I have transfused as many as 12 units of whole blood during the initial 24 hour period in several patients with alcoholic gastritis who were successfully managed nonoperatively. This regimen is almost always successful if the patient is watched closely, replaced unit for unit, and is not allowed to become hypovolemic or hypotensive. Inability to maintain normal vital signs during this 24 hour period mandates operative intervention. Bleeding from alcoholic gastritis is much more severe in patients with associated Laennec's cirrhosis. One well known cirrhotic patient at Detroit General Hospital received approximately 148 transfusions for 13 different episodes of alcoholic gastritis over an 18 month period before consenting to operation; he survived a total gastrectomy and returned to his old ways although his capacity to consume alcohol is reduced.

Acute erosive gastritis due to antiinflammatory drugs, such as aspirin, is also a self-limiting process in most patients, but the bleeding often continues for 3-5 days. Ongoing blood replacement of 6-8 units per day is acceptable in selected instances as long as vital signs are maintained. Many patients with aspirin gastritis, however, have a deeper stress ulceration mixed with the gastritis and are candidates for earlier operative intervention. This can be confirmed at the time of endoscopy. Furthermore, the underlying problem for which aspirin is prescribed is often chronic such as is seen in the arthritic patient, so that recurrent bleeding is likely. Assuming that drug therapy will be maintained, an operation designed to eliminate acid secretion will significantly reduce the problem of acid back diffusion through an aspirin damaged mucosa. Patients with active bleeding from acute erosive gastritis due to sepsis, or burns respond best to supportive care, correction of the underlying insult, and appropriate blood and coagulation factor replacement. Avoidance of iatrogenic sepsis, appropriate antibiotic coverage and drainage of trapped pus are essential. When these factors are followed the number of transfusions given as part of a nonoperative regimen can usually be restricted to six units per 24 hours. When bleeding exceeds that rate, operative intervention is appropriate depending upon the patient's general status and associated problems.

Acute erosive gastritis in association with trauma and hypovolemic shock is usually self-limiting as long as sepsis does not supervene. Shock initiates a low perfusion and ischemic state to the proximal stomach (fundic mucosa) where superficial red-based erosions become manifest within 24 hours of insult [1]. Deeper black-based erosions extending throughout the fundic mucosa evolve over the next 24-96 hours and may cause bleeding requiring transfusion. Resolution begins, however, at about this time. As long as blood and coagulation factor replacement is provided, operative intervention is seldom indicated [10]. When sepsis supervenes increased bleeding is common; six or more transfusions per day may be needed to provide adequate replacement therapy while the sepsis is brought under control. Patients with head injury or uremia, or recovering from cardiopulmonary bypass follow the same sequence as the injured patient. If sepsis develops, the pattern of gastitis will correspond to that seen in other septic patients. Each type of gastritis follows a predictable pattern. When a patient with acute erosive gastritis develops a pattern of clinical bleeding which is not typically seen with that specific etiology, repeat endoscopy is indicated.

Case Report

A 41-year-old man presented to the hospital with acute upper gastrointestinal bleeding of 18 hours duration. Initial resuscitation with salt and blood restored vital signs to normal. Bleeding continued despite vigorous saline lavage. Endoscopy showed diffuse acute erosive gastritis located primarily in the antrum, thus confirming a suspected diagnosis of alcoholic gastritis. He received eight transfusions during the first day. Bleeding slowed and only 2 transfusions were needed on day two. The nasogastric tube became occluded on the second night when he vomited clots and began rebleeding which required 7 transfusions over the next eleven hours. Since alcoholic gastritis seldom follows this course, repeat endoscopy was done; this showed a fresh Mallory-Weiss tear which was treated by gastric balloon tamponade. Two separate inflations of the gastric balloon were required over the next 48 hours (hospital days 4-5). This controlled bleeding temporarily but bleeding recurred on day six and repeat endoscopy revealed superficial mucosal necrosis at the site of the previous gastric balloon tamponade. All tubes were removed and he was successfully managed with antacids as mucosal regeneration occurred.

OPERATIVE INTERVENTION

Once one accepts that nonoperative therapy has failed the patient must be prepared for operative control of bleeding. The optimal procedure varies according to the underlying insult, the severity of bleeding, and the ability of the patient to withstand a second operation if the first operation fails to completely control bleeding [9] (Table 6). Vagotomy should be an essential part of all operative procedures for acute erosive gastritis and stress ulceration. Vagal denervation not only causes a temporary reduction in gastric mucosal blood flow or, most specifically, a shunting of blood away from the superficial gastric mucosa, but it also eliminates the cephalic phase of acid secretion. This is especially important in septic, burned, injured, and postcardiopulmonary bypass patients. Vagotomy is also beneficial in patients with normal acid secretion but impaired mucosal barrier defense leading to increased acid back diffusion as is seen with aspirin and other antiinflammatory drug-induced gastritis. Since the

Table 6
Operative Therapy for Continued Bleeding

Vagotomy for all causes
   Temporarily decreases or shunts mucosal perfusion
   Decreases postoperative acid secretion

Pyloroplasty
   Alcoholic AEG — most patients
   Aspirin AEG without SU
   Shock, septic, and burn AEG if insult controlled

Distal gastrectomy
   Aspirin AEG with deeper SU
   Shock, septic, and burn AEG if insult uncontrolled
   Renal failure or nephrectomy

Total gastrectomy
   Failure of previous operation
   Very high acid secretion
   Zollinger-Ellison syndrome

AEG, acute erosive gastritis; SU, stress ulceration.

increase in back diffusion represents a percentage of total acid secretion, the total amount of acid back diffusion will be significantly reduced by vagotomy in such patients. This affords protection against acid damage in the postoperative phase.

The decision to do a pyloroplasty, partial gastrectomy, or total gastrectomy relates primarily to the underlying disease process. Patients being operated upon for alcoholic gastritis respond best to vagotomy and pyloroplasty. Significant rebleeding requiring reoperation is uncommon. The addition of Laennec's cirrhosis to the alcoholic gastritis, however, increases the likelihood of rebleeding and such patients may require gastric resection. Gastrectomy in patients with alcoholic gastritis may be difficult if the full-thickness gastric wall edema causes increased friability. Total gastrectomy is rarely indicated for alcoholic gastritis.

Following vagotomy in patients with aspirin-induced gastritis, pyloroplasty is indicated if all of the erosions are shallow based. Acute stress ulceration and more chronic appearing gastric ulcers often accompany aspirin induced gastritis. This combination is best treated by adding a distal gastrectomy incorporating the stress ulceration lesions which have been identified endoscopically to extend below the muscularis mucosa.

When operating upon a patient with gastritis due to sepsis, respiratory failure, uremia or burns, the decision between pyloroplasty and gastric resection varies according to the physician's ability to successfully manage the underlying septic process in the early postoperative period. When the underlying septic process appears to be easily controllable immediately following operation, vagotomy with pyloroplasty is preferred. This might occur in a patient having incision and drainage of a well loculated abscess in conjunction with the operation for bleeding gastritis. When the underlying septic process is not readily correctable within the first 24-48 hour postoperative phase, distal gastrectomy is added to vagotomy. Examples of septic processes which are not easy to control in the immediate postoperative period include (1) respiratory and ventilatory failure due to sepsis, (2) intraparenchymal pulmonary abscess, (3) multiple intraabdominal loop abscesses, and (4) uncontrolled visceral cutaneous fistula. When gastrectomy is selected for such patients, gastroduodenostomy reconstruction whenever possible is preferred. When the septic process arises from within the abdomen, performance of more than a 60% distal gastrectomy is technically difficult because of associated septic jaundice with hepatomegaly, increased gastric wall edema, and perigastric inflammatory reaction which makes mobilization of the stomach and duodenum difficult. Because of this, such patients are reconstructed by way of a gastrojejunostomy in order to preclude any problems related to tension on the gastroduodenal anastomosis because of a noncompliant proximal stomach. Distal gastrectomy is also preferred for patients with bleeding gastritis due to renal failure and uremia since the failing kidneys are no longer able to effectively degradate circulating gastrin. Total gastrectomy is seldom indicated as the initial operative procedure for gastritis. This procedure is formidable in the actively bleeding, critically ill patient and is best reserved for those patients who have had failure of a lesser procedure to control bleeding, or for those patients who have very high acid secretion (>10 mEq free HCl/hr) or hypergastrinemia compatible with the Zollinger-Ellison syndrome.

Survival following operative intervention is to be expected in patients with alcoholic, aspirin, or antiinflammatory drug-induced gastritis as long as rebleeding does not occur following operation. The prime exception to this generalization occurs in patients with associated Laennec's cirrhosis. Survival following operative intervention for acute alcoholic gastritis and stress ulceration due to burns, sepsis, renal failure with uremia, shock and other critical illness is more likely to be related to the natural history of that particular illness. Because of this, success of operative intervention should be judged by its effectiveness in preventing postoperative rebleeding. Using that reference point vagotomy and partial gastrectomy are far superior for control of bleeding even though they are usually reserved for those patients who have the most severe underlying insult and would therefore be expected to have the highest probability for postoperative rebleeding [9]. Whenever, in the opinion of the operating surgeon, the underlying septic insult can be successfully reversed and survival therefore would be a function of the postoperative rebleeding, the procedure of choice is a vagotomy and partial gastrectomy [10].

INTEROPERATIVE ENDOSCOPY

The diagnostic success of early endoscopy for acute upper gastrointestinal bleeding has allowed for rational therapy to be implemented based upon a confirmed diagnosis. When uncontrollable factors such as patient uncooperativeness due to hypoxia or ethanol intoxication, massive hemorrage with vomiting and potential aspiration, hypovolemia and hypotension, diffuse gastric clots which can't be removed, or general patient instability preclude safe preoperative diagnostic endoscopy, the patient is a candidate for emergency intraoperative endoscopy performed under general anesthesia [8]. When a decision has been made to provide operative correction for the cause of bleeding, this intraoperative endoscopy should be performed after the patient has been anesthetized. General anesthesia fortuitously decreases splanchnic blood flow and thereby slows the active bleeding from whatever cause. After the patient is anesthetized, the balloon on the endotracheal tube is temporarily deflated as the endoscope is passed through the esophagus into the stomach at which time the endotracheal balloon is reinflated. The proximal jejunum is occluded with a rubber shod clamp in order to prevent the air which is instilled during endoscopy from being passed through the duodenum into the small bowel thereby making the subsequent dissection more difficult and more hazardous. Diagnostic endoscopy in this circumstance provides for an accurate observation of the site of bleeding even when the stomach contains significant clot. This technique eliminates the need for intraoperative gastrotomy with all of its frustration, contamination, bleeding, and expenditure of time. Furthermore, the control of peritoneal soilage afforded by this technique facilitates an easier operation and a more benign postoperative course without the superimposed threat of sepsis. This procedure is best performed with an end view esophagogastroduodenoscope. The time has come for the surgeon to either familiarize himself with the modern endoscopes or else invite his medical colleague to the operating room to provide diagnostic endoscopy during laparotomy in these critically ill patients who cannot tolerate preoperative endoscopy.

REFERENCES

1. Buckley G, Goldman H, Trecis L, et al: Gastric microcirculatory changes in hemorrhagic shock. Surg Forum 21:27, 1979
2. Bowen JC: Persistent gastric mucosa hypoxia and interstitial edema after hemorrhagic shock; prevention with steroid therapy. Surgery 85:268, 1979
3. Carrasquillia C, Weaver A, Amarasinghe DC, et al: Gastroesophageal erosions and ulcerations. Arch Surg 107:447, 1973
4. Davenport HW: "Back diffusion of acid through the gastric mucosa and its physiological consequences." In Glass GBJ (Ed): Progress in Gastroenterology. New York, Grune & Stratton, 1970, p 42
5. Kivilaakso E, Silen W: Pathogenesis of experimental gastric-mucosal injury. N Engl J Med 301:364, 1979
6. Kohler TR, Dellinger EP, Simonowitz DA, et al: Cimetidine pharmacopinetics in trauma patients. Surg Forum 30:12, 1979
7. Lucas CE: Unpublished data.
8. Lucas CE, Sugawa C: Diagnostic endoscopy during laparotomy for acute hemorrhage from the upper part of the gastrointestinal tract. Surg Gynecol Obstet 135:285, 1972
9. Lucas CE, Sugawa C, Friend W, et al: Therapeutic implications of disturbed gastric physiology in patients with stress ulcerations. Am J Surg 123:25, 1971
10. Lucas CE, Sugawa C, Riddle J, et al: Natural history and surgical dilemma of "Stress" gastric bleeding. Arch Surg 102:266, 1971
11. Lucas CE, Ravikant T, Walt AJ: Gastritis and gastric blood flow in hyperdynamic septic pigs. Am J Surg 131:73, 1976
12. McElwee HP, Sirinek KR, Levine BA: Cimetidine affords protection equal to antacids in prevention of stress ulceration following thermal injury. Surgery 86:620, 1979
13. Ritchie WP Jr: Acute gastric mucosal damage induced by bile salts, acids and ischemia. Gastroenterology 68:699, 1975
14. Schiessel R, Bargilai AH, Silen, W: Effect of prostaglandin E_2 on amphibian gastric mucosa. Surg Forum 30:330, 1979

15. Skillman JJ, Bushnell IS, Goldman H, et al: Respiratory failure, hypotension, sepsis and jaundice: A clinical syndrome associated with lethal hemorrhage from acute stress ulceration of the stomach. Am J Surg 117:523, 1969
16. Stremple JF, Mori H, Lev R, et al: The stress ulcer syndrome. Curr Prob Surg, April 1973
17. Sugawa C, Lucas CE, Walt AJ: Effects of histamine and aspirin on healing of standardized gastric ulcers in dogs. Surgery 70:590, 1971
18. Sugawa C, Shier M, Lucas CE, et al: Electrocoagulation of bleeding in the upper part of the gastrointestinal tract. Arch Surg 110:975, 1975
19. Sugawa C, Werner MH, Hayes DF, et al: Early endoscopy: a guide to therapy for acute hemorrahge in the upper gastrointestinal tract. Arch Surg 107:133, 1973

Robert L. Protell, M.D.
Fred E. Silverstein, M.D.

Therapeutic Endoscopy: Photocoagulation and Electrocoagulation

ABSTRACT

This report reviews a number of available endoscopic methods to control gastrointestinal hemorrhage in experimental animals and man. Many factors must be considered before an optimal technique can be selected for use. Laser photocoagulation is not generally available, is expensive and is potentially hazardous for the operator [4, 19]. Nonetheless, both argon and Nd:YAG laser photocoagulation are highly effective. Electrocoagulation is a technique which is both widely available and relatively inexpensive. However, it poses some electrical hazards to the patient and to the operator. Of the available types of electrocoagulation, bipolar appears to cause less tissue injury in the experimental situation but much additional work needs to be done before this technique is ready for clinical use.

, Fiberoptic endoscopy is a highly accurate diagnostic procedure in the evaluation of patients with upper and lower gastrointestinal bleeding [6, 22]. However, mortality from serious upper gastrointestinal hemorrhage has been unchanged for the past three decades [1, 20, 26]. In fact, emergency endoscopy for upper gastrointestinal hemorrhage has not been shown to be of benefit to the patient [11, 18]. However, this may change with the development of safe, effective hemostatic techniques that can be delivered through use of the fiberendoscope [2].

Robert L. Protell, M.D.: Assistant Professor of Internal Medicine, Department of Medicine, University of Washington, and Director, Harborview Medical Center Endoscopy Clinic; Fred E. Silverstein, M.D.: Associate Professor of Medicine, Department of Medicine, University of Washington, Seattle, Washington.

This study was supported by United States Public Health Service, Contract 1-AM-5-2211, and Clinical Investigator Award 1 K08-AM 00406.

, In this chapter we shall review the two most extensively studied endoscopic hemostatic methods: laser photocoagulation and electrocoagulation. The two lasers which are suitable for use with modern fiberendoscopes, the argon and neodymium YAG (Nd:YAG) lasers, will be discussed. In addition, the three forms of electrocoagulation, monopolar, bipolar, and electrofulguration, will be considered. For each modality we shall describe some engineering and safety considerations, animal experiments and human clinical experience.

LASER PHOTOCOAGULATION

Engineering and Safety Considerations

Laser beams are a spatially coherent, intense form of light energy. The word laser is an acronym for *l*ight *a*mplification by *s*timulated *e*mission of *r*adiation. When this light is absorbed and converted to thermal energy, coagulation of blood and tissue protein results. Succcessful endoscopic therapy for gastrointestinal hemorrhage depends upon the ability of a given modality to deposit sufficient thermal energy to the bleeding site to denature protein and to form a coagulum.

There are two lasers that are currently suitable for endoscopic therapy, the argon laser and the neodymium YAG laser. The blue-green argon laser light (wavelength 0.44-0.52 μm) is selectively absorbed by red and well absorbed by a layer of blood 100 μm thick. In contrast, the neodymium YAG laser has a longer wavelength in the near infrared range (1.06 μm) and is not well absorbed until it has passed through a layer of blood 300 μm thick. The absorption coefficient of laser radiation is thus a function of the laser's wavelength. The overall thermal profile for absorbed laser light also depends upon the distribution within the tissue matrix of blood and other substances that preferentially absorb a particular laser's energy.

Lasers are effective photocoagulating instruments because of the high degree of spatial coherence of the laser beam. This quality allows the laser beam to be focused efficiently onto a tiny filament. Such filaments can be used as waveguides to carry the laser beam down fiberendoscopes, provided they can conduct the laser light without significant loss of energy.

Argon laser light is highly coherent and can be focused to a spot 10 μm in diameter. Quartz waveguide fibers of 80-140 μm are satisfactory for transmission of argon laser light. The neodymium YAG laser light is less coherent and requires quartz fiber diameters of 200-400 μm for effective waveguide transmission. A triconical quartz waveguide with funnel-shaped proximal and distal ends has been developed by Nath et al [28]. This provides focusing of the output beam for Nd:YAG laser work.

Many factors influence the effectiveness of laser photocoagulation. The laser type and power, duration of laser exposure, and modifiers such as the presence of an irrigating solution or a coaxial jet of CO_2 gas are all important. One of the most important variables in photocoagulation is the output angle of light emerging from the laser waveguide. This exit angle and the distance from the waveguide tip to the target tissue determine the laser spot size. This is the area over which laser energy is deposited; it is described in energy density (joules/cm^2) or power density (watts/cm^2). Wide output angles require the laser catheter to be positioned close to the target in order to achieve a small enough spot size for an adequate power density. Narrow output angles allow one to move farther from the target while maintaining a small spot size and adequate power densities for effective photocoagulation. A small spot size is less effective than a larger spot size of the same power density if other variables are held constant. In endoscopy output angles of less than 20° are most practical because working distances from bleeding lesions generally range between 1 and 4 cm.

A typical setup for endoscopic laser photocoagulation is diagrammed in Fig. 1. A shutter/beamsplitter allows 0.1% of the laser light to be focused on the input tip of a flexible endoscopically passable waveguide. This is used for aiming and does not emit sufficient laser energy to be harmful. When an invisible laser beam like the Nd:YAG is used, a separate low power visible laser is used for

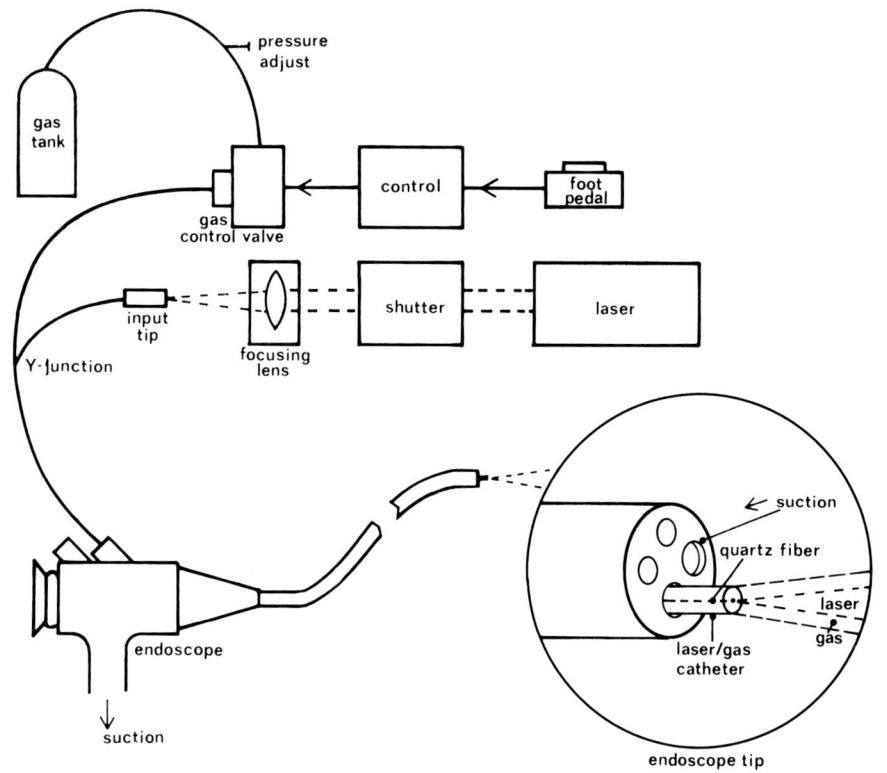

Fig. 1. Typical setup of endoscopic laser photocoagulation.

aiming by directing it along the path of the invisible beam. When the laser is fired at full power, the beamsplitter moves aside and all of the laser light is directed into the waveguide. Laser power can be adjusted as desired and the duration of laser firing can be preset. A coaxial jet of CO_2, a gas which does not support combustion, can be delivered using the endoscopic waveguide along with the laser light. CO_2 gas removes obscuring blood and transiently back-pressurizes bleeding vessels, thereby slowing the rate of hemorrhage. This has been shown to improve the efficiency of argon laser photocoagulation of experimental bleeding ulcers [39]. Similar effects on Nd:YAG photocoagulation may occur but this has not yet been formally tested.

Safety precautions are very important in endoscopic laser work. Lasers that are powerful enough to photocoagulate bleeding arteries can produce serious skin burns and even cause blindness from accidental retinal exposure. To minimize the dangers to the patient the laser beam is interrupted when the waveguide is not in the endoscope. The foot pedal that controls full power firing is deactivated until just prior to use. All participants in the procedure, including the patient, wear protective filter goggles.

The endoscopist's eye is protected by a failsafe electronic shutter interposed between the eye and the endoscope eyepiece [3]. This filter moves into position before the laser will fire and remains in place until the laser is off. An effective filter for argon laser work is yellow-orange in color (Wratten No. 22). The near infrared Nd:YAG laser radiation can be attenuated with filters of high visual transmittance; these can be permanently inserted into the endoscope eyepiece without disturbing the endoscopic view.

Animal Studies and Clinical Experience

ARGON LASER

Experimental endoscopic laser photocoagulation was first described in 1973. Nath et al reported a flexible fiber waveguide for argon laser transmission [28]. Frühmorgen and his colleagues soon published a description of their endoscopic argon laser system [16]; in addition, they reported their studies of low to moderate power argon photocoagulation on intact esophagus, stomach, duodenum and colon of experimental animals [15]. Fruhmorgen et al concluded that argon laser photocoagulation could be used successfully throughout the gastrointestinal tract without danger of excessive tissue damage.

Several American investigators began to report their early results with argon laser photocoagulation at approximately the same time. Dwyer et al [9] and Waitman et al [45] reported hemostasis of bleeding gastric lesions in dogs following photocoagulation with argon lasers of low power, 0.35-0.7 watts. These early studies were performed in nonheparinized animals; the type of lesions created often ceased bleeding spontaneously.

In 1974 our endoscopic research group at the University of Washington first described an argon laser photocoagulator [2]. Later we reported successful argon laser photocoagulation of bleeding gastric erosions in heparinized dogs with laser powers of 7-8 watts [36]. The laser power was higher than that reported to date by other groups. Once a reproducible model of massively bleeding acute gastric ulcers was developed [35] we compared high-power argon laser photocoagulation (7 watts), low-power argon laser photocoagulation (1 watt) and no treatment for severely bleeding experimental gastric ulcers in heparinized dogs [40]. This controlled randomized experiment showed that while all control ulcers and those treated with low-power argon laser photocoagulation continued to bleed, 83% of ulcers treated with the high-power argon laser stopped after a mean of 14 five-second applications. In a separate part of the study, done to assess the depth of tissue damage following high-power argon laser photocoagulation, 3 of 28 treated ulcers showed microscopic evidence of full thickness damage through the gastric wall 7 to 28 days from the time of laser therapy.

The addition of a coaxial jet of CO_2 to the argon laser catheter markedly increased the efficacy of photocoagulation. This development was reported simultaneously by Fruhmorgen [14] and by our group [37]. We performed a series of experiments to evaluate the benefit of a coaxial jet of CO_2 with argon laser photocoagulation in experimental bleeding gastric ulcers [39]. In controlled randomized experiments it was discovered that 6-7 watts of argon laser power with coaxial CO_2 gas flow at 75 cc/sec produced the most effective homostasis (2.5 five-second applications) with no full thickness injury to the gastric wall.

Using the CO_2-assisted argon laser photocoagulation, Fruhmorgen et al have treated patients with 270 bleeding or potentially bleeding gastrointestinal lesions [13]. They report a 95% success rate in stopping bleeding and have had no complications attributable to laser therapy. Unfortunately, this study is neither controlled nor randomized. Thus the effectiveness of this method compared to spontaneous bleeding cessation is unknown. Two other American investigators have performed uncontrolled pilot experiments using argon laser photocoagulation without gas assistance to control gastrointestinal bleeding [10, 44]. Three American groups including our own are currently evaluating gas-assisted argon laser photocoagulation of bleeding upper gastrointestinal lesions in randomized, controlled clinical studies.

Nd:YAG LASER

Much of the early work with the endoscopically deliverable Nd:YAG laser was performed by Kiefhaber and Nath [24]. Following animal experiments with low-power argon laser photocoagulation without gas jet assistance, Kiefhaber et al have compared this low-power argon laser photocoagulation with Nd:YAG laser photocoagulation in an animal model of acute gastric ulcer bleeding [26].

The argon laser had an energy density of 200 joules/cm^2; the Nd:YAG laser, an energy density of 600 joules/cm^2. It was reasoned that this was a valid comparison because the Nd:YAG laser radiation penetrated tissues 3-5 times more deeply than the argon laser and would thus require a greater energy density to produce comparable tissue heating. The results of this study showed Nd:YAG laser photocoagulation to be superior. However, the power of the argon laser was approximately 2 watts while that of the Nd:YAG laser was 50 watts. Therefore, the area of tissue that was exposed during laser photocoagulation was very much smaller with the argon than with the Nd:YAG laser.

Based on the results of these experiments, Kiefhaber and his group have begun treating patients with severe upper gastrointestinal bleeding. They use Nd:YAG laser photocoagulation and have thus far reported an uncontrolled series of 106 bleeding patients [26]. They report a 93% success rate but have had 2 perforations related to Nd:YAG laser therapy. Dr. Kiefhaber had extended his experience to almost 600 patients at the time of this publication.

These studies are uncontrolled so that the expected rate of spontaneous cessation of bleeding is not known. No postmortem histologic data are available on patients who died after Nd:YAG laser photocoagulation.

Several research groups [8] including our own are experimenting with high-power Nd:YAG lasers. In a controlled randomized study, we compared the 55 watt Nd:YAG laser photocoagulator with the 7 watt CO_2-assisted argon laser photocoagulator in the treatment of massively bleeding acute canine gastric ulcers in heparinized dogs [38]. Although both lasers were 100% effective, the Nd:YAG laser produced full-thickness damage to the gastric wall in approximately 80% of treated ulcers. No full-thickness injuries were noted with the argon laser photocoagulator. Additional experiments were undertaken in an attempt to decrease the depth of tissue damage produced by Nd:YAG laser photocoagulation. Changes in the power, duration and presence of coaxial CO_2 failed to significantly decrease the tissue injury produced in this model by Nd:YAG laser photocoagulation. Studies are continuing in an attempt to make the Nd:YAG laser less damaging while preserving its tremendous hemostatic efficiency.

ELECTROCOAGULATION

Monopolar Electrocoagulation

For the past 50 years monopolar electrocoagulation has been a valuable adjunct to the operating surgeon. With this modality electrical current passes from a small active electrode through the patient to a wide dispersal plate (Fig. 2A). The high energy density at the small active electrode can heat tissue and produce coagulation.

Electrosurgical generators produce two types of current: coagulating current and cutting current. In the latter a continuous sine wave current causes rapid

A	B	C
Monopolar	Bipolar	Fulguration

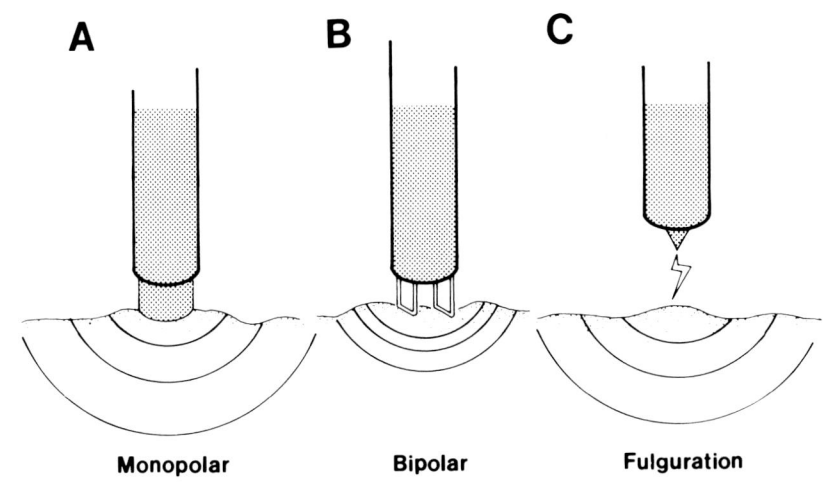

Fig. 2. Electrocoagulation.

tissue heating and dessication, favoring tissue incision without coagulation. In the former, repeated short bursts of high voltage current favor tissue dessication and coagulation without cutting. The coagulating wave form is most commonly used for hemostasis and was utilized in all of the studies which will be described.

Endoscopically deliverable monopolar electrocoagulation was first studied in 1974 by Blackwood et al [5]. They reported using a ball-tipped monopolar electrode to produce standard-sized lesions in canine intestinal tissue. These investigators felt that the diameter of mucosal blanching secondary to electrocoagulation was directly related to the depth of tissue necrosis. A similar study with a different electrode was performed by Papp et al on the esophageal, gastric and duodenal mucosa of dogs [30, 31]. This group concluded that the tissue damage produced by endoscopic monopolar electrocoagulation was directly related to the duration and pressure of electrode application, but that the diameter of mucosal blanching did not correlate with depth of tissue damage.

Neither group was able to precisely control or monitor the pressure or duration of electrode application, Also, these authors used different monopolar electrodes. The current density of the electrode tip, a parameter which may affect tissue damage, is related to the shape of the electrode and to the area in contact with the mucosa. In addition, these investigators were unable to measure the total energy delivered to the tissue during electrocoagulation. Different electrosurgical generators of the same model from the same manufacturer have different power outputs at identical settings [12].

In order to overcome these difficulties, Piercey et al reported the development and use of an analogue computer for experimental electrocoagulation [32]. The computer interfaces with a standard electrosurgical generator and is capable of monitoring the power, energy and duration of electrode application. Alternately, the computer can deliver a predetermined amount of energy by continuously adjusting the electrosurgical generator's voltage to compensate for changes in tissue impedance during electrocoagulation (Fig. 3).

This computer was used for a series of experiments in heparinized dogs undergoing laparotomy. An endoscopic monopolar electrode was modified to provide a reproducible area of tissue-electrode contact, and a hand-held force gauge was used to insure a reproducible electrode application pressure. In controlled randomized experiments using a standard-sized bleeding ulcer model [35], monopolar electrocoagulation was shown to be an effective hemostatic technique. However, the tissue damage produced was unpredictable; it was not related to the total energy (joules) applied to the ulcer, the number of electrode applications, or the rate of ulcer bleeding.

Clinical experience with endoscopic monopolar electrocoagulation has been limited. All reported studies are uncontrolled and nonrandomized. Gaisford [17], Papp [29], Sugawa et al [42], and Volpicelli et al [43] each report endoscopic monopolar electrocoagulation; hemostasis has been achieved in 87%-96% of bleeding upper gastrointestinal lesions. These authors report no complications, in contrast to a survey of German endoscopists showing an 80%-95% success rate for endoscopic monopolar electrocoagulation with a 1.8% perforation rate [41].

Monopolar Electrofulguration

In electrofulguration the monopolar electrode is in close proximity but does not touch the tissue. A spark jumps across a small gap to the surface being coagulated (Fig. 2C). Thermal energy may be deposited more superficially than with other electrocoagulation techniques because the electrode tip is not in contact with the tissue. The only randomized controlled experimental study of monopolar electrofulguration was reported by Dennis et al [7]. In a canine laparotomy model of acute gastric ulcer bleeding, electrofulguration treatment was compared at three different settings of the electrosurgical generator. The previously described analogue computer was used. During electrofulguration a jet of CO_2 gas was employed to blow away obscuring blood. At the three generator settings all treated ulcers stopped bleeding. After seven days when examined histologically, the mean injury to the muscularis externa following electrofulguration was 30%.

Dennis et al then performed an experiment to see whether they could reduce the depth of tissue damage from electrofulguration [7]. Because the fulguration spark is produced by ionization of the gas between the electrode and the tissue, a more easily ionizable gas might allow a spark to be generated with less power. Theoretically this might result in less damage during electrofulguration. Therefore, electrofulguration with CO_2 gas was compared to that with a 50/50 mixture of CO_2 and argon gas. Both produced effective hemostasis but there was

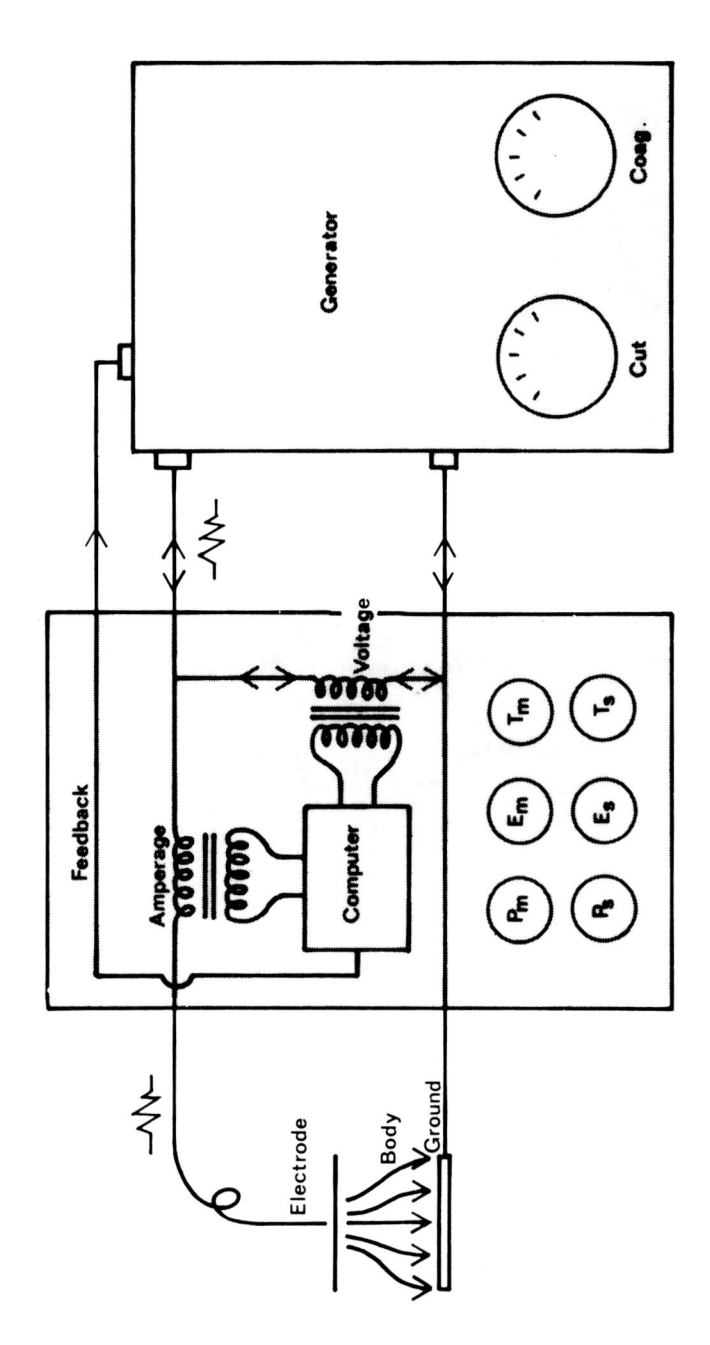

Fig. 3. Analogue computer for experimental electrocoagulation.

no significant reduction in the extent of tissue damage from adding argon to the CO_2 gas jet.

These authors concluded from their animal studies that electrofulguration is effective but that the tissue damage produced is unpredictable and deeper than with other available endoscopic methods. Electrofulguration is presently not being considered for clinical use.

Bipolar Electrocoagulation

In bipolar electrocoagulation two close active electrodes touch the tissue (Fig. 2B). Current passes between the two electrodes (≤3 mm apart for endoscopic use). Theoretically this provides more localized pathways and is the basis for the hypothesis that bipolar electrocoagulation may produce less tissue damage.

Published reports of endoscopically deliverable bipolar electrocoagulation use the Medi-tech electrode. In 1978 the effect of bipolar electrocoagulation on canine gastric mucosa was evaluated by Moore et al [27]. They studied normal gastric mucosa, gastric mucosa ulcerated 3 days earlier, and standard sized acute gastric ulcers made at laparotomy in heparinized dogs. The irrigant flow rate from the central channel of the bipolar electrode and pressure of the electrode application were not controlled, and the energy delivered to the tissue could not be quantified. Nevertheless, only 2 instances of full thickness damage to the gastric wall were observed in 87 lesions treated. This group also did uncontrolled nonrandomized experimental endoscopic comparisons of bipolar with monopolar electrocoagulation that showed monopolar electrocoagulation produced deeper tissue damage.

We have used the analogue computer to study the efficacy and resulting depth of tissue damage from endoscopically deliverable bipolar electrocoagulation [34]. Heparinized foxhounds were studied at laparotomy using the previously described acute bleeding gastric ulcer model. Pressure, duration of electrode application and energy per application were controlled. All ulcers treated with bipolar electrocoagulation stopped bleeding while the untreated controls did not. However, bipolar electrocoagulation produced occasional deep tissue damage. These investigators are now prospectively comparing bipolar and monopolar electrocoagulation using the same ulcer model and the analogue computer [33].

Experimental bipolar electrocoagulation has also been compared with argon laser photocoagulation in the treatment of bleeding canine gastric ulcers [21]. In randomized controlled laparotomy experiments all ulcers treated with either technique stopped bleeding. Chronic studies performed to compare the tissue damage produced by these two techniques suggested that bipolar electrocoagulation produced more histologic injury than argon laser photocoagulation. Energy delivered to the tissue during bipolar electrocoagulation was not monitored.

There are currently no reports of clinical endoscopic bipolar electrocoagulation using the flexible fiberendoscope.

REFERENCES

1. Allan R, Dykes P: A study of the factors influencing mortality rates from gastrointestinal haemorrhage. Q J Med 45:533, 1976
2. Auth DC, Lam TY, Mohr R, et al: A high-power gastric photocoagulator for endoscopy in Proceedings of the 27th Annual Conference on Engineering in Medicine and Biology. Philadelphia, 1974, p 84
3. Auth DC, Mohr RW: Safety considerations in endoscopic argon laser coagulation. In Proceedings of the 28th Annual Conference on Engineering in Medicine and Biology. New Orleans, 1975, p 518
4. Becker CD: Accident victim's view. Laser Focus, August 6, 1977
5. Blackwood WD, Silvis SE: Standardization of electrosurgical lesions. Gastrointest Endosc 21:22, 1974
6. Dehyle P, Blum AI, Nuesch HJ, et al: Emergency colonoscopy in the management of the acute peranal hemorrhage. Endoscopy 6:229, 1974
7. Dennis MB, Peoples J, Hulett R, et al: Evaluation of electrofulguration in control of bleeding experimental gastric ulcers. Dig Dis Sci 24:845, 1979
8. Dixon JA, Berenson MM, McCloskey DW: Neodymium-YAG laser treatment of experimental canine gastric bleeding. Acute and chronic studies of photocoagulation, penetration and perforation. Gastroenterology 77:647, 1979
9. Dwyer RM, Haberback BJ, Bass M, et al: Laser-induced hemostasis in the canine stomach. Use of a flexible fiberoptic delivery system. JAMA 231:486, 1975
10. Dwyer RM, Yellin AE, Craig J, et al: Gastric hemostasis by laser phototherapy in man. JAMA 236:1383, 1976
11. Eastwood GL: Does early endoscopy benefit the patient with active upper gastrointestinal bleeding? Gastroenterology 72:737, 1977
12. Ellefson DM: Development of an analog computing monitor for high frequency electrosurgery, MSEE Thesis, University of Washington, 1978
13. Fruhmorgen P, Bodem F, Reidenbach HD, et al: Endoscopic photocoagulation by laser irradiation in the gastrointestinal tract of man. Acta Hepatogastroenterol 25:1, 1978
14. Fruhmorgen P, Bodem F, Reidenbach HD, et al: The first successful endoscopic laser coagulations of bleeding and potential bleeding lesions in the human gastrointestinal tract (Abstr). Gastrointest Endosc 22:225, 1976
15. Fruhmorgen P, Kaduk B, Reidenbach HD, et al: Long-term observations in endoscopic laser coagulations in the gastrointestinal tract. Endoscopy 7:181, 1975
16. Fruhmorgen P, Reidenbach HD, Bodem F, et al: Experimental examinations on laser endoscopy. Endoscopy 6:116, 1974

17. Gaisford WD: Endoscopic electrohemostasis of active upper gastrointestinal bleeding. Am J Surg 137:47, 1979
18. Graham DY: The value of endoscopy in the management of acute upper gastrointestinal bleeding: A prospective controlled randomized study (Abstr). Gastroenterology 74:1125, 1978
19. Gulacsik C, Auth DC, Silverstein FE: Ophthalmic hazards associated with laser endoscopy. Appl Optics 18:1816, 1979
20. Himal HS, Watson WW, Jones CW, et al: The management of upper gastrointestinal hemorrhage: a multiparametric computer analysis. Ann Surg 179:489, 1974
21. Johnston JH, Jensen DM, Mautner W: A comparison of bipolar electrocoagulation and argon laser photocoagulation with coaxial CO_2 in the treatment of bleeding canine gastric ulcer (Abstr). Gastrointest Endosc 24:200, 1978
22. Katon RM: Experimental control of gastrointestinal hemorrhage via the endoscope: a new era dawns. Gastroenterology 70:272, 1976
23. Katon RM, Smith FW: Panendoscopy in the early diagnosis of acute upper gastrointestinal bleeding. Gastroenterology 65:728, 1973
24. Kiefhaber P, Nath G, Moritz K: Eigenschaften und Eignung verschiedener Laser-transmissions-systeme fur die endoskopische Blutstillung. In Proceedings of 7, Kongress fur gastroenterologische Endoskopie. Wien, September 1975, p 1
25. Kiefhaber P, Nath G, Moritz K: Endoscopical control of massive gastrointestinal hemorrhage by irradiation with a high-power neodymium YAG laser. Prog Surg 15:140, 1977
26. Kim V, Dreiling DA, Kark AE, et al: Factors influencing mortality in surgical treatment for massive gastroduodenal hemorrhage. Am J Gastroenterol 62:24, 1974
27. Moore JP, Silvis SE, Vennes JA: Evaluation of bipolar electrocoagulation in canine stomachs. Gastrointest Endosc 24:148, 1978
28. Nath G, Gorisch W, Kiefhaber P: First laser endoscopy via a fiberoptic transmission system. Endoscopy 5:208, 1973
29. Papp JP: Endoscopic electrocoagulation of upper gastrointestinal hemorrhage. JAMA 236:2076, 1976
30. Papp JP, Fox JM, Walbandian RM: Experimental electrocoagulation of dog esophageal and duodenal mucosa. Gastrointest Endosc 23:27, 1976
31. Papp JP, Fox JM, Wicks, HS: Experimental electrocoagulation of dog gastric mucosa. Gastrointest Endosc 22:27, 1975
32. Piercey JRA, Auth DC, Silverstein FE, et al: Electrosurgical treatment of experimental bleeding canine gastric ulcers. Development and testing of a computer control and a better electrode. Gastroenterology 74:527, 1978
33. Protell RL, Gilbert DA, Jensen DM, et al: Computer-assisted electrocoagulation: bipolar vs monopolar in the treatment of experimental gastric ulcer bleeding (Abstr). Gastroenterology 76:1221, 1979
34. Protell R, Jensen D, Silverstein F, et al: Efficacy and safety of computer-controlled bipolar electrocoagulation in experimental acute gastric ulcer bleeding (Abstr). Clin Res 26:151A, 1978

35. Protell RL, Silverstein FE, Piercey J, et al: A reproducible animal model of acute bleeding ulcer – the ulcer maker. Gastroenterology 71:961, 1976
36. Silverstein FE, Auth DC, Rubin CE, et al: High power argon laser treatment via standard endoscopes – I. A preliminary study of efficacy in control of experimental erosive bleeding. Gastroenterology 71:558, 1976
37. Silverstein F, Protell R, Auth D, et al: Comparison of high-power and low-power argon laser photocoagulation using an animal model of acute bleeding ulcer (Abstr). Gastroenterology 70:938, 1976
38. Silverstein FE, Protell RL, Gilbert DA, et al: Argon vs neodymium YAG laser photocoagulation of experimental canine gastric ulcers. Gastroenterology 77:491, 1979
39. Silverstein FE, Protell RL, Gulacsik C, et al: Endoscopic laser treatment III: the development and testing of a gas-jet-assisted argon laser waveguide in control of bleeding experimental ulcers. Gastroenterology 74:232, 1978
40. Silverstein FE, Protell RL, Piercey J, et al: Endoscopic laser treatment II: comparison of the efficacy of high and low power photocoagulation in control of severely bleeding experimental ulcers in dogs. Gastroenterology 73:481, 1977
41. Stadelmann O, Weisbart D, Zeus U: Blutende Lasionen im Gastrointestinaltrakt Elektrokoagulation. Symposium, Operative Endoscopie. Erlangen, 1977
42. Sugawa C, Shier M, Lucas CE, et al: Electrocoagulation of bleeding in the upper part of the gastrointestinal tract: a preliminary experimental clinical report. Arch Surg 10:975, 1975
43. Volpicelli MA, McCarthy JD, Bartlett JD, et al: Endoscopic electrocoagulation: an alternative to operative therapy in bleeding peptic ulcer disease. Arch Surg 113:483, 1978
44. Waitman AM, Spira I, Chryssanthou CP, et al: Endoscopic argon laser photocoagulation in the control of experimental gastric bleeding (Abstr). Gastrointest Endosc 22:236, 1976
45. Waitman AM, Spira I, Chryssanthou CP, et al: Fiberoptic coupled argon laser in the control of experimentally produced gastric bleeding. Gastrointest Endosc 22:7881, 1975

Kyung J. Cho, M.D.
Douglass F. Adams, M.D.

Therapeutic Angiography in Gastrointestinal Hemorrhage

ABSTRACT

Therapeutic angiography for gastrointestinal hemorrhage has made significant progress in the past several years. It is becoming an accepted therapeutic modality for many etiologies of gastrointestinal hemorrhage.

Vasopressin infusion and selective arterial embolization are the standard techniques that have been used. Intraarterial vasopressin infusion has successfully controlled bleeding from gastroesophageal varices, hemorrhagic gastritis, Mallory-Weiss tears and colonic diverticula. Selective arterial embolization is more effective in arresting bleeding from peptic ulcers or tumors.

Reported complications of selective embolization and of vasopressin infusion have been few. An interdisciplinary approach and total commitment of the angiographer are prerequisites to successful management of the patient with massive gastrointestinal hemorrhage.

With the technical improvements of selective angiography in recent years, superselective catheterization of visceral arteries has become possible. Utilizing this subselective technique, either embolic materials or vasoconstrictive agents can now be selectively delivered to the vessels supplying sites of gastrointestinal hemorrhage. The basic angiographic methods that have been used for control of gastrointestinal hemorrhage are: (1) infusion of a vasoconstrictive agent, generally vasopressin; (2) selective embolization; and (3) other occlusive methods including balloon catheterization and electrocoagulation. Over the past several years considerable clinical experience has accumulated in regard to the selection of the proper angiographic method and therapeutic agents [10, 28, 30, 33, 45].

Kyung J. Cho, M.D.: Associate Professor, Department of Radiology, and Director, Division of Cardiovascular Radiology, University of Michigan Medical Center; Douglass F. Adams, M.D.: Professor and Chairman, Department of Radiology, University of Michigan Medical Center, Ann Arbor, Michigan.

The guidelines for selection of vasopressin infusion or embolization in the management of gastrointestinal hemorrhage have been outlined [3]. This chapter will present an overview of clinical indications, angiographic techniques, results and complications of therapeutic angiography in gastrointestinal hemorrhage.

ANGIOGRAPHIC METHODS FOR CONTROL OF UPPER GASTROINTESTINAL HEMORRHAGE

Intraarterial Vasopressin Infusion

Vasoconstrictive agents that have been used for infusion therapy are vasopressin and epinephrine [40, 48]. Vasopressin constricts small arteries and arterioles by direct action on the smooth muscle of the vessels. Continuous intraarterial infusion at a low dosage produces persistent mesenteric arterial vasoconstriction without significant ischemic complications. Epinephrine is a potent vasoconstrictor for the celiac artery and its branches, but it is less effective in the mesenteric circulation because of the vasodilatory beta receptor effect. Vascular dilatation caused by the beta effect of epinephrine can be blocked by preinfusion or simultaneous administration of propranolol [48]. Because of the cardiac effect of epinephrine and propranolol, vasopressin has become the drug of choice for intraarterial vasoconstrictive therapy for gastrointestinal hemorrhage.

It has been shown that both intravenous and mesenteric arterial vasopressin infusion at the same dose have similar effects on mesenteric and portal flow [5, 24]. This has led to the current trend of the use of intravenous prior to intraarterial vasopressin infusion in the management of variceal bleeding. Intraarterial infusion as close as possible to the bleeding artery is beneficial to achieve successful control of nonvariceal, arterial or mucosal bleeding [48].

The infusion technique for vasopressin has been well established [3, 6, 7]. The generally accepted dosage of vasopressin is 0.2 U/min. Repeat angiography 20-30 minutes after infusion of vasopressin at 0.2 U/min is performed to evaluate the status of bleeding and the degree of vasoconstriction. The dosage is then adjusted accordingly. The dose of vasopressin can be increased to 0.3 or 0.4 U/min if bleeding persists. When bleeding persists at the dose of 0.4 U/min, or higher, an alternate procedure, either embolization or operation, should be considered. The duration of infusion at the adjusted dose is generally from 12 to 24 hours. When clinical signs indicate the cessation of hemorrhage, the dose rate is reduced to half of the initial dose for the next 12 hours and is replaced by infusion of normal saline for the following 6-12 hours before the catheter is removed.

Patients who are being treated with vasopressin should be closely monitored in the intensive care unit for any sign of complication. Angiographers should have a primary responsibility in the care of the infusion catheter and in the adjustment of the vasoconstrictor dosage during the entire course of infusion therapy. When intestinal ischemia is suspected or bleeding recurs, repeat angiography should be immediately performed for reassessment of bleeding and catheter position. If recurrent bleeding occurs during adequate infusion, an alternative treatment is indicated.

The location, degree and etiology of bleeding are important factors in the success of vasopressin in gastrointestinal hemorrhage. Coagulation defect has a definite role in the success and survival rate of the patient with variceal bleeding who undergoes infusion therapy [32].

Vasopressin has been most successful in controlling hemorrhage from hemorrhagic gastritis, stress ulcers and Mallory-Weiss tears (Figs. 1 and 2). Intraarterial vasopressin has controlled bleeding in 17 of the 22 reported cases (77%) of Mallory-Weiss tears [2-4, 19, 24, 38, 40] and in 40 of the 49 cases (82%) of acute gastric mucosal hemorrhage previously reported [2, 19, 38, 48].

Vasopressin therapy is less effective when the bleeding artery is large. This method has controlled bleeding in 7 of the 23 cases (30%) of peptic ulcers [20, 38, 48]. The bleeding artery in peptic ulcer disease responds poorly to vasopressin because it is generally large and is often associated with inflammatory reaction. A recent report by Waltman et al [56] also indicated a low control rate (31%) in pyloroduodenal peptic ulcer bleeding by intraarterial vasopressin. Ring, et al [46] emphasized the rationale of frequent therapeutic failures by vasopressin infusion when bleeding arises from a branch of dual blood supply such as duodenum or splenic flexure of the colon. When infusion of one limb of a vascular arcade fails, both limbs may have to be infused to achieve successful arrest of hemorrhage.

Vasopressin therapy has some disadvantages when compared with embolization. An intraarterial catheter has to be placed for several hours to several days, which may cause arterial thrombosis or hematoma at the puncture site. Repeat angiographic examinations are frequently required to secure catheter position and to prevent infusion of unintended vessels. Fortunately, the incidence of side effects from the pharmacologic action of vasopressin is low and can be easily managed by medical treatment or minimized by reducing dosage. Ischemic complication is unlikely to occur if excessive vasoconstriction is avoided by adjusting the dose of vasopressin.

The advantages of vasopressin are that subselective catheterization may not be necessary and ischemic complications rarely occur. Vasopressin infusion into celiac or common hepatic arteries can be performed since the hepatic artery is known to escape from the vasoconstrictive effect of vasopressin [21].

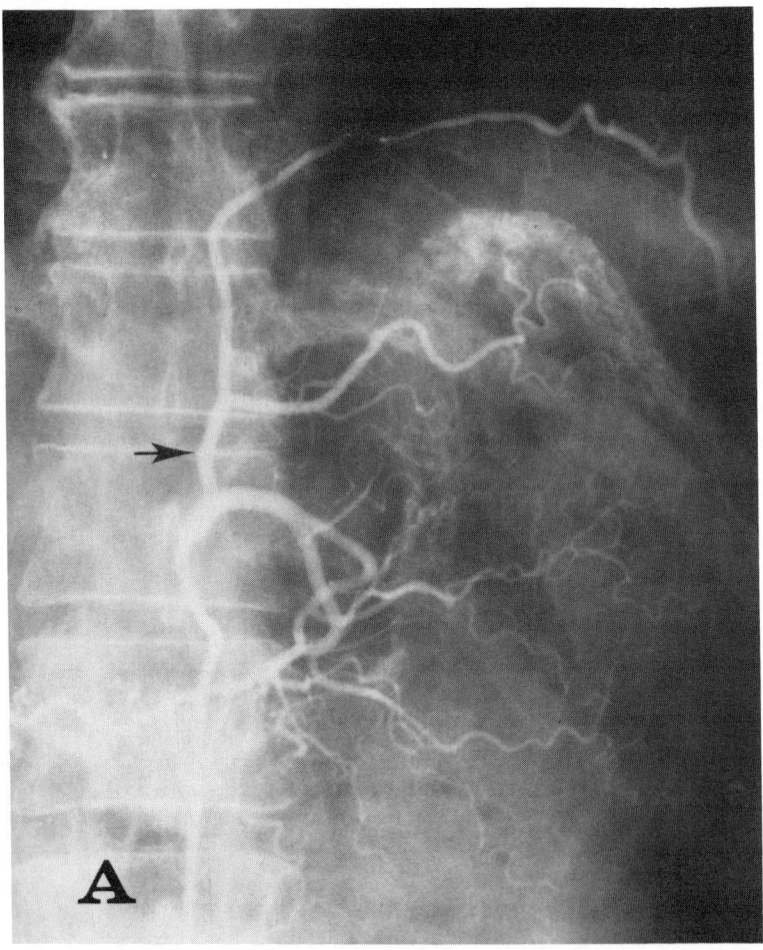

Fig. 1. Gastric hemorrhage in 56-year-old man with gastric mucosal erosion controlled with intraarterial vasopressin infusion. (A) Left gastric arteriogram (arterial phase) shows irregular gastric arterial branches with increased contrast accumulation. Left inferior phrenic artery originates from the left gastric artery (arrow). (B, right) Repeat angiogram, 20 minutes postintraarterial vasopressin infusion (0.2 U/min), shows marked arterial vasoconstriction of left gastric arterial branches without contrast stain in gastric wall. The inferior phrenic artery shows no vasoconstrictive response to vasopressin.

THERAPEUTIC ANGIOGRAPHY

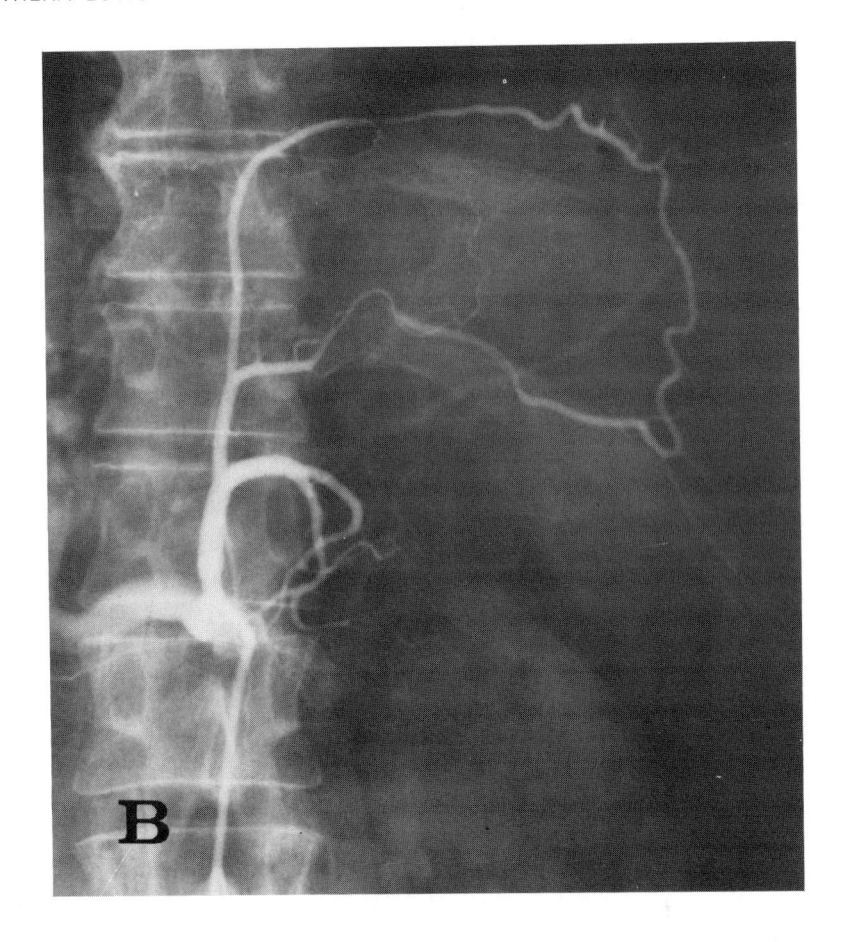

Selective Arterial Embolization

Selective arterial embolization technique was first introduced by Rösch et al in 1972 [49]. Since then the technique has become a well accepted method for control of massive gastrointestinal hemorrhage and used as an alternative to vasopressin infusion [10, 16, 28, 29, 33, 45]. Therapeutic arterial embolization should be performed in organs with rich collateral circulation, such as the stomach and duodenum. Combined therapy with embolization and vasopressin should be avoided, particularly in patients who have had resection, since such a combination has caused tissue necrosis [12, 43]. Embolization of a vessel should not be performed unless a discrete extravasation of contrast medium is demonstrated on angiogram.

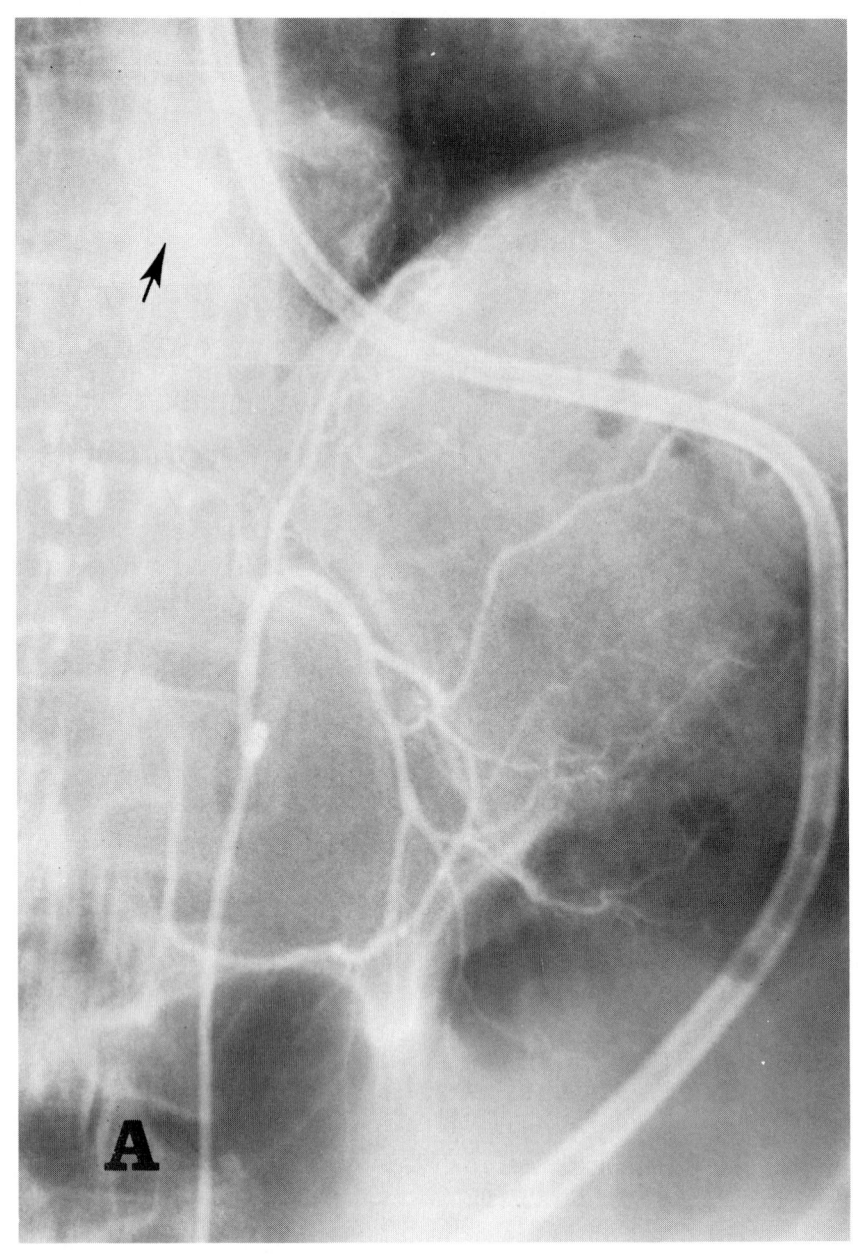

Fig. 2A. Selective left gastric arteriogram in 37-year-old man with chronic renal disease and esophageal mucosal erosion demonstrates extravasation of contrast medium in the distal esophagus (arrow).

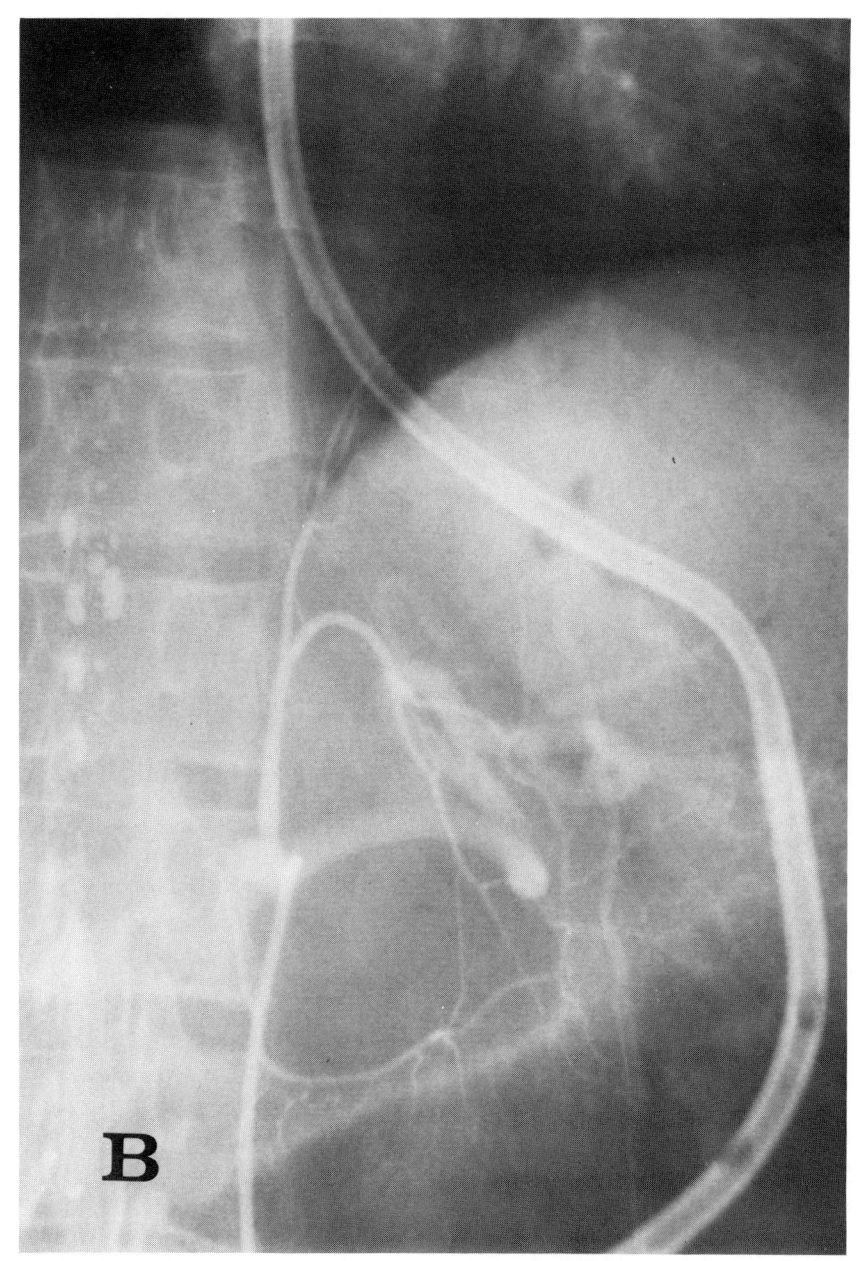

Fig. 2B. Repeat angiogram 15 minutes post-intraarterial vasopressin infusion (0.1 U/min) reveals arrest of hemorrhage. Left gastric arterial branches are moderately constricted.

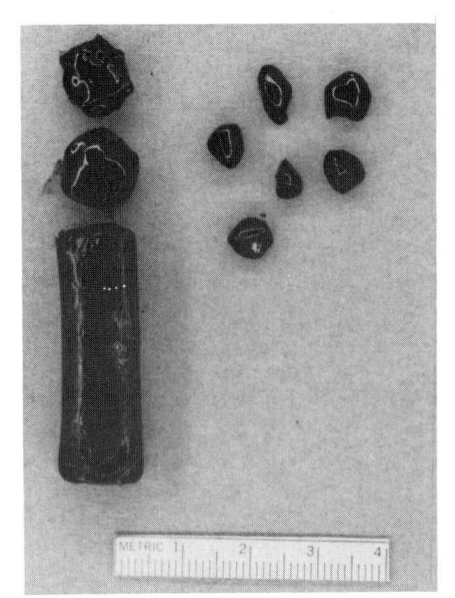

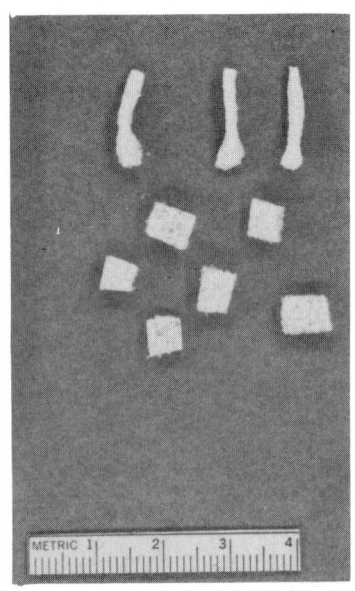

Fig. 3. (A, left) Autogenous clots (Amicar clot) used for selective arterial embolization. Clot (left) was made by withdrawing 9 cc of the patient's blood into a 10 cc glass syringe containing 1.0 cc of epsilon aminocaproic acid (Amicar). Clot is removed from syringe and cut into 5 mm pieces (right) which are then loaded into a 1.0 ml tuberculin syringe for embolization. Approximately 0.3-0.5 ml of the clot is initially injected into selectively placed angiographic catheter. Contrast medium is used to push the clot into bleeding artery using the same tuberculin syringe under close fluoroscopic monitor. (B, right) Absorbable gelatin sponge (Gelfoam) and its pellets used for arterial and variceal embolization. Gelfoam strip is removed from package and cut into small pieces of various sizes and shapes (right). One or a few pellets are loaded in 1.0 ml tuberculin syringe and injected into vessel to be occluded with contrast medium. Judicious injection of Gelfoam in as small amount as possible is made under constant fluoroscopic monitor to avoid reflux of embolic agent.

Various materials have been used for embolic occlusion of the bleeding artery including autologous clot, absorbable gelatine sponge (Gelfoam), Oxycel, polyvinyl alcohol (Ivalon) and isobutyl 2-cyanoacrylate (Bucrylate). Autologous clot (Fig. 3A) is a short acting agent generally used for small arterial hemorrhage; its rapid lysis in 30 minutes to 2 hours may cause rebleeding. Gelfoam (Fig. 3B) is an ideal material when the bleeding artery is large or when longer duration of occlusion is desired. It has been particularly useful for embolization of bleeding tumors [31].

Patients with gastrointestinal hemorrhage embolized at the University of Michigan Medical Center from 1973 to 1978 are summarized in Table 1.

Table 1
Patients With Gastrointestinal Hemorrhage Treated With Embolization
at University of Michigan Medical Center (1973 − 1978)

Source	No. of Patients Embolized	Successful Control
Mallory-Weiss tears	3	3
Hemorrhagic gastritis	5	1
Gastroduodenal bleeding (mostly ulcers, 1 leiomyoma)	19	18
Jejunal bleeding	4	4
Colonic bleeding (abscess, tumor)	2	2
Variceal bleeding	5	5
Total	38	33

Selective embolization has controlled bleeding in 14 of the 15 reported (93%) of Mallory-Weiss tears [10, 14, 23, 28, 29, 33, 45]. This is higher than the control rate of vasopressin infusion (77%). Vasopressin infusion should be attempted first for bleeding Mallory-Weiss tears. Embolic technique, which is reserved for those patients who did not respond to vasopressin therapy, has been successful in controlling bleeding from peptic ulcers (90%) [10, 25, 27-29, 33] (Figs. 4 and 5), whereas it arrested bleeding in 6 of the 11 patients (55%) with acute gastric mucosal hemorrhage [29, 33, 45].

Because of frequent failure of vasopressin infusion to control bleeding from gastrointestinal neoplasms, transcatheter arterial embolization has been particularly useful in such patients (30). We have successfully embolized the anterior superior pancreaticoduodenal artery for a bleeding duodenal leiomyoma and inferior mesenteric artery for a bleeding colonic metastatic tumor. Gelfoam was the embolic material used in both patients, and no ischemic complication was encountered.

Selective hepatic artery embolization for control of hemobilia has been reported [55]. Reports have indicated that hepatic artery embolization can be performed without significant parenchymal damage [17, 54].

Balloon Catheter

The use of a balloon catheter for control of hemorrhage has been described [57]. Over the past several years the technology of balloon catheters has advanced and they are manufactured in various sizes. The balloon catheter can be introduced selectively using the conventional angiographic technique. Balloons as small as a No. 3 or 4 French have become available and they can be used coaxially to achieve occlusion of smaller arterial branches. One of the advantages of the balloon catheter is that immediate occlusion of a large artery can be easily accomplished. However, the development of collateral vessels distal to balloon occlusion may lead to recurrence of bleeding.

Electrocoagulation

Transarterial electrocoagulation is the most recently introduced technique for arterial occlusive therapy [26]. Electrocoagulation of the vessel is accomplished through a guidewire introduced into the angiographic catheter and an alternating current is used. The effectiveness and safety of the technique have not been established and clinical experience is limited.

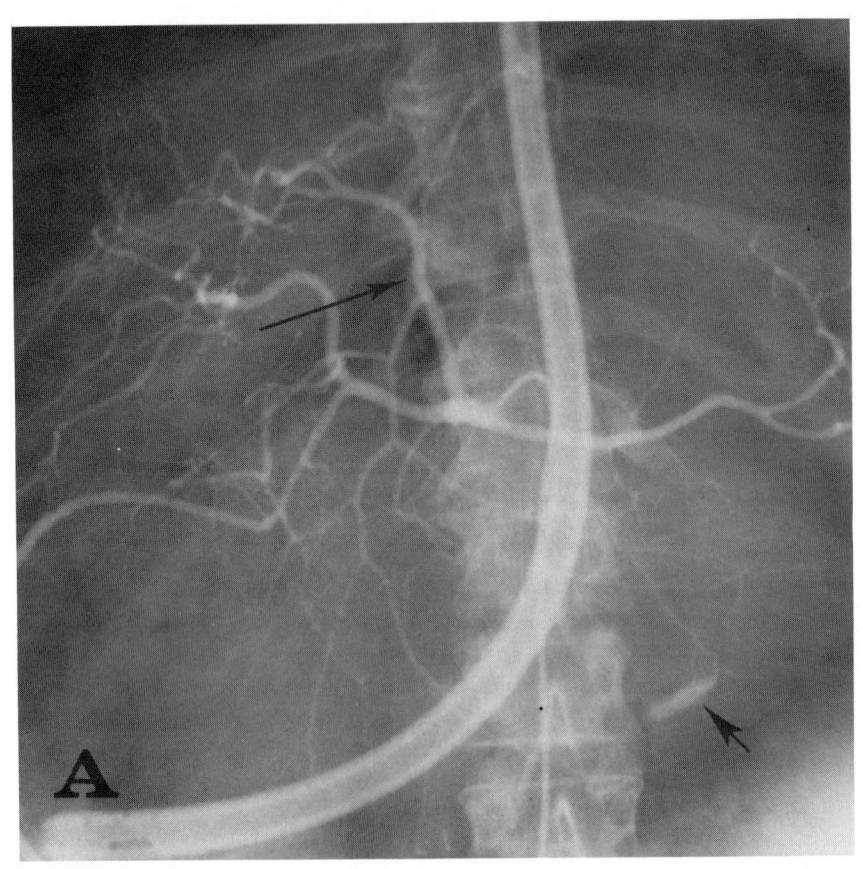

Fig. 4. A 50-year-old woman with 20% burn and massive gastric hemorrhage. (A) Selective celiac angiogram shows extravasation of contrast medium (short arrow) in gastric body. Left hepatic artery (long arrow) arises from left gastric artery. (B, right) Repeat angiogram after embolization with Gelfoam demonstrates complete control of hemorrhage with occlusion of multiple gastric branches (arrows). Bleeding did not recur for two months, when patient died of systemic disease.

B

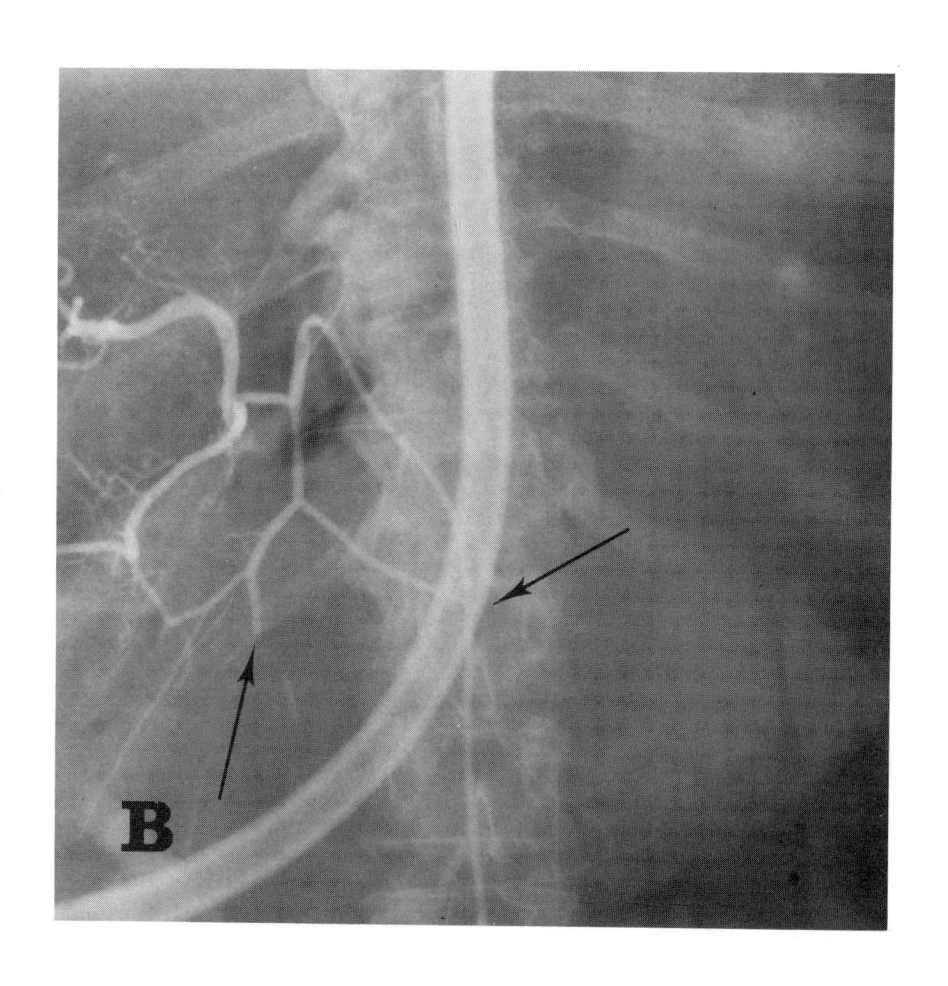

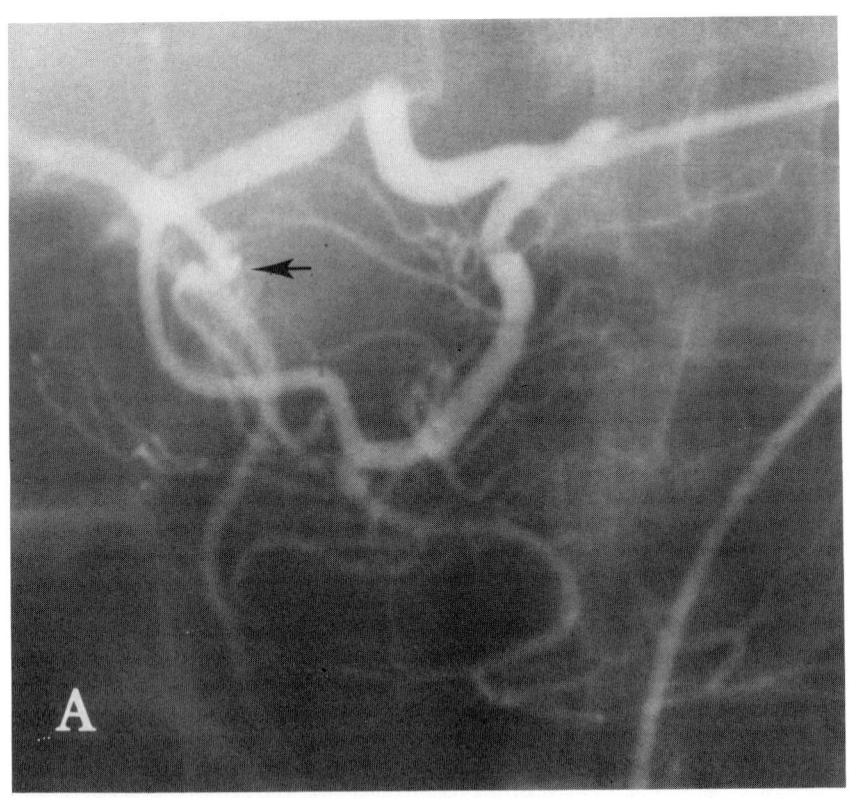

Fig. 5A. Selective gastroduodenal arteriogram in 68-year-old man with massive upper gastrointestinal hemorrhage demonstrates extravasation of contrast medium in proximal duodenum (arrow).

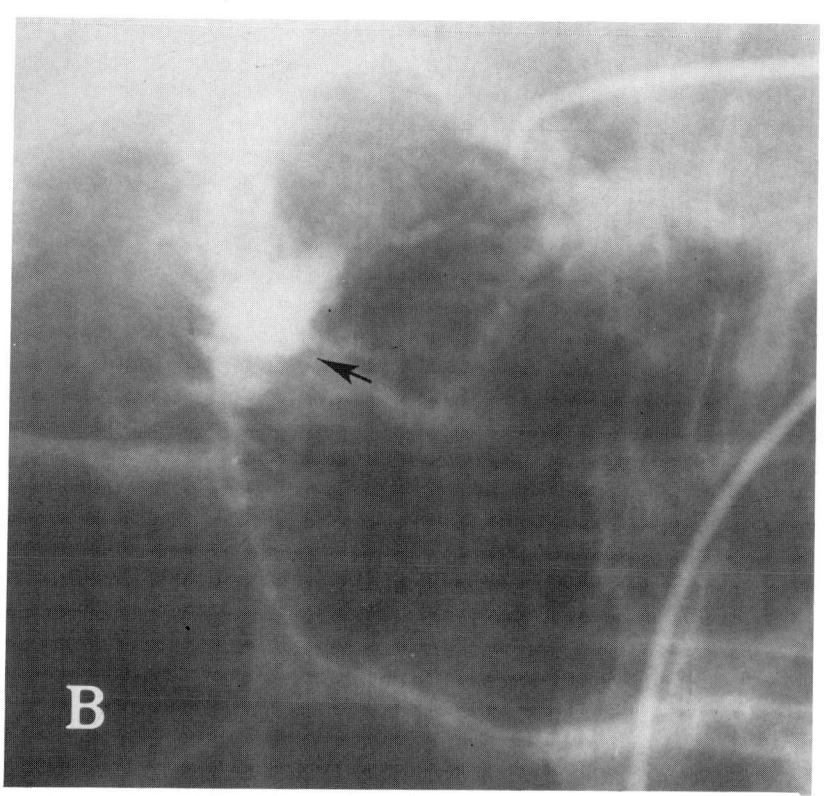

Fig. 5B. Venous phase of the same angiogram shows duodenal mucosal fold outlined by extravasated contrast medium (arrow).

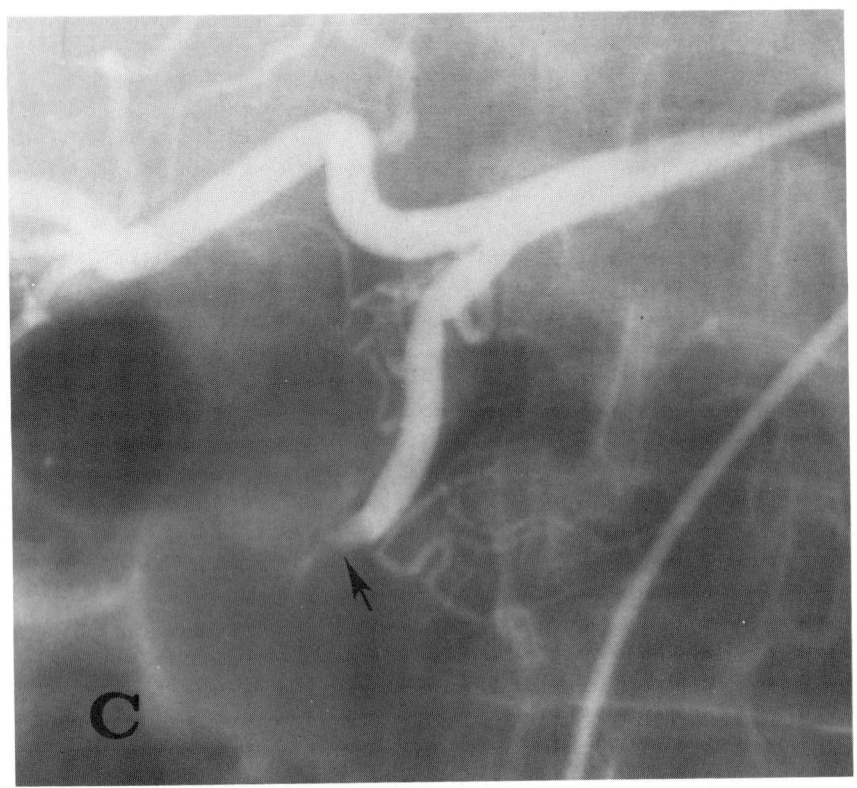

Fig. 5C. Repeat angiogram following embolization with autogenous clot shows cessation of hemorrhage and occlusion of the distal gastroduodenal artery (arrow).

Control of Variceal Bleeding by Coronary Vein Embolization

Percutaneous transhepatic portal vein catheterization and obliteration of gastroesophageal varices is an effective method for control of active bleeding from varices [34, 36, 53]. This technique is indicated for those who fail to respond to conventional treatment and for those who are not surgical candidates for portasystemic shunt procedure (Fig. 6).

Viamonte et al [53] reported successful obliteration of varices in all of 32 patients bleeding actively. Successful control was achieved in 5 of the 6 patients by Lunderquist et al [35]. This method is generally considered as a palliative, temporarily effective treatment for patients with bleeding varices. Following embolic obliteration of varices, hemorrhage may recur because of recanalization of the embolized varices or development of collaterals [28, 35].

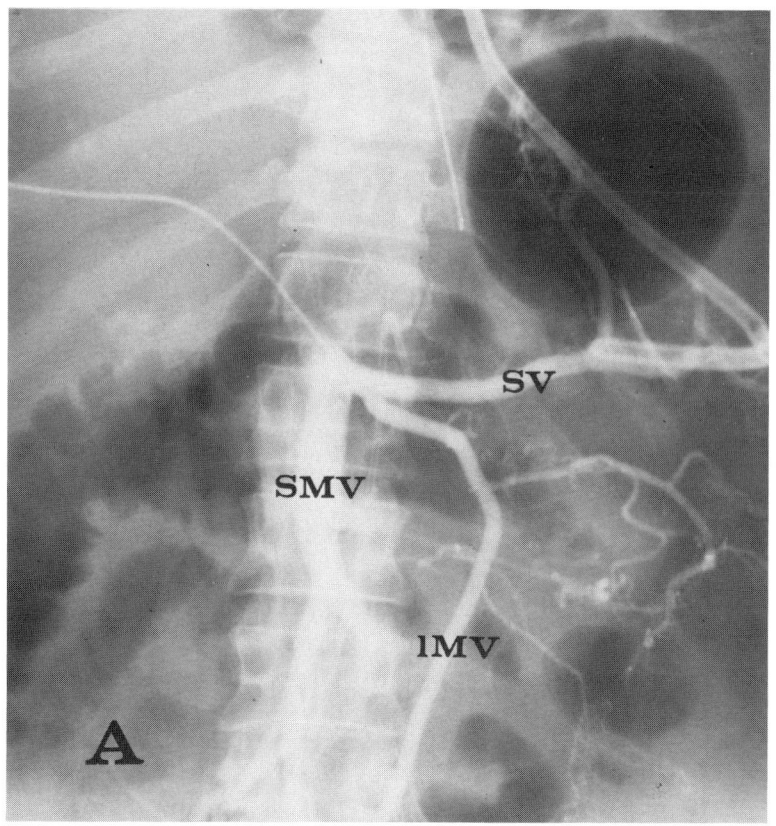

Fig. 6. Percutaneous transhepatic coronary vein embolization in 47-year-old man with massive gastroesophageal variceal bleeding who failed to respond to therapy with Sengstaken-Blakemore tube and intravenous vasopressin infusion. (A) Transhepatic portography demonstrates retrograde filling of superior mesenteric (SMV), inferior mesenteric (IMV) and splenic (SV) veins. Portal vein is not opacified due to reversed portal venous flow. (B) Selective injection of coronary vein following deflation of balloons shows visualization of large gastroesophageal varices. (C) Portography after embolization with Gelfoam, 50% glucose and 1.0 cc thrombin shows complete obliteration of the varices. Portal vein is partially thrombosed. Previously visualized inferior mesenteric vein is not filled, suggesting occlusion. Intrahepatic portal vein radicles are seen following coronary vein embolization.

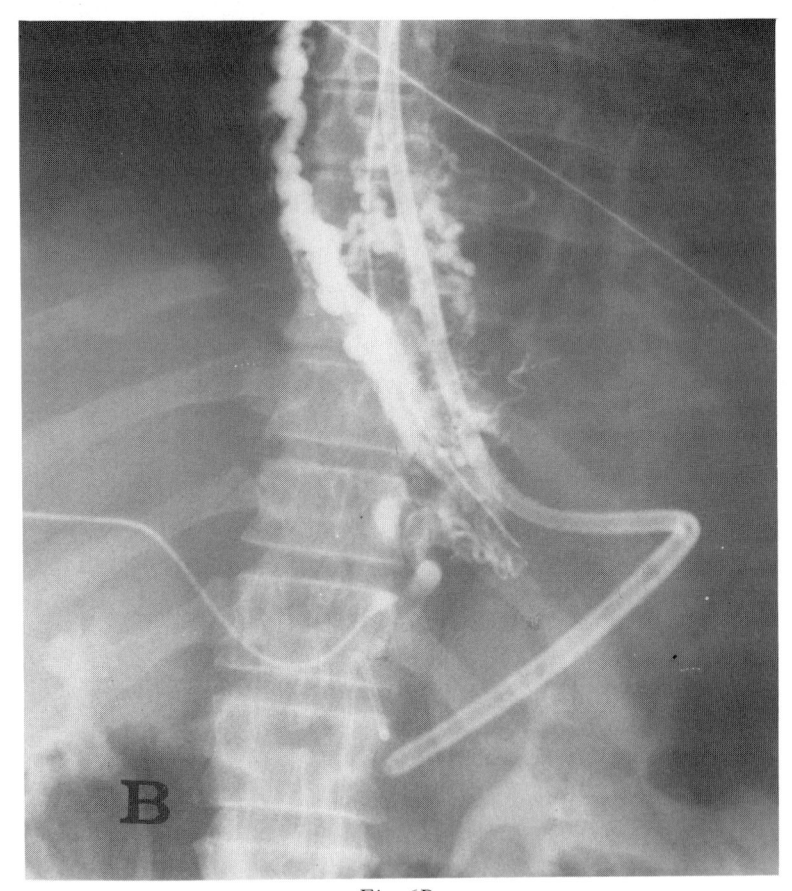

Fig. 6B.

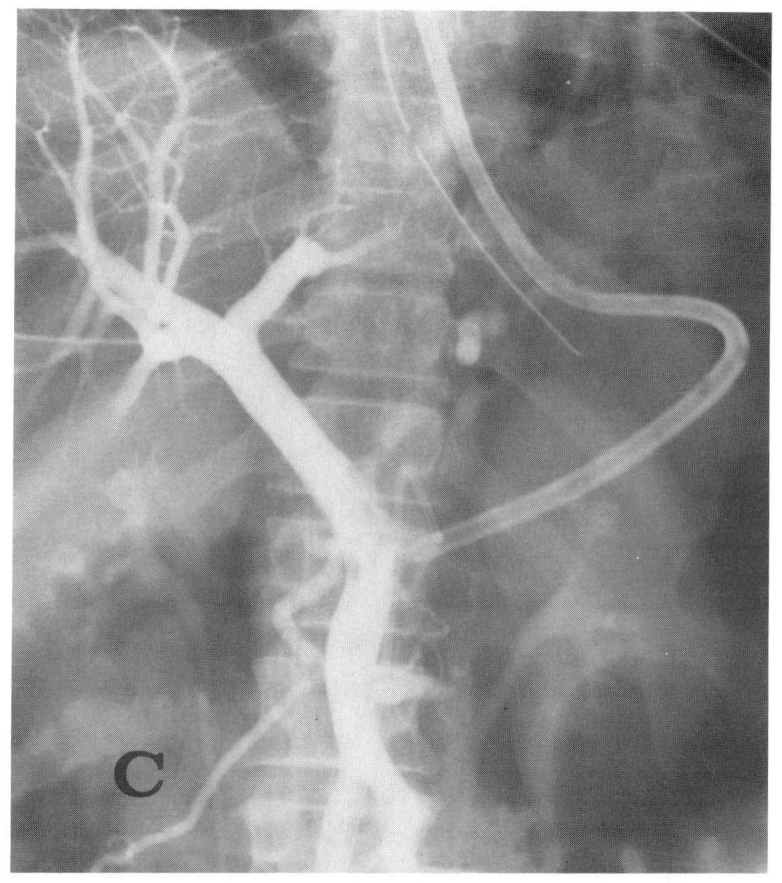

Fig. 6C.

Follow-up studies 1 month to 3 years after embolization showed persistent occlusion in all of the 10 patients studied in one series [53], while recanalization of the previously occluded varices was observed in 13 of the 16 patients in another series [35]. A recent report also indicated that follow-up examination 1-12 months later showed recanalization in 6 of the 8 patients embolized with isobutyl 2-cyanoacrylate [34]. The difference in the incidence of recanalization in two previous reports is probably secondary to different materials being used for variceal obliteration.

The inactive bleeders who are poor surgical risks or who refuse operation have been treated with transhepatic coronary vein embolization. Patients treated with this technique may undergo elective portasystemic shunt procedure or may be followed. For those who had recurrent bleeding after embolization, repeat embolization can be performed.

Transhepatic, umbilical and transjugular routes have been used to catheterize the portal vein and its tributaries. The transhepatic approach from the midaxillary line is preferred. The portal vein can easily be catheterized through a portacaval or a mesocaval shunt. We have successfully embolized a coronary vein through a stenotic mesocaval graft from a percutaneous transfemoral approach in 2 patients (Fig. 7). Various materials have been used for obliteration of gastroesophageal varices including autogenous clots, Gelfoam, thrombin, balloons, Bucrylate, and sclerosing agents (50% dextrose, Keflin and Sotradecol). Bucrylate seems to be an ideal agent but requires angiographic experience for use. In addition, the agent is still considered to be an experimental drug and is not readily available. Gelfoam soaked with sclerosing agent (Sotradecol) has

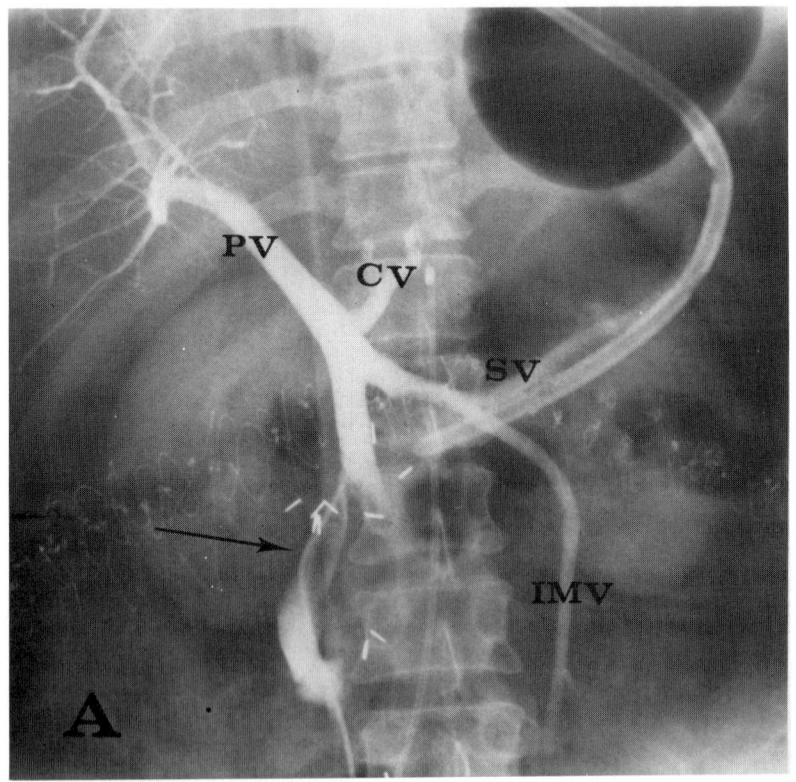

Fig. 7A. Portogram through the stenotic mesocaval shunt (arrow) in 41-year-old man with variceal bleeding, after mesocaval shunt demonstrates retrograde opacification of coronary (CV), splenic (SV) and inferior mesenteric (IMV) veins. The twisted mesocaval graft caused incomplete decompression of portal hypertension (portal vein pressure 49.0 cm saline). PV, portal vein.

THERAPEUTIC ANGIOGRAPHY 221

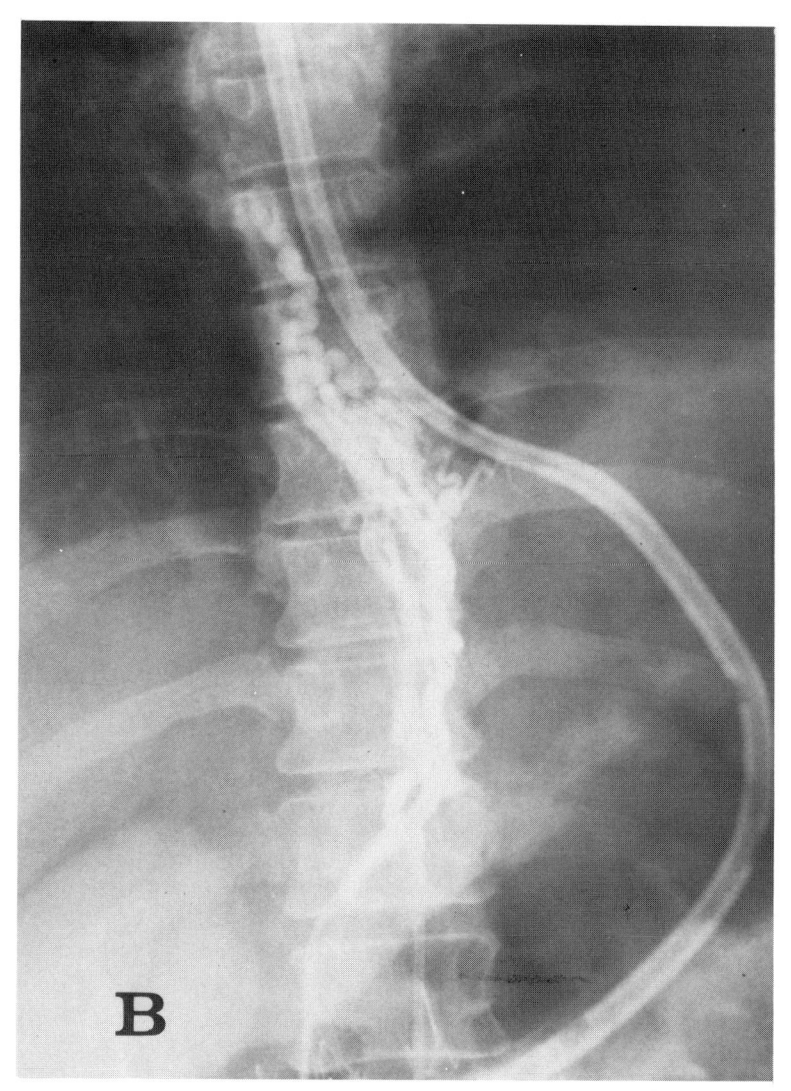

Fig. 7B. Selective injection into coronary vein shows large gastroesophageal varices.

been the most commonly used embolic agent and also proved to be effective [53].

Contraindications of the transhepatic approach include severe coagulopathy (prolonged prothrombin time, platelet count below 50,000), massive ascites and vascular tumor along the path of the catheter.

Transhepatic coronary vein embolization has proved to be an effective angiographic method for temporary control of variceal bleeding. It can be

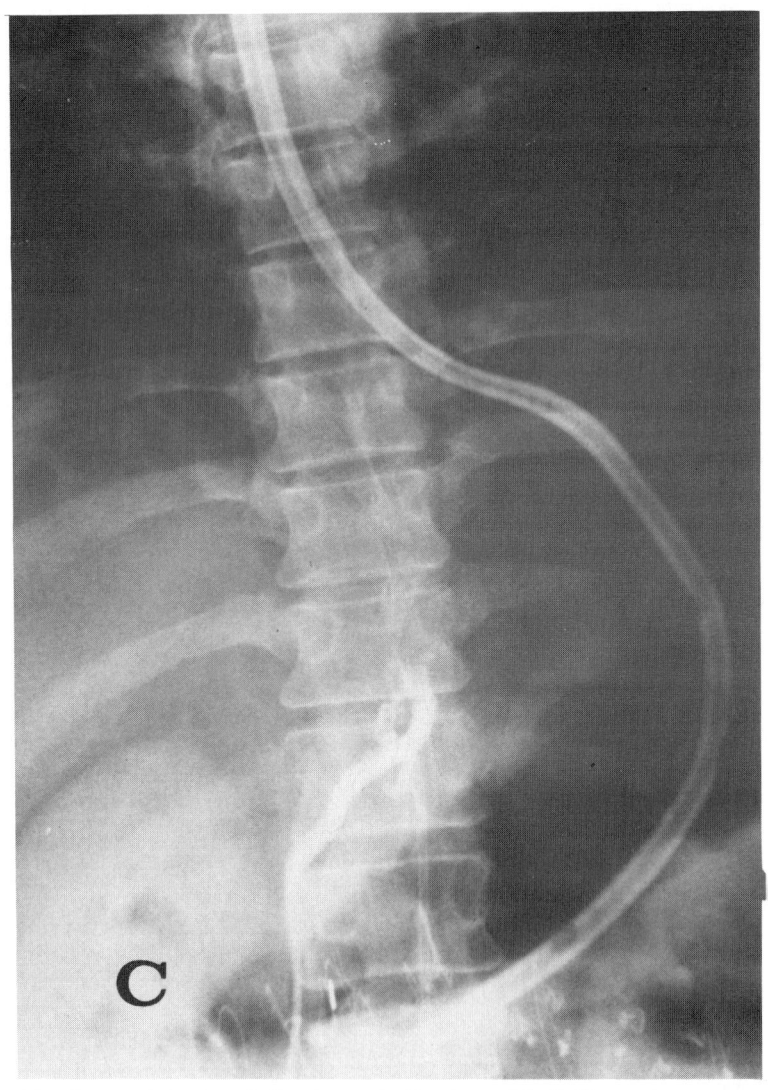

Fig. 7C. Repeat injection following embolization with Gelfoam shows complete obliteration of the gastroesophageal varices and bleeding successfully controlled.

performed on both active and inactive bleeders. Long-term follow-up studies in patients treated with embolization of coronary vein are limited and its role in managing variceal bleeding compared with portasystemic shunt is not definitely defined.

ANGIOGRAPHIC METHODS FOR CONTROL OF LOWER GASTROINTESTINAL HEMORRHAGE

Intraarterial Vasopressin

Vasopressin infusion is the primary angiographic method used to control bleeding from the small intestine and colon (Fig. 8). When a bleeding point is demonstrated on angiography, a catheter is placed in the superior mesenteric or

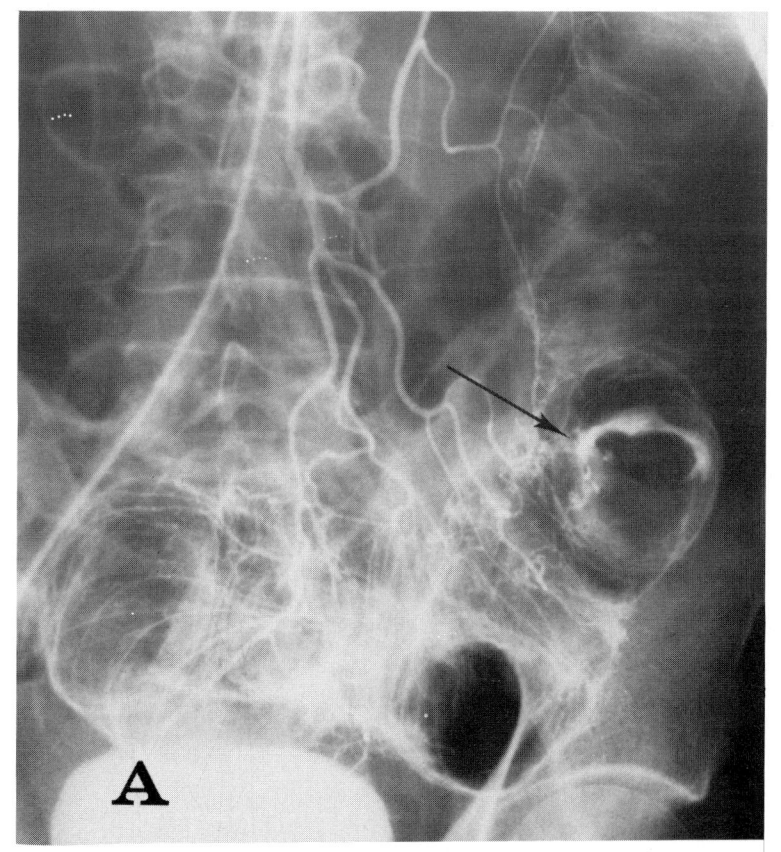

Fig. 8A. Inferior mesenteric angiogram in patient with massive rectal hemorrhage following colonoscopic polypectomy shows active extravasation of contrast medium in the distal descending colon (arrow).

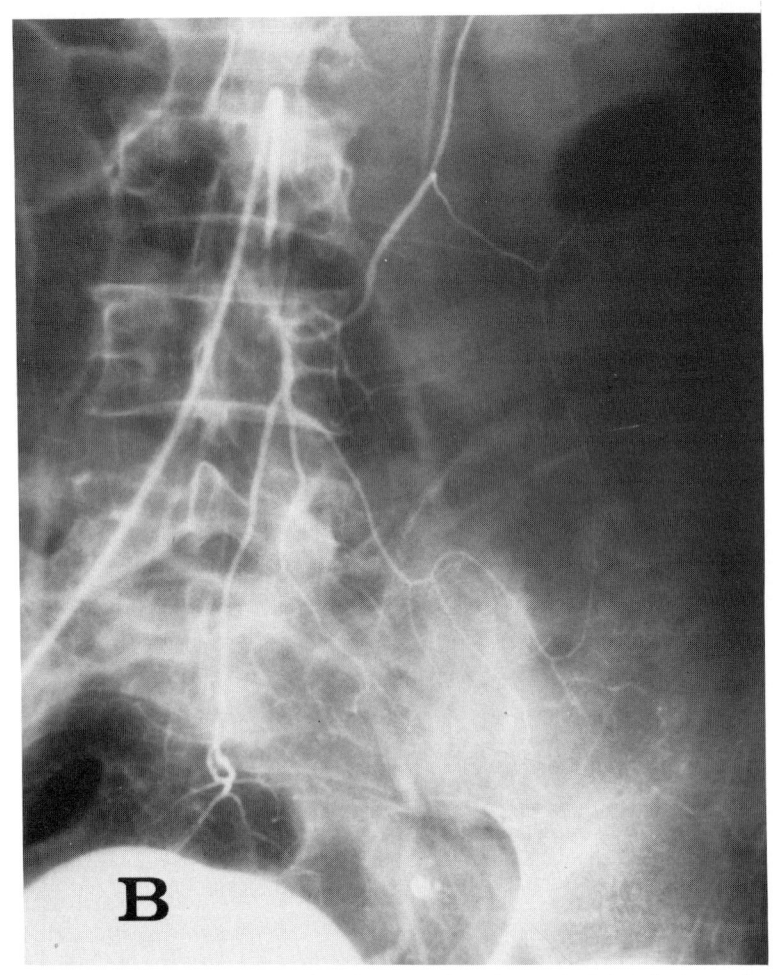

Fig. 8B. Repeat angiogram 30 minutes after intraarterial infusion of vasopressin, 0.2 U/min shows arrest of the bleeding.

inferior mesenteric artery depending on the location of the bleeding. The infusion technique is the same as described for upper gastrointestinal hemorrhage. Subselective infusion of the mesenteric branch is not generally necessary.

The most important use of intraarterial vasopressin in lower gastrointestinal hemorrhage has been control of diverticular hemorrhage of the colon. Vasopressin has controlled hemorrhage in 30 of the 33 patients (91%) with colonic diverticula [1, 6, 38, 48]. This high control rate of vasopressin therapy has virtually eliminated emergency surgery in diverticular bleeding, and, thus, elective surgery with segmental resection can be performed. Rebleeding after initial control of diverticular hemorrhage by vasopressin is reported to occur in one-fourth of patients [1]. This has led to elective operation following initial control of the bleeding by vasopressin or to the use of the embolic method.

Several cases of massive hemorrhage following endoscopic polypectomy of the colon have been successfully treated with vasopressin [4, 13]. Patients with bleeding from inflammatory bowel disease may respond poorly to vasopressin. Massive hemorrhage from ulcerative colitis and Crohn's disease reported in the literature responded to intraarterial vasopressin infusion [5, 42]. Our 2 patients with massive hemorrhage from Crohn's disease and ulcerative colitis also responded to intraarterial vasopressin.

Selective Arterial Embolization

Because of the occasional failure of vasopressin infusion to permanently or temporarily arrest hemorrhage, transcatheter embolization has been successfully performed in 3 patients with diverticular hemorrhage [11]. Selective mesenteric branch embolization has also controlled the bleeding from 3 cases of arteriovenous malformation, 1 ischemic colitis, 2 benign ulcers and 1 colonic tumor [11, 16, 31, 50]. Vasopressin infusion is usually ineffective in controlling bleeding from tumors and from larger arteries of the small intestine and colon.

Clinical and experimental studies have indicated that bowel ischemia and stricture are potential complications following mesenteric branch embolization, particularly when a longer acting material such as Gelfoam or Oxycel is used [10, 18]. Greater experience with long-term follow-up is necessary before mesenteric embolization can be safely used as an alternative to operation or vasopressin therapy.

COMPLICATIONS OF THERAPEUTIC ANGIOGRAPHY IN GASTROINTESTINAL HEMORRHAGE

Complications of Vasopressin Infusion

Complications secondary to vasopressin infusion have rarely occurred [2, 7]. Complications associated with an infusion catheter may include sepsis, femoral artery thrombosis and pseudoaneurysm. Complications from the pharmacological effect of vasopressin seem to be related to the dose of the drug. Early experiences in both humans and animals indicated no evidence of mesenteric ischemia following intraarterial vasopressin infusion [7]. However, with increased use of infusion therapy it has become evident that mesenteric arterial infusion can, on rare occasions, cause bowel damage [47]. Reported complications included hypertension, myocardial ischemia, portal and mesenteric vein thrombosis, mesenteric arterial thrombosis and gangrene of the feet [7, 8, 20, 32, 44, 52]. The cardiac complications included bradycardia, ventricular fibrillation, cardiac infarction and arrest. Water retention and hyponatremia also occur because of increased water absorption by the antidiuretic effect of the drug [37].

Since vasoconstrictive complications of vasopressin seem to be associated with the dose administered, the smallest possible dose of vasopressin should be used. When a larger dose is required for control of hemorrhage, close clinical observation is important and frequent angiographic follow-up is necessary to evaluate the degree of vasoconstriction and bleeding. Alternatives such as embolization or surgical intervention should be considered when the bleeding is not easily arrested with infusion therapy.

Complications of Selective Arterial Embolization

Embolic complications in general include those related to occlusion of the embolized vessels and those caused by inadvertent embolization. Complications of the former are rare because embolization is generally performed in organs with abundant collateral circulation. Gastric infarction following left gastric embolization has been reported in 2 instances [12, 43]. Ischemic complications of the duodenum and the afferent loop of jejunum were encountered following embolization of gastroduodenal and jejunal arteries with Oxycel, respectively [10]. Prior operation and simultaneous vasopressin infusion increase the likelihood of ischemic complication of embolization.

Inadvertent embolization secondary to reflux of excessive embolic agent has caused infarction of the liver and kidney, and gangrene of the feet [51, 58]. Careful injection of a small amount of embolic materials through a catheter placed as close as possible to the bleeding point should alleviate a complication of the latter type. Safe and successful embolization requires an experienced angiographer. In our institution, where more than 50 cases have been embolized for various diseases, no recognizable inadvertent embolization has occurred.

Complications of Transhepatic Obliteration of Gastroesophageal Varices

The complications of transhepatic obliteration of gastroesophageal varices can be divided into three categories: (1) traumatic complications from the catheterization procedure; (2) toxic effect from injection of excessive amount of contrast material; and (3) inadvertent embolization.

The most common traumatic complications are hepatic subcapsular hematomas, occurring in about 50% of the patients [53]. They are generally asymptomatic and do not require specific treatment. Bleeding or bile leakage into the peritoneal cavity is a serious complication but occurs rarely. This complication is unlikely to occur if the catheter tract is obliterated by injecting a piece of Gelfoam or Ivalon near the hepatic capsule.

Renal failure secondary to the administration of contrast medium is a potential problem in cirrhotic patients with ascites in whom renal function might have been already compromised. Embolic materials, if small, may pass through gastroesophageal varices and result in pulmonary embolism. No such serious complications have been reported. Balloon occlusion of the azygos vein was used to prevent pulmonary embolism from coronary vein embolization. This technique has not been generally used and the effectiveness of the method is not known. A recent study demonstrated that ^{99m}Tc labeled Gelfoam injected into large coronary veins was detected in the lung by gamma camera [22].

REFERENCES

1. Athanasoulis CA, Baum S, Rösch J, et al: Mesenteric arterial infusions of vasopressin for hemorrhage from colonic diverticulosis. Am J Surg 129:212, 1975
2. Athanasoulis CA, Baum S, Waltman AC, et al: Control of acute gastric mucosal hemorrhage: intraarterial infusion of posterior pituitary extract. N Engl J Med 290:597, 1974
3. Athanasoulis CA, Waltman AC, Novelline RA, et al: Angiography: its contribution to the emergency management of gastrointestinal hemorrhage. Radiol Clin N Am 14:265, 1976
4. Athanasoulis CA, Waltman AC, Ring EJ, et al: Angiographic management of postoperative bleeding. Radiology 113:37, 1974
5. Barr JW, Lakin RC, Rösch J: Similarity of arterial and intravenous vasopressin on portal and systemic hemodynamics. Gastroenterology 69:13, 1975
6. Baum S, Athanasoulis CA, Waltman AC: Angiographic diagnosis and control of large bowel bleeding. Dis Colon Rectum 17:447, 1974
7. Baum S, Nusbaum M: The control of gastrointestinal hemorrhage by selective mesenteric arterial infusion of vasopressin. Radiology 98:497, 1971
8. Beller BM, Trevino A, Urban E: Pitressin-induced myocardial injury and depression in a young woman. Am J Med 51:675, 1971
9. Berardi RS: Vascular complications of superior mesenteric artery infusion with Pitressin in treatment of bleeding esophageal varices. Am J Surg 127:757, 1974
10. Bookstein JJ, Chlosta EM, Foley D, et al: Transcatheter hemostasis of gastrointestinal bleeding using modified autogenous clot. Radiology 113:277, 1974
11. Bookstein JJ, Naderi MJ, Walter JF: Transcatheter embolization for lower gastrointestinal bleeding. Radiology 127:345, 1978
12. Bradley EL III, Goldman ML: Gastric infarction after therapeutic embolization. Surgery 79:421, 1976
13. Carlyle DR, Goldstein HM: Angiographic management of bleeding following transcolonoscopic polypectomy. Am J Dig Dis 20:1196, 1975
14. Carsen GM, Casarella WJ, Spiegel RM: Transcatheter embolization for treatment of Mallory-Weiss tears of the esophagogastric junction. Radiology 128:309, 1978

15. Cavaluzzi JA, Kaufman SL, White RI Jr: Vasopressin control of massive hemorrhage in chronic ulcerative colitis. Am J Roentgenol 127:672, 1976
16. Cho KJ, Reuter SR: Embolic control of superior mesenteric artery hemorrhage caused by abdominal abscesses. Am J Roentgenol 128:1041, 1977
17. Cho KJ, Reuter SR, Schmidt R: Effects of experimental hepatic artery embolization on hepatic function. Am J Roentgenol 127:563, 1976
18. Cho KJ, Schmidt RW, Lenz J: Effects of experimental embolization of superior mesenteric artery branch on the intestine. Invest Radiol 14:207, 1979
19. Clark RA: Intraarterial vasopressin infusion for treatment of Mallory-Weiss tears of the esophagogastric junction. Am J Roentgenol 133:449, 1979
20. Conn HO, Ramsby GR, Storer EH: Selective intraarterial vasopressin in the treatment of upper gastrointestinal hemorrhage. Gastroenterology 63:634, 1972
21. Conn HO, Ramsby GR, Storer EH: Hepatic arterial escape from vasopressin-induced vasoconstriction: an angiographic investigation. Am J Roentgenol 119:102, 1973
22. Conroy RM, Lyons KP, Kuperus JH, et al: New technique for localization of therapeutic emboli using radionuclide labeling. Am J Roentgenol 130:523, 1978
23. Davis GB, Bookstein JJ, Coel MN: Advantage of intraarterial over intravenous vasopressin infusion in gastrointestinal hemorrhage. Am J Roentgenol 128:733, 1977
24. Davis GB, Bookstein JJ, Hagan PL: The relative effects of selective intraarterial and intravenous infusion. Radiology 120:537, 1976
25. Eisenberg H, Steer ML: The nonoperative treatment of massive pyloroduodenal hemorrhage by retracted autologous clot embolization. Surgery 79:414, 1976
26. Gold RE, Blair DC, Finlay JB, et al: Transarterial electrocoagulation therapy of a pseudoaneurysm in the head of the pancreas. Am J Roentgenol 125:422, 1975
27. Goldin AR: Control of duodenal hemorrhage with cyanoacrylate. Br J Radiol 49:583, 1976
28. Goldman ML, Freeny PC, Tallman JM, et al: Transcatheter vascular occlusion therapy with isobutyl 2-cyanoacrylate (Bucrylate) for control of massive upper gastrointestinal bleeding. Radiology 129:41, 1978
29. Goldman ML, Land WC Jr, Bradley EL III, et al: Transcatheter therapeutic embolization in the management of massive upper gastrointestinal bleeding. Radiology 120:513, 1976
30. Goldstein HM, Medellin H, Yoram Ben-Menachem, et al: Transcatheter arterial embolization in the management of bleeding in the cancer patient. Radiology 115:603, 1975
31. Goldstein HM, Wallace S, Anderson JH, et al: Transcatheter occlusion of abdominal tumors. Radiology 120:539, 1976
32. Johnson WC, Widrich WC: Efficacy of selective splanchnic arteriography and vasopressin perfusion in diagnosis and treatment of gastrointestinal hemorrhage. Am J Surg 131:481, 1976

33. Katzen BT, Rossi P, Passariello R, et al: Transcatheter therapeutic arterial embolization. Radiology 120:523, 1976
34. Lunderquist A, Börjesson B, Owman T, et al: Isobutyl 2-cyanoacrylate (Bucrylate) in obliteration of gastric coronary vein and esophageal varices. Am J Roentgenol 130:1, 1978
35. Lunderquist A, Simert G, Tylen U, et al: Follow-up of patients with portal hypertension and esophageal varices treated with percutaneous obliteration of gastric coronary vein. Radiology 122:59, 1977
36. Lunderquist A, Vang J: Transhepatic catheterization and obliteration of the coronary vein in patients with portal hypertension and esophageal varices. N Engl J Med 291:646, 1974
37. Marubbio AT Jr, Lombardo RP, Holt PR: Control of variceal bleeding by superior mesenteric artery pitressin perfusions — complications and indications. Am J Dig Dis 18:539, 1973
38. Melson GL, Geisse G, Stanley RJ: Selective intraarterial infusion of vasopressin for control of gastrointestinal bleeding: experience with 35 cases. Gastrointest Radiol 1:59, 1976
39. Nusbaum M, Baum S, Kuroda K, et al: Control of portal hypertension by selective mesenteric arterial infusion. Arch Surg 97:1005, 1968
40. Nusbaum M, Baum S, Blakemore WS: Clinical experience with the diagnosis and management of gastrointestinal hemorrhage by selective mesenteric catheterization. Ann Surg 170:506, 1969
41. Pereiras R, Viamonte M Jr, Russell E, et al: New techniques for interruption of gastroesophageal venous blood flow. Radiology 124:313, 1977
42. Podolny GA: Crohn's disease presenting with massive lower gastrointestinal hemorrhage. Am J Roentgenol 130:368, 1978
43. Prochaska JM, Flye MW, Johnsrude IS: Left gastric artery embolization for control of gastric bleeding: a complication. Radiology 107:521, 1973
44. Renert WA, Button KF, Fuld SL, et al: Mesenteric venous thrombosis and small bowel infarction following infusion of vasopressin into the superior mesenteric artery. Radiology 102:299, 1972
45. Reuter SR, Chuang VP, Bree RL: Selective arterial embolization for control of massive upper gastrointestinal bleeding. Am J Roentgenol 125:119, 1975
46. Ring EJ, Oleaga JA, Freiman D, et al: Pitfalls in the angiographic management of hemorrhage: hemodynamic considerations. Am J Roentgenol 129:1007, 1977
47. Roberts C, Maddison FE: Partial mesenteric arterial occlusion with subsequent ischemic bowel damage due to pitressin infusion. Am J Roentgenol 126:829, 1976
48. Rösch J, Dotter CT, Antonovic R: Selective vasoconstrictor infusion in the management of arteriocapillary gastrointestinal hemorrhage. Am J Roentgenol 116:279, 1972
49. Rösch J, Dotter CT, Brown MJ: Selective arterial embolization: a new method for control of acute gastrointestinal bleeding. Radiology 102:303, 1972
50. Sniderman KW, Franklin J Jr, Sos TA: Successful transcatheter Gelfoam

embolization of a bleeding cecal vascular ectasia. Am J Roentgenol 131:157, 1978
51. Tegtmeyer CJ, Smith TH, Shaw A, et al: Renal infarctions: a complication of Gelfoam embolization of a hemangioendothelioma of the liver. Am J Roentgenol 128:305, 1977
52. Twiford TW Jr, Granmayeh M, Tucker MJ: Gangrene of the feet associated with mesenteric intraarterial vasopressin. Am J Roentgenol 130:558, 1978
53. Viamonte M Jr, Pereiras R, Russell E, et al: Transhepatic obliteration of gastroesophageal varices: results in acute and nonacute bleeders. Am J Roentgenol 129:237, 1977
54. Wallace S, Gianturco C, Anderson JH, et al: Therapeutic vascular occlusion utilizing steel coil technique: clinical applications. Am J Roentgenol 127:381, 1976
55. Walter JF, Paaso BT, Cannon WB: Successful transcatheter embolic control of massive hematobilia secondary to liver biopsy. Am J Roentgenol 127:847, 1976
56. Waltman AC, Greenfield AJ, Novelline RA, et al: Pyloroduodenal bleeding and intraarterial vasopressin: clinical results. Am J Roentgenol 133:643, 1979
57. Wholey MH, Stockdale R, Hung TK: A percutaneous balloon catheter for the immediate control of hemorrhage. Radiology 95:65, 1970
58. Woodside J, Schwarz H, Gergreen P: Peripheral embolization complicating bilateral renal infarction with Gelfoam. Am J Roentgenol 126:1033, 1976

Variceal Bleeding

Thomas C. Chalmers, M.D.
Henry Sacks, Ph.D., M.D.

Prognosis in the Cirrhotic With Gastrointestinal Hemorrhage

ABSTRACT

Gastrointestinal hemorrhage is the commonest terminal episode in patients with cirrhosis of the liver. Although the modern era of high technology medicine has brought about many changes in the diagnosis and therapy of this condition, there is little evidence that patients have been benefited. There are two possible explanations for this: Either portal hypertension has reached an irreversible state by the time the patient bleeds, such that early correct diagnosis and any conceivable therapy will be ineffective, or incorrect application of the scientific method to clinical management has perpetuated confusion.

It is likely that the former is only partly true, and the latter a certainty. The means employed over the last 40 years to evaluate new diagnostic methods and preventive and therapeutic measures will be examined in this presentation. The frequency of randomized control trials of each new procedure will be presented. The quality of the few randomized control trials that have been performed will be graded according to a new quality scoring system, and the conclusions examined from the standpoint of patient selection and quality of the study. So far only one principle has been established: the radiologists prefer to diagnose and treat by radiologic methods, the endoscopists prefer the endoscopic approach, and the surgeons are in favor of surgery. The comparative efficacy of each approach is still obscure.

Thomas C. Chalmers, M.D.: President and Dean, Mount Sinai School of Medicine; Henry Sacks, Ph.D., M.D.: Instructor, Departments of Medicine and Biostatistics, Mount Sinai School of Medicine, New York, New York.

Frederic E. Eckhauser, M.D.
William E. Strodel, M.D.
Jeremiah G. Turcotte, M.D.

Hemodynamics in Portal Hypertension

ABSTRACT

Current operative therapy for the cirrhotic patient with portal hypertension and bleeding esophageal varices is not ideal. Portasystemic shunt procedures although effective in reducing portal pressure and the risk of recurrent, life-threatening hemorrhage, are nonphysiological. Total diversion of portal flow (standard portacaval, splenorenal or mesocaval shunts) may result in the serious complications of encephalopathy and liver failure. Selective or partial portal flow diversion (distal splenorenal shunt) is associated with a decreased incidence of postshunt encephalopathy, but late effects upon patient survival and variceal rebleeding are unknown.

In order to better select candidates for operative portal decompression, a variety of risk classifications have been developed. Of these, evaluation of cardiovascular hemodynamics appears to provide "dynamic" information for early risk discrimination in the bleeding patient before differences in liver function tests become readily apparent. Established risk classifications based upon clinical, biochemical, angiographic or hepatic histological criteria are useful, but provide insufficient information upon which to base therapeutic decisions during episodes of acute bleeding. Cirrhosis is emerging as a disorder not only of portal hemodynamics but of systemic physiology as well.

Varicose veins of the esophagus I have never met with before, nor have I found any similar case recorded; they may sometimes exist to a lesser degree, but I doubt whether their presence to such an extent, and death caused by

---

Frederic E. Eckhauser, M.D.: Assistant Professor of Surgery, Department of Surgery, University of Michigan Medical Center, and Assistant Chief, Surgical Service, Ann Arbor Veterans Administration Medical Center; William E. Strodel, M.D.: Instructor in Surgery, Department of Surgery, University of Michigan Medical Center, and Staff Surgeon, Ann Arbor Veterans Administration Medical Center; Jeremiah G. Turcotte, M.D.: Professor of Surgery, Chairman, Department of Surgery, University of Michigan Medical Center, Ann Arbor, Michigan.

their rupture, be not something as yet unheard of in pathological anatomy [37].

It has now been nearly a century and a half since W. Power (1840) described the first reported death from bleeding esophageal varices in this country. Despite a tremendous clinical experience with portasystemic shunting over the past 40 years, the precise indication for this procedure in clinical practice remains controversial.

The objectives of this chapter are twofold: (1) to review the evolution of our present concepts of the hemodynamic pathophysiology of cirrhosis and portal hypertension; and (2) to evaluate the utility of hemodynamic criteria as survival determinants in patients with portal hypertension and bleeding esophageal varices.

HISTORICAL SUMMARY

Nicolai Eck first demonstrated in 1877 that portacaval anastomosis in the dog was both technically feasible and compatible with survival of the animal [12]. Seventy years elapsed before Dr. Allen Whipple demonstrated elevations of portal venous pressure in patients with Banti's syndrome [66]. The combination of frequent gastroesophageal hemorrhage in these patients and dissatisfaction with the surgical control afforded by splenectomy alone prompted investigators to reconsider Eck's original dog model. By the mid 1940s Whipple and others had demonstrated the clinical potential of portasystemic shunting procedures to reduce portal pressures [66]. Since exsanguinating hemorrhage from gastroesophageal varices was a leading cause of death in untreated patients with portal hypertension, with reported mortality rates of 60-90% [1, 26], the protection from rebleeding afforded by a successful portasystemic shunt was hailed as a therapeutic milestone.

Within a decade, however, it became apparent to Blakemore and others that the death rate among patients surviving portasystemic shunt procedures continued to be distressingly high [4]. This was attributed to progression of the natural disease only; little if any consideration was given to the potentially deleterious effects of portal blood flow diversion on liver function.

Evidence from ongoing investigation suggested that portal venous flow diversion might cause significant abnormalities in hepatic metabolism [2, 14, 28]. Clinical appreciation of two potential postshunt sequelae, encephalopathy and liver failure, was retarded initially by enthusiasm for operative portal decompression as a means of preventing recurrent, life-threatening hemorrhage from gastroesophageal varices.

Postshunt encephalopathy was not a new concept, it was observed experimentally in the mid 1890s. Several reports of the clinical association between protein intolerance and encephalopathy in cirrhotic patients appeared sporadically during the 1950s [28, 35], and were supplemented by the experimental work of Riddell and others implicating ammonia and other nitrogen-containing substances as possible etiologic factors [42]. By the late 1960s most investigators had come to accept hepatic encephalopathy as a significant complication associated with portasystemic shunting [26, 69].

Investigation of the potential role of portal hemodynamics in liver maintenance was prompted by evidence suggesting that in the absence of degenerative liver disease or portal obstruction, encephalopathy and hepatic deterioration occurred frequently following the systemic diversion of portal venous blood [28]. Child and later Ono demonstrated that these potential complications could be prevented by transposing the portal and systemic venous circulations (portasystemic transposition) [9, 34]. Cirrhosis appears to be a "dynamic" process and may result in both progressive increases in portal pressure and progressive decreases in prograde portal perfusion. The extent of liver damage in cirrhosis varies and this may account for the observation that encephalopathy and liver failure occur with unpredictable frequency following the construction of a portasystemic anastomosis. Dissatisfaction with the predictive specificity of clinical and biochemical staging criteria prompted investigation of other forms of patient selection based upon hemodynamic criteria.

PATHOGENESIS AND NATURAL HISTORY OF PORTAL HYPERTENSION

Portal hypertension may result from either an increase in prograde portal flow (inflow theory) or an increase in resistance to flow (outflow resistance theory) anywhere within the portal system. The majority of common etiologies fall under the latter category and result in anatomic or functional obstruction to the flow of venous blood within the portal system. Current classifications of portal hypertension are based on the anatomical site of obstruction relative to the hepatic sinusoid [40].

Portal hypertension in the United States is usually due to cirrhosis, either nutritional or postnecrotic. The initiating insult in the cirrhotic patient is hepatic cell necrosis [30]. Regenerating nodules develop from parenchymal cell remnants which persist after liver injury or from small clusters of hepatocytes within connective tissue septae. These nodules gradually expand and eventually compress surrounding tissues, including the various intrahepatic arteries, veins and bile ducts. The net result is obstruction to hepatic venous outflow and hypertension within the hepatic sinusoid.

Hepatic sinusoids may become entrapped within connective tissue envelopes that form in response to parenchymal necrosis. Capillaries may arborize throughout these collagenous septae, eventually making direct contact with entrapped sinusoids. This "capillarization" process creates direct channels between the intrahepatic branches of the portal and hepatic veins (venovenous shunts). Blood flowing within these venous channels may bypass large numbers of hepatocytes, effectively depriving them of nutrient blood flow. Communications may similarly develop between branches of hepatic arterioles and portal venules partially transmitting arterial pressure into the portal venous system [15]. As the scarring process worsens, portal venules within the substance of the liver may become compressed or even obliterated; this seems to further reduce prograde flow of portal venous blood. As pressure in the portal system increases, collateral channels develop between the portal and systemic venous circulations. Of particular importance are the veins which lie in the submucosa of the gastric cardia and esophagus. These veins are thin-walled and in response to increases in portal pressure may undergo dilatation, resulting in the formation of gastroesophageal varices.

Hypertension within the hepatic sinusoid leads to an increase in hepatic lymph production. Lieberman and Reynolds measured plasma volumes in patients with cirrhosis and found them to be significantly greater [25] than similar values in noncirrhotic patients. They concluded that the increased plasma volumes observed in cirrhotics were due to an increase in hepatic lymph production. Expansion of the plasma volume may ultimately result in an increase in the volume of the splanchnic venous bed. The concomitant deterioration of hepatocyte function may result in a decreased capability to degrade certain humoral and vasoactive substances delivered through the portal circulation [48, 50]. These vasoactive substances, by virtue of their potential action on vascular smooth muscle, may further increase pressure in the portal and mesenteric venous circulations. Figures 1 and 2 demonstrate the various mechanisms which have been implicated in the pathogenesis of portal hypertension.

The natural history of portal hypertension includes the development of significant complications, notably hemorrhage from esophageal varices and the development of ascites, hypersplenism or both.

It is estimated that 1 in 3 cirrhotic patients will experience a significant episode of variceal bleeding during the course of his illness. The vast majority of cirrhotics die as a result of hepatic failure, malnutrition and infection. The prognosis per bleed for cirrhotic patients with variceal hemorrhage is poor, with reported mortality rates of 40-70%. The risk of rebleeding within two years may be as high as 75-80%. Long term prognosis for these patients is poor; estimates of five year survival range from 6% to 35% [17, 36, 38].

Portal cirrhosis is a disease of some magnitude in this country with nearly 30,000 deaths annually. Cirrhosis is now included within the top 15 leading causes of death in the United States. Hemorrhage from esophageal varices presents as a dramatic complication of portal hypertension. Over the years, our approach to the cirrhotic patient with portal hypertension and bleeding

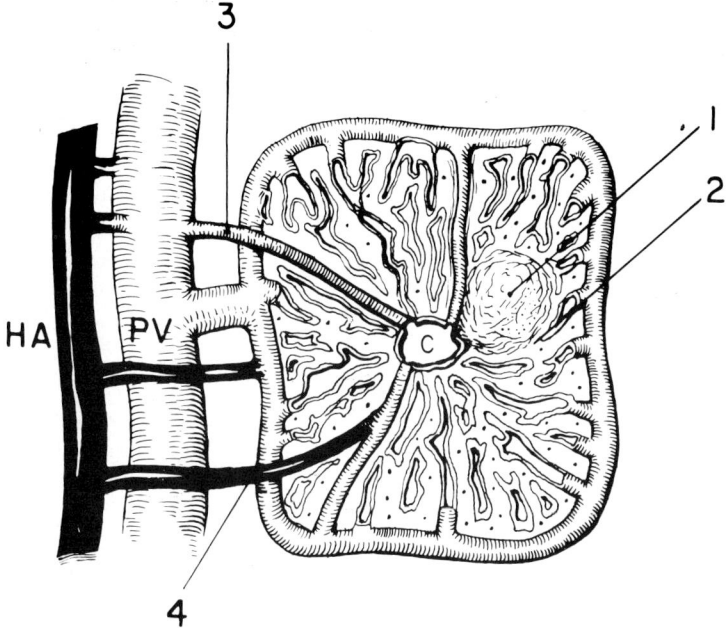

Fig. 1. Changes in hepatic lobular architecture with advanced portal cirrhosis: (1) regenerating nodule, (2) compressed hepatic parenchyma, (3) venovenous anastomosis, (4) arteriovenous anastomosis. HA, hepatic artery; PV, portal vein; C, central vein.

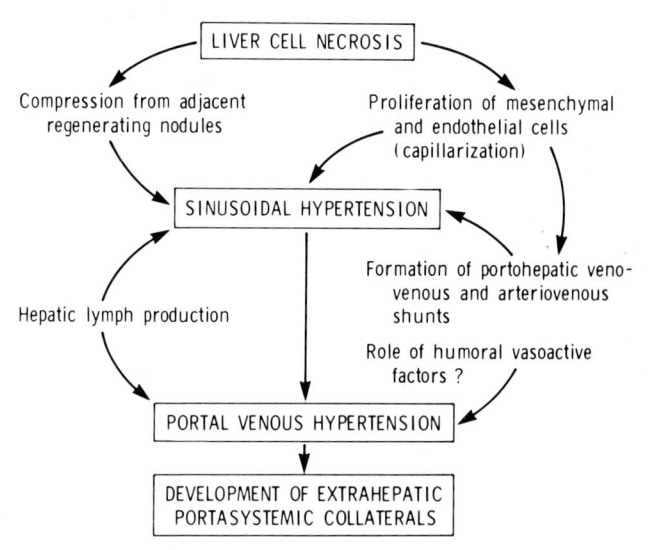

Fig. 2. Pathogenesis of portal hypertension – postulated mechanisms.

esophageal varices has changed due to an improved understanding of the coexisting abnormalities in splanchnic and cardiovascular hemodynamics.

SPLANCHNIC HEMODYNAMICS

Portal pressure and flow are determined by splanchnic inflow, resistance to hepatic outflow, and pressure in the inferior vena cava. Each should be evaluated accurately in every cirrhotic patient with portal hypertension. Operative portal decompression, athough clearly effective in preventing recurrent variceal hemorrhage, is associated with diversion of the portal component of liver blood flow and is therefore nonphysiological. The inability to predict in advance those patients who would develop postshunt encephalopathy and liver failure prompted investigation of portal and splanchnic pressures and flows in patients with cirrhosis and portal hypertension.

Experimental evidence suggested that maintenance of prograde portal perfusion might prevent postshunt encephalopathy and hepatic deterioration [9, 34]. Several investigators postulated that preoperative assessment of splanchnic pressures and flows might better define those poor risk patients who would not benefit from portacaval shunting. Early efforts to evaluate splanchnic hemodynamics were hampered by a lack of sophisticated techniques for diagnosis and investigation. A number of recently developed radiographic and radioisotopic techniques now allow estimation of total hepatic blood flow, the relative contributions of the portal vein and hepatic artery to total liver blood flow, portal and splanchnic pressures within the system, and the location and extent of portasystemic collateral pathways.

Hepatic vein catheterization often is performed as a part of mesenteric angiography [41]. It was hoped initially that measurements of wedged hepatic vein pressure would be of prognostic value. This has been subsequently disproved. A direct outgrowth of this investigation, however, has been Viallet's demonstration of the direct relationship between wedged hepatic vein pressure and the free portal vein pressure [58]. Measurements of portal vein pressure may be obtained by direct catheterization of the umbilical vein or transhepatic puncture of portal vein radicles [20, 68, 69]. Corrected portal vein or sinusoidal pressure (CPP or CSP) may be calculated by subtracting the pressure obtained in the inferior vena cava from the wedged hepatic vein pressure. Several investigators have observed that measurement of corrected sinusoidal pressure in patients with upper gastrointestinal hemorrhage, esophageal varices, and equivocal endoscopic evidence regarding the source of bleeding may provide useful information [41, 59]. Low corrected sinusoidal pressure values are rarely observed in patients with variceal bleeding associated with portal cirrhosis. Esophagogastroscopy, however, may demonstrate bleeding from gastroesophageal varices in patients without any objective clinical evidence of chronic liver disease. In the absence of sinusoidal hypertension (portal cirrhosis), low values of corrected sinusoidal pressure may occasionally be recorded. This finding suggests extrahepatic obstruction of the portal vein. Additional studies such as splenoportography, umbilical vein portography or venous phase mesenteric arteriography may aid in confirming this diagnosis.

Currently, the least invasive techniques for measuring hepatic blood flow employ either dye indicators or radioactive colloid tracers. Using these indirect and other direct techniques, the hepatic artery has been shown to provide 25%-33% of total liver blood flow. The remainder consists of portal blood flow. Several investigators have shown that total liver blood flow gradually decreases with progressive portal hypertension of intrahepatic etiology [62]. The bulk of this decrease in flow is due to a reduction in flow through the portal vein. Hepatic artery flow increases but cannot completely compensate, and overall liver blood flow decreases. Estimates of overall hepatic blood flow in patients with portal cirrhosis may not reflect true "sinusoidal" blood flow.

Even when overall blood flow is not reduced, effective or nutrient sinusoidal blood flow may be diminished secondary to increased veno-venous and arteriovenous shunting. Warren and colleagues used measurements of estimated hepatic blood flow in an attempt to predict those groups of patients likely to develop postshunt encephalopathy. They observed that patients with normal or near normal preshunt liver blood flow and those with extremely low preoperative values did poorly following the construction of a portasystemic shunt [16, 63]. In an attempt to better define the causes of elevated portal pressure in cirrhosis and their relationship to variceal hemorrhage, patterns of splanchnic and portal venous pressures in cirrhotic patients were evaluated. Free and clamp-occluded portal pressures have been measured intraoperatively in large numbers of patients undergoing portasystemic shunts [16, 33, 41, 56]. Figure 3 illustrates the terminology used to define the various aspects of splanchnic and portal pressure. Warren and others reaffirmed that obstruction to portal flow appears to be the most valid explanation of the elevated portal pressures observed in patients with portal cirrhosis, and largely disclaimed the influence of arteriovenous shunts in the development of portal hypertension [22, 61].

Maximum perfusion pressure is a term derived from the difference between pressure measured on the intestinal and hepatic sides of a clamp-occluded portal vein. Using these data, Warren et al suggested that the major hemodynamic effect of cirrhosis was the development of sinusoidal hypertension and that with pathoprogression of the underlying liver disease, pressure in the sinusoids might actually exceed pressure within the portal vein. Ultimately this might result in spontaneous reversal of portal flow [61]. The concept of "hepatofugal portal flow" was consistent with previous observations that cirrhosis might result in a progressive reduction of prograde portal perfusion, and for that reason was widely accepted. It was not until 1974 that Moreno et al presented an impressive

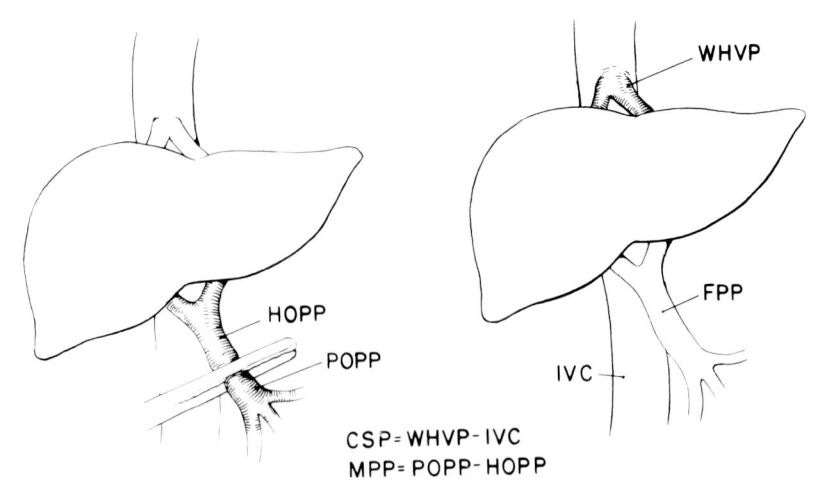

Fig. 3. Terminology used in measurement of portal and splanchnic pressure: HOPP, hepatic-occluded portal pressure; POPP, peripheral-occluded portal pressure; FPP, free portal pressure; WHVP, wedge hepatic vein pressure; CSP, corrected sinusoidal pressure; MPP, maximum perfusion pressure; IVC, inferior vena cava pressure.

argument against this concept [31]. They noted that among 273 cirrhotic patients evaluated for spontaneous reversal of portal flow using a variety of radiologic techniques, true documentation was lacking in all. Using data obtained from a hydrodynamic model, they further suggested that measurements of static-occluded portal pressures could not and should not be used to construct hydraulic gradients for portal flow. It is of interest, however, that one clinical entity may be associated with spontaneous portal flow reversal. Anatomical obstruction of the major hepatic veins (Budd-Chiari syndrome) may cause high grade or complete obstruction of the hepatic venous outflow tract. In this setting, hepatic outflow resistance might exceed resistance in the portasystemic collateral bed and result in true spontaneous reversal of flow within the portal vein.

A number of investigators have recently questioned the utility of splanchnic pressure measurements in predicting outcome after portasystemic shunting. Smith evaluated hemodynamic staging in 130 cirrhotic patients with portal hypertension [56]. He concluded that among selected groups of patients, operative therapy based upon hemodynamic staging did not result in a decreased incidence of encephalopathy or of death from liver failure. Bismuth and associates attempted to reduce the extent of portal flow diversion by constructing portacaval anastomoses of differing calibers [3]. They observed no differences between side-to-side portacaval anastomoses of different calibers and patient mortality or long-term survival. Finally, Burchell's group obtained direct measurements of portal flow at the time of portasystemic shunting and compared these values with measurements of maximum perfusion pressure and the completeness of portal vein filling on splenoportography [7]. No correlation was found between direct and inferential estimations of portal flow and patient survival. It has become increasingly apparent that operative determination of static portal pressures and flows is of little real prognostic significance in the bleeding patient.

One additional hemodynamic measurement may be of prognostic importance. The hepatic artery flow is thought to normally contribute 25%-33% of total liver blood flow. Experimental evidence suggests that following occlusion of the portal vein or diversion of portal flow there is a constant increase in hepatic artery flow [46]. The extent to which increases in hepatic artery flow occur following the construction of a portasystemic shunt is apparently determined by several factors. Arteries are more resistant than veins to compression and distortion by adjacent areas of regenerating liver tissue. The vascular reactivity or compliance of the hepatic arterial circulation might be severely compromised by extensive fibrosis within the liver. Furthermore, the construction of portasystemic shunts that decompress both the hepatic and intestinal ends of the portal vein (side-to-side portacaval or interposition mesocaval shunts) may actually augment hepatic artery flow through preformed intrahepatic arteriovenous anastomoses. Retrograde flow of portal blood through the hepatic limb of a side-to-side portacaval shunt has been demonstrated [61]. Warren and others, however, disproved the latter speculation by demonstrating that blood leaving the portal vein after a side-to-side portacaval shunt is not exclusively arterial in nature [61, 63]. These observations suggest that postshunt increases in hepatic arterial flow are not simply the result of enhanced arteriovenous shunt flow and that this increased flow is of nutrient value to hepatocytes.

Zimmon and Burchell have investigated the prognostic importance of hepatic arterial reactivity in cirrhotic patients undergoing operative portal decompression. Zimmon et al using an umbilical vein catheterization technique, observed that in normal patients and some cirrhotics there is negligible change in wedged hepatic venous pressure despite large volume changes within the portal venous system; this response suggested normal arterial reactivity. Conversely, wide fluctuations in wedged hepatic venous pressure resulting from changes in the portal venous volume appeared to reflect abnormal compliance of the hepatic arterial tree [67, 68]. These and other investigators noted that prognosis after portasystemic shunt operation correlated with preoperative assessment of the responsiveness of the hepatic arterial bed to changes in portal volume [21]. Burchell et al further noted a relationship between increases in hepatic artery flow following side-to-side portacaval shunt and improved patient survival following operation [7].

Portasystemic shunting procedures are nonphysiological in that they direct metabolic substrates and humoral substances necessary for maintenance of normal function from the liver. More recently alternative procedures have been developed to selectively reduce variceal pressure while maintaining prograde portal perfusion (distal splenorenal shunt) [6, 45]. While it is generally accepted that the incidence of postoperative encephalopathy is decreased following this type of procedure [39, 64], the issue of potential late rebleeding has not been settled. The latter operation is certainly attractive in physiologic terms, yet the potential to form new collaterals between the right and left halves of the portal system and thereby obviate any hemodynamic advantage of this shunt exists and has been demonstrated angiographically in several patients [27].

CARDIOVASCULAR HEMODYNAMICS

The concept that degnerative liver disease may lead to multiple cardiorespiratory and hemodynamic abnormalities has gained increasing acceptance in recent years.

Cirrhosis may frequently be associated with a hyperdynamic circulatory state [24]. Increases in resting cardiac output have been reported in 25%-50% of patients with chronic liver disease [11, 24, 51], and may represent a compensatory response to decreases in vascular resistance. The frequent occurrence in cirrhotics of palmar erythema, warm extremities, prominent capillary pulsations and spider angiomata may serve to confirm this explanation. Peripheral blood flow increases without simultaneous changes in the splanchnic, coronary or cerebral circulations [23]. The finding by Silverstein et al of increases in peripheral venous oxygen saturation in patients with portal cirrhosis implies that the observed increases in peripheral blood flow are secondary to abnormal shunting through precapillary arteriovenous anastomoses [55]. Elevated levels of blood lactate have been measured in cirrhotic patients with hyperdynamic circulations and reduced peripheral resistance [23]. These observations suggest that increases in peripheral blood flow functionally bypass perfusing capillary beds and result in altered tissue metabolism.

Increases in plasma volume and arterial desaturation have been observed in patients with portal cirrhosis [25]. The cardiac output changes seen in hyperdynamic cirrhotics appear to correlate with the extent of portasystemic collaterals. Similar collaterals may be observed in association with extrahepatic obstruction of the portal vein, yet in the absence of coexisting liver disease, abnormal circulatory patterns are infrequent. Arterial oxygen desaturation is frequently associated with clinical signs of digital clubbing and cyanosis, and suggests the presence of systemic venoarterial shunting. Abnormal shunting of systemic venous blood through preformed pulmonary arteriovenous fistulas has been previously reported [32, 44] yet alternative sites of shunting through portopulmonary and intracardiac anastomoses may be of additional importance [10, 30]. It is difficult to outline completely the multiple factors that contribute to the development of a hyperdynamic circulation in patients with portal cirrhosis, but available evidence suggests that ongoing liver injury is requisite. The elevated cardiac output and expanded plasma volume seen in hyperdynamic cirrhotics are analogous to features of large systemic arteriovenous fistulas [5, 13, 60]. Similar findings may be observed in patients with beriberi [65]. During recent years, two theories have been postulated to explain the circulatory abnormalities observed in patients with cirrhosis and portal hypertension.

Proponents of the "humoral theory" have suggested that hormone-like substances with vasodilator properties may be found in increased concentrations in the blood of patients with chronic liver disease [48, 50]. The failing liver may elaborate an abnormal vasoactive substance or fail to detoxify a normally circulating compound of similar nature. The failure of the liver to inactivate normally circulating vasoactive peptides may result from hepatocyte dysfunction or from diversion of blood through portasystemic collaterals effectively bypassing the liver. Available evidence suggests that changes in regional vascular perfusion are selective; peripheral blood flow appears to increase preferentially without simultaneous changes in other circulatory beds and suggests indirectly that a hormone-mediated phenomenon may not entirely explain the observed changes in circulatory patterns.

Physiologic studies have shown that increases in transmural pressure across the great vessels of the thorax may cause a reflex inhibition of peripheral vasoconstrictor tone and result in increases in skeletal muscle blood flow [49]. Segal et al investigated a group of hyperdynamic patients with portal cirrhosis and demonstrated that elevations in pulmonary wedge and right heart pressures were common to all [47]. Although the neural and hormonal theories are both plausible, they are by no means exclusive. Hypocapnia is a frequent clinical finding in patients with cirrhosis, and may increase both cardiac output and skeletal muscle blood flow [8, 43]. Hyperventilation in these patients may occur as a response to acidic tissue metabolites which accumulate because of inadequate nutrient blood flow through perfusing capillary beds.

The ability of the hyperdynamic cirrhotic patient to tolerate the stresses of hemorrhage and operation is determined by the magnitude of circulatory abnormalities and the effectiveness of compensatory mechanisms. Recent studies have shown that preoperative assessment of cardiorespiratory functions may provide important prognostic information in cirrhotic patients with portal hypertension (Table 1). This work has been based on earlier observations that cirrhotic patients with hyperdynamic circulations appear to do poorly following operative portal decompression [10, 24]. Siegel and Williams identified among cirrhotics three patterns of cardiovascular response to hemorrhage or surgical stress. These classifications proved to have prognostic significance [54]. Figure 4 summarizes these abnormal hemodynamic and metabolic patterns.

Basal state cirrhotics generally demonstrate mild abnormalities in hepatic function (similar to Child Class A and B patients) and minimal alterations in

Table 1
Assessment of Prognosis in Patients With Portal Hypertension

Physiological Phenomena	Measurements
Vascular tone	Cardiac index Systemic vascular resistance
Effective oxygen transport	Oxygen consumption Cardiac index
Relative peripheral shunting	Systemic vascular resistance Effective oxygen transport
Ventricular function	Central venous pressure Ventricular stroke work

vascular tone. Under situations of imposed stress, marked increases in cardiac output and heart rate may occur without concomitant reduction in mean arterial blood pressure; this suggests a reduction in peripheral vascular resistance. However, mixed venous oxygen saturation, arteriovenous oxygen difference, and oxygen consumption remain relatively unchanged, suggesting that myocardial reserve is adequate to meet the increased peripheral demands for oxygen and metabolic substrates. This compensated hyperdynamic pattern is common following acute hemorrhage and is frequently observed in patients surviving operative portal decompression [18, 51, 52].

The progression to a decompensated hyperdynamic state is usually accompanied by significant deterioration of liver function. Several of the features of

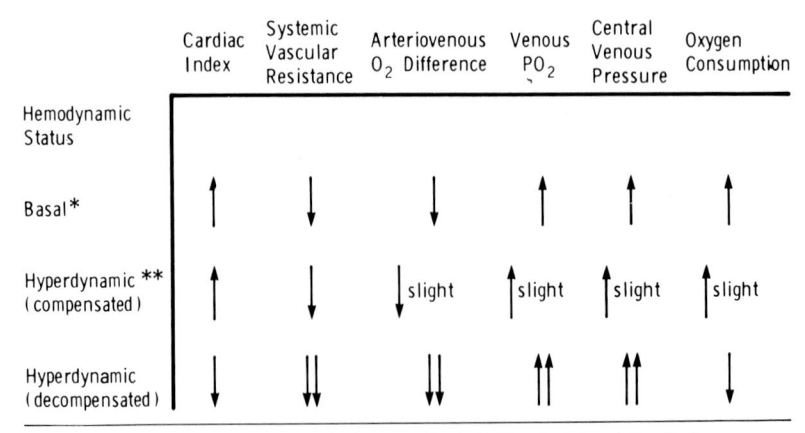

Hemodynamic Status	Cardiac Index	Systemic Vascular Resistance	Arteriovenous O_2 Difference	Venous PO_2	Central Venous Pressure	Oxygen Consumption
Basal*	↑	↓	↓	↑	↑	↑
Hyperdynamic** (compensated)	↑	↓	↓ slight	↑ slight	↑ slight	↑ slight
Hyperdynamic (decompensated)	↓	↓↓	↓↓	↑↑	↑↑	↓

* Values recorded in basal state cirrhotics deviate minimally from non-cirrhotic normals.

** Values compared to basal state cirrhotics.

Fig. 4. Hemodynamic and metabolic patterns observed in patients with portal cirrhosis.

this decompensated hemodynamic state are similar to those seen in septic shock [53]. These may include increased cardiac output, narrowing of the arteriovenous oxygen difference and elevation of central venous oxygen saturation. This decompensated hemodynamic state is characterized by a worsening disparity between nutrient and non-nutrient peripheral perfusion; further increases in myocardial contractility cannot effectively meet metabolic needs. Without expeditious cardiotropic support, high output congestive failure, cardiogenic shock and death frequently ensue [5, 52]. This already grave situation may be further complicated by the frequent coexistence of occult myocardiopathies in patients with alcoholic cirrhosis. Two factors appear to determine the progression from a compensated to decompensated hyperdynamic state. The first and most important is adequacy of myocardial reserve. The second is less obvious and is based largely on recent studies which have shown that reductions in vascular tone may occur independent of the level of cardiac output [52]. This observation suggests paralysis of vascular neuro-regulatory mechanisms (similar to septic shock) and further implies that the failing liver may elaborate a toxic factor similar to endotoxin [53].

Preoperative determination in cirrhotics of abnormal cardiorespiratory and metabolic patterns may be of prognostic importance. These factors appear to correlate with patient survival and may be expressed as a survival index (Fig. 5) [11, 54]. In the final analysis, hyperdynamic cirrhotic patients with severe abnormalities in vascular tone (increased arteriovenous shunt flow and decreased

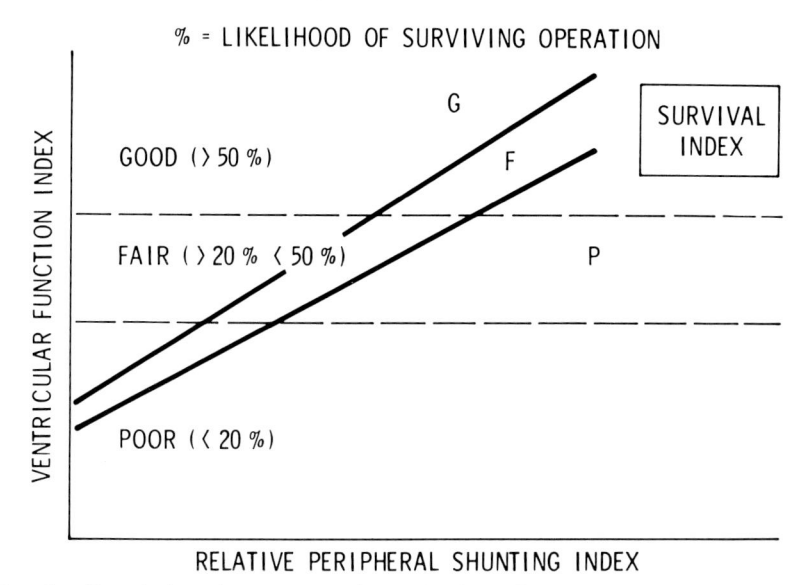

Fig. 5. Correlation between predetermined cardiorespiratory hemodynamics and patient survival following operative portal decompression. The three regions of survival index based on studies of Siegel et al [61] are shown.

effective capillary or nutrient blood flow), require substantial myocardial reserve to adequately meet the metabolic demands of operative portal decompression. Conversely the prognosis for patients with fewer circulatory abnormalities is better. The prognostic significance of this hemodynamic classification system cannot be ignored. Clinical and histological patient selection criteria are useful, but only in a general sense. It has become increasingly clear that cirrhosis is a "systemic" disorder associated with major disturbances in circulatory physiology; as such it can best be assessed by evaluating parameters of cardiorespiratory physiology. Twenty years ago, Murray observed that cardiac output in hyperdynamic patients with cirrhosis and portal hypertension returned to normal as liver function improved [32]. More recently DiCarlo et al have demonstrated a strong correlation between the magnitude of observed hemodynamic abnormalities and the extent of histologic pathology seen on liver biopsy [11]. Recognition of specific hyperdynamic patterns has profound therapeutic and therefore prognostic implications for the cirrhotic with bleeding varices. Indeed, the near fatal association between operative portal decompression and a decompensated hyperdynamic response state suggests that these patients should not be considered surgical candidates [11, 51]. Alternative methods of controlling varix hemorrhage such as injection sclerotherapy or transhepatic coronary vein embolization should be considered.

REFERENCES

1. Baker AL, Smith C, Lieberman G: Natural history of esophageal varices. Am J Med 26:288, 1959
2. Beknoe S, Mijock B, Rone A, et al: Comparison of liver mitochondrial function after end-to-end and end-to-side portacaval shunting. Am J Surg 123:43, 1972
3. Bismuth H, Franco D, Hepp J: Portal systemic shunt in hepatic cirrhosis: does the type of shunt decisively influence the clinical results? Ann Surg 179:209, 1974
4. Blakemore AH: Portacaval shunting for portal hypertension. Surg Gynecol Obstet 941:443, 1952
5. Border JR, Gallo E, Schenk WG: Systemic arteriovenous shunts in patients under severe stress: a common cause of high output cardiac failure. Surgery 60:225, 1966
6. Britton RC, Voorhees AB, Price JB: Selective portal decompression. Surgery 67:104, 1970
7. Burchell AR, Moreno AH, Panke WF, et al: Hemodynamic variables and prognosis following portacaval shunts. Surg Gynecol Obstet 138:359, 1974
8. Burnam JF, Hickman JB, McIntosh HD: Effect of hypocapnia on arterial blood pressure. Circulation 9:89, 1954
9. Child CG III, Barr D, Holswade GR, et al: Liver regeneration following

portacaval transposition in dogs. Ann Surg 138:600, 1953
10. Del Guercio LRM, Coomaraswamy RP, Feins NR, et al: Pulmonary arteriovenous admixture and the hyperdynamic cardiovascular state in surgery for portal hypertension. Surgery 56:74, 1964
11. DiCarlo V, Staudacher C, Chiesa R, et al: The role of cardiovascular hemodynamics and liver histology in evaluating bleeding cirrhotic patients. Ann Surg 190:218, 1979
12. Eck NV: Ligature of the portal vein. Voen Med J St Petersburg 130:1, 1877 [Translated and discussed by Child CG III: Eck's fistula. Surg Gynecol Obstet 96:375, 1953]
13. Epstein FH, Shadle OW, Ferguson TB, et al: Cardiac output and intracardiac pressures in patients with arteriovenous fistulas. J Clin Invest 32:543, 1953
14. Fischer JE, Myers A, James H: Ornithine decarboxylase: a defect in liver regeneration following portacaval shunt. Surgery 70:182, 1971
15. Foley WJ, Turcotte JG, Haskins PA, et al: Intrahepatic arteriovenous fistulas between the hepatic artery and portal vein. Ann Surg 174:849, 1971
16. Fomon JJ, Warren WD: Hemodynamic studies in portal hypertension. Ann Res Med 20:277, 1969
17. Garceau AJ, Chalmers TC, The Boston Inter-hospital Liver Group: The natural history of cirrhosis I: survival with esophageal varices. N Engl J Med 268:469, 1963
18. Greenspan M, Del Guercio LRM: Cardiorespiratory determinants of survival in cirrhotic patients requiring surgery for portal hypertension. Am J Surg 115:43, 1968
19. Hinshaw LB, Blake CM, Emerson TE: Biochemical and pathologic alterations in endotoxin shock, In Mills LC (ed): Shock and Hypotension. New York, Grune and Stratton, 1965, p 431
20. Hoiisawa M, Boyer TD, Redeker AG, et al: Direct measurement of portal and hepatic vein pressures using thin transhepatic needle (Abstr). Gastroenterology 69:830, 1975
21. Kessler RE, Tice DA, Solowey AC, et al: Clinical vs hemodynamic classification of cirrhosis. Surg Forum 26:417, 1975
22. Kessler RE, Tice DA, Zimmon DS: Retrograde flow of portal vein blood in patients with cirrhosis. Radiology 92:1038, 1969
23. Kontos HA, Shapiro W, Mauck HP, et al: General and regional circulatory alterations in cirrhosis of the liver. Am J Med 37:526, 1964
24. Kowalski HJ, Abelmann WH: The cardiac output at rest in Laennec's cirrhosis. J Clin Invest 32:1025, 1953
25. Lieberman FL, Reynolds TB: Plasma volume in cirrhosis of the liver: its relation to portal hypertension, ascites and renal failure. J Clin Invest 46:1297, 1967
26. Ludington LG: A study of 158 cases of esophageal varices. Surg Gynecol Obstet 106:519, 1958
27. Maillard JN, Flamant YM, Hay JM, et al: Selectivity of the distal splenorenal shunt. Surgery 86:663, 1979

28. McDermott WV Jr, Adams RD: Episodic stupor associated with an Eck fistula in the human with particular reference to the metabolism of ammonia. J Clin Invest 33:1, 1954
29. McDermott WV Jr, Barnes BA, Nardi GL, et al: Postshunt encephalopathy. Surg Gynecol Obstet 126:585, 1962
30. Mellemgaard K, Winkler K, Tygstrup N, et al: Sources of venoarterial admixture in portal hypertension. J Clin Invest 42:1399, 1963
31. Moreno AH, Burchell AR, Reddy RV, et al: Spontaneous reversal of portal blood flow: the case for and against its occurrence in patients with cirrhosis of the liver. Ann Surg 181:346, 1975
32. Murray JF, Dawson AM, Sherlock S: Circulatory changes in chronic liver disease. Am J Med 24:358, 1958
33. Nabseth DC, Widrick WC, O'Hara ET, et al: Flow and pressure characteristics of the portal system before and after splenorenal shunts. Surgery 78:739, 1975
34. Ono H, Kojima Y, Ackroyd FW, et al: Longterm results in portarenal transposition in dogs. Surgery 64:214, 1968
35. Phillips GB, Schwartz R, Gabuzda JR Jr, et al: Syndrome of impending hepatic coma in patients with cirrhosis of the liver given certain nitrogenous compounds. N Engl J Med 247:239, 1952
36. Powell WJ, Klatskin G: Duration of survival in patients with Laennec's cirrhosis. Am J Med 44:406, 1968
37. Power W: Contributions to pathology. Maryland Med Surg J 1:306, 1840
38. Ratnoff OD, Patek AJ: The natural history of Laennec's cirrhosis of the liver: an analysis of 386 cases. Medicine 21:207, 1942
39. Reichle FA, Fahrmy WF, Golsorkhi M: Prospective comparative clinical trials with distal splenorenal and mesocaval shunts. Am J Surg 137:13, 1979
40. Resnick RH: Portal hypertension. Med Clin N Am 59:945, 1975
41. Reynolds TB: The role of hemodynamic measurements in portosystemic shunt surgery. Arch Surg 108:276, 1974
42. Riddell AG, Kopple PN, McDermott WV Jr: Etiology of "meat intoxication" in Eck fistula dog. Surgery 36:675, 1954
43. Roddie IC, Shepherd JT, Whelan RF: Humoral vasodilation in the forearm during voluntary hyperventilation. J Physiol 137:80, 1957
44. Rydell R, Hoffbauer FW: Multiple pulmonary arteriovenous fistulas in juvenile cirrhosis. Am J Med 21:450, 1956
45. Salam AA, Warren WD, LePage JR, et al: Hemodynamic contrasts between selective and total portal-systemic decompression. Ann Surg 173:827, 1971
46. Schenk WG, McDonald JC, McDonald K, et al: Direct measurement of hepatic blood flow in surgical patients: with related observations on hepatic flow dynamics in experimental animals. Ann Surg 156:463, 1962
47. Segal N, Bayley TJ, Paton A, et al: The effects of synthetic vasopressin and angiotensin on the circulation in cirrhosis of the liver. Clin Sci 25:43, 1963
48. Shaldon C: Dynamic aspects of portal hypertension. Ann R Coll Surgeons Engl 31:308, 1962
49. Shepherd JT: Physiology of the Circulation in Human Limbs in Health and Disease. Philadelphia, Saunders, 1963

50. Shorr E, Zweifarch BW, Furchgott EF, et al: Hepatorenal factors in circulatory homeostasis. Circulation 3:42, 1951
51. Siegel JH, Goldwyn RM, Farrell EJ, et al: Hyperdynamic states and the physiologic determinants of survival. Arch Surg 108:282, 1974
52. Siegel JH, Greenspan M, Cohn JD, et al: The prognostic implications of altered physiology in operations for portal hypertension. Surg Gynecol Obstet 126:249, 1968
53. Siegel JH, Greenspan M, Del Guercio LRM: Abnormal vascular tone, defective oxygen transport and myocardial failure in human septic shock. Ann Surg 165:504, 1967
54. Siegel JH, Williams JB: A computer based index for the prediction of operative survival in patients with cirrhosis and portal hypertension. Ann Surg 169:191, 1969
55. Silverstein E: Peripheral venous oxygen saturation in patients with and without liver disease. J Lab Clin Med 47, 513, 1956
56. Smith GW: Use of hemodynamic selection criteria in the management of cirrhotic patients with portal hypertension. Ann Surg 179:782, 1974
57. Turcotte JG, Lambert MJ: Variceal hemorrhage, hepatic cirrhosis and portacaval shunts. Surgery 78:810, 1973
58. Viallet H, Joly J, Marleau D, et al: Comparison of free portal venous pressure and wedged hepatic venous pressure in patients with cirrhosis of the liver. Gastroenterology 59:372, 1970
59. Viallet A, Marleau D, Huet M, et al: Hemodynamic evaluation of patients with intrahepatic portal hypertension. Gastroenterology 69:1297, 1975
60. Warren JV, Elkin DC, Nickerson JL: The blood volume in patients with arteriovenous fistulas. J Clin Invest 30:220, 1951
61. Warren WD, Foman JJ, Viamonte M, et al: Spontaneous reversal of portal blood flow in cirrhosis. Surg Gynecol Obstet 126:315, 1968
62. Warren WD, Mueller WH: A clarification of some hemodynamic changes in cirrhosis and their surgical significance. Ann Surg 150:413, 1959
63. Warren WD, Restrepo JE, Respees JC, et al: The importance of hemodynamic studies in management of portal hypertension. Ann Surg 158:387, 1963
64. Warren WD, Rudman D, Millikan W, et al: The metabolic basis of portasystemic encephalopathy and the effect of selective vs nonselective shunts. Ann Surg 180:573, 1974
65. Weiss S, Wilkins RW: The nature of the cardiovascular disturbances in nutritional deficiency states (beriberi). Ann Int Med 11:104, 1937
66. Whipple AO: The problem of portal hypertension in relation to hepatosplenopathies. Ann Surg 122:449, 1945
67. Zimmon DS, Kessler RE: Regulation of portal pressure in man. Gastroenterology 60:169, 1971
68. Zimmon DS, Kessler RE: The portal pressure-blood volume relationship in cirrhosis. Gut 15:99, 1974
69. Zuidema GD, Kirsh MM: Hepatic encephalopathy following portal decompression: evaluation of end-to-side and side-to-side anastomosis. Am Surg 31:567, 1965

Keith S. Henley, M.D.
H. Clifford Lane, M.D.
Timothy T. Nostrant, M.D.

Gastrointestinal Hemorrhage, Portacaval Shunts, and Hepatic Reserve

ABSTRACT

Examination of the records of the University of Michigan Hospitals shows that there was considerable difficulty in fitting patients into the classical Child's predictors of operative risk and long term survival. In medically treated patients presumed to be suffering from bleeding varices, long-term survival was best in those in whom the bleeding site could not be identified with confidence and poorest in those who were demonstrably bleeding from varices. Survival of surgically treated patients appeared to be independent of the confidence with which the bleeding source could be identified. We would like to suggest that the failure of prospective studies to establish the benefit of the surgical treatment of portal hypertension may be related, in part, to the short life expectancy of these patients and to the inevitable inclusion in those studies of patients who did not bleed from varices.
, Patients in whom varices have been seen to bleed, who have a portahepatic gradient of more than 12 mm Hg who do not have significant collateral flow and who do not have abundant Mallory bodies in their liver biopsies are the subgroup of cirrhotic patients most likely to benefit from operations for portal venous decompression. This suggestion needs to be verified prospectively before it is accepted or acted upon.

In the late 1950s, the surgical treatment of gastrointestinal bleeding secondary to portal hypertension came to be widely practiced. As with any

---

Keith S. Henley, M.D.: Professor of Internal Medicine, Head, Section of Gastroenterology, University of Michigan Medical Center, Ann Arbor, Michigan; H. Clifford Lane, M.D.: Clinical Associate, Division of Allergy and Infectious Diseases, National Institutes of Health, Washington, D.C.; Timothy T. Nostrant, M.D.: Instructor, Section of Gastroenterology, Department of Internal Medicine, University of Michigan Medical Center, Ann Arbor, Michigan.

major operative procedure, surgical mortality occurred. This was recognized by many but it was thanks to the leadership of Child that a serious attempt was made to match preoperative findings with mortality, morbidity and clinical achievement [3]. This led to the formulation of the Child criteria, according to which patients would be judged to be good, fair or poor risks, (A, B, and C, respectively). These criteria are described in Table 1.

Child insisted that these criteria be based on the best information which could be readily obtained and that they not be expected to provide more than a modest measure of guidance. The criteria have subsequently been used with much less flexibility than was originally intended.

More than 20 years later we want to determine whether it is valid to assign patients to one of these three groups, whether, if valid, such assignment is useful, and if not, to suggest alternative approaches to resolve some of the many issues in the surgical management of variceal bleeding.

Inspection of the criteria listed in Table 1 suggests that many patients may not readily fall into any of the three categories. We have all seen jaundiced patients (criterion C), without ascites, in good nutrition, with normal serum albumin concentration, and who have never been in coma (criterion A). Other patients may have poorly controlled ascites (criterion C), with normal serum bilirubin concentrations (criterion A). Furthermore, the presence of ascites is associated in part with the serum albumin concentration [1], and these are therefore not independent measurements. To determine whether these reservations are correct, we have examined the records of 16 randomly selected patients with cirrhosis (excluding patients with primary biliary cirrhosis), and tried to classify them according to the Child criteria. Patients who died during their first admission or who were not followed up in the Medical GI Clinic were excluded. The selection, therefore, favored patients with compensated disease. Some of the patients had undergone shunt operation, some had not and some had never been considered for such an operation because they had never bled. The point of assessment was the earliest clinic visit for which complete data were available.

Table 1
Clinical and Laboratory Classification of Patients
With Cirrhosis in Terms of Hepatic Functional Reserve

Group Designation	A (Minimal)	B (Moderate)	C (Advanced)
Serum bilrubin* (mg%)	Below 2.0	2.0 – 3.0	Over 3.0
Serum albumin (gm%)	Over 3.5	3.0 – 3.5	Under 3.0
Ascites	None	Easily controlled	Poorly controlled
Neurological disorder	None	Minimal	Advanced coma
Nutrition	Excellent	Good	Poor, wasting

*Equivocal in biliary cirrhosis.

The distribution of the 16 patients is shown in Table 2. It is obvious that assignment to A, B, or C risk categories should be made with complete confidence in only 1 patient and with some confidence in 3 others. In the remainder, no meaningful assessment could be made. It would be incorrect to average these data. A patient who has a serum bilirubin of 4.5 mg% (criterion C), but has never shown evidence of neurological problems (criterion A), cannot be considered as being equivalent to a criterion B patient with lower but still abnormal serum bilirubin, who suffers from minor neurological difficulties. These observations agree with published data. Thus, Mikkelsen [10] described a series of class A risk patients. In this group, the *mean* concentration of albumin in serum was quoted as 3.4 gm%, i.e., a criterion for a criterion B patient.

While there are difficulties in assigning patients to the Child criteria, it may be argued that the criteria did correlate with both the immediate and long term results of operations for the relief of portal hypertension [14]. Alternatively, a retrospective analysis may sharpen these criteria [9], but there is serious doubt whether this is a meaningful undertaking. No matter what series of prognostic indicators are developed, they will, at best, provide the essentially trivial information that patients with advanced disease do poorly, whereas patients with less advanced disease do better. If criteria of severity of disease were found to disagree with the outcome of a therapeutic program, this would not necessarily invalidate the program. The program may be correct but the criteria may be wrong. The Child criteria were developed out of a need to substitute objective predictors of outcome for subjective assessment. We may now wonder whether such an assessment is feasible or necessary.

Among the cirrhotic patients suffering from gastrointestinal hemorrhage, there is still a need to identify those who will benefit from a portal decompression operation. Before this is done, it is crucial to establish that varices are the source of bleeding because the operation cannot be expected to arrest bleeding from any other source. It should be recalled that roughly one half of, cirrhotic patients with varices and bleeding from their gastrointestinal tract will bleed from sources other than varices [2, 6].

Examination of the data from the University of Michigan suggests that prognosis depends on the confidence with which the bleeding site is identified. The records of 153 patients seen between 1969 and 1977, suffering from 200

Table 2
Attempted Assignment of Patients to Child's Criteria

Patients meeting same criteria in all five categories	1
Patients meeting same criteria in four out of five categories	3
Three to two split (i.e., 3 B and 2 A)	8
Divergence, (categories A and C coexist)	4
Total	16

episodes of gastrointestinal hemorrhage, were collected. Charts were then reviewed to determine whether a patient was bleeding from varices, (i.e., varices seen to bleed endoscopically, and occasionally demonstrated to do so by the venous phase of angiography), was probably bleeding from varices, (i.e., varices documented and no other bleeding source identified), or possibly bleeding from varices (patients with liver disease but with more than one potential bleeding site). Each group was then classified, depending on whether they received surgical or medical treatment, and their survival ascertained. The distribution of these patients is given in Table 3. While the method of collection of the data does not permit meaningful statistical analysis, it appears from Fig. 1 that the outcome of hospitalization may depend on the confidence with which a variceal bleed could be demonstrated. The prognosis appeared to be worst in patients with a demonstrated variceal bleed, regardless of therapy.

As expected, patients receiving medical therapy for uncertain cause of gastrointestinal hemorrhage tended to survive longer than those who were treated surgically for relief of portal hypertension. It should be noted that these data were generated at a time when routine endoscopy was used less liberally than it is now, and independent of any measurement of hepatic reserve. These data help to explain the inconclusive results of the controlled trials of shunt therapy reported from this country [7, 10, 12].

In the first instance, we are dealing with a group of patients whose life expectancy is short. This is evident from the figure and makes it very difficult to demonstrate, on statistical grounds, the benefit of any operative procedure which is not curative or free from operative risk. The almost certain "pollution" of all published controlled studies in this field by non-variceal bleeders would further minimize the chance of demonstrating a statistically valid benefit of portal decompression operations. Since the U.S. studies show better survival in the operated patients, even if this is not statistically convincing, it appears that the operations have a place. It is for surgeons to define that place more precisely than has been possible in the past. This will require the inclusion in any prospective trial of unoperated controls.

The objective then is to find those patients who are known to have bled from varices and who may benefit by an operation. In the remainder of this discussion, we would like to suggest how such a population can be identified. It is in such a population that we can *test* whether our suggestion is correct. It

Table 3
Analysis of 153 Patients With Discharge Diagnosis of Bleeding Varices

	Variceal Bleeding		
	Definite	*Probable*	*Possible*
Medical treatment	17	33	48
Surgical treatment	15	39	48

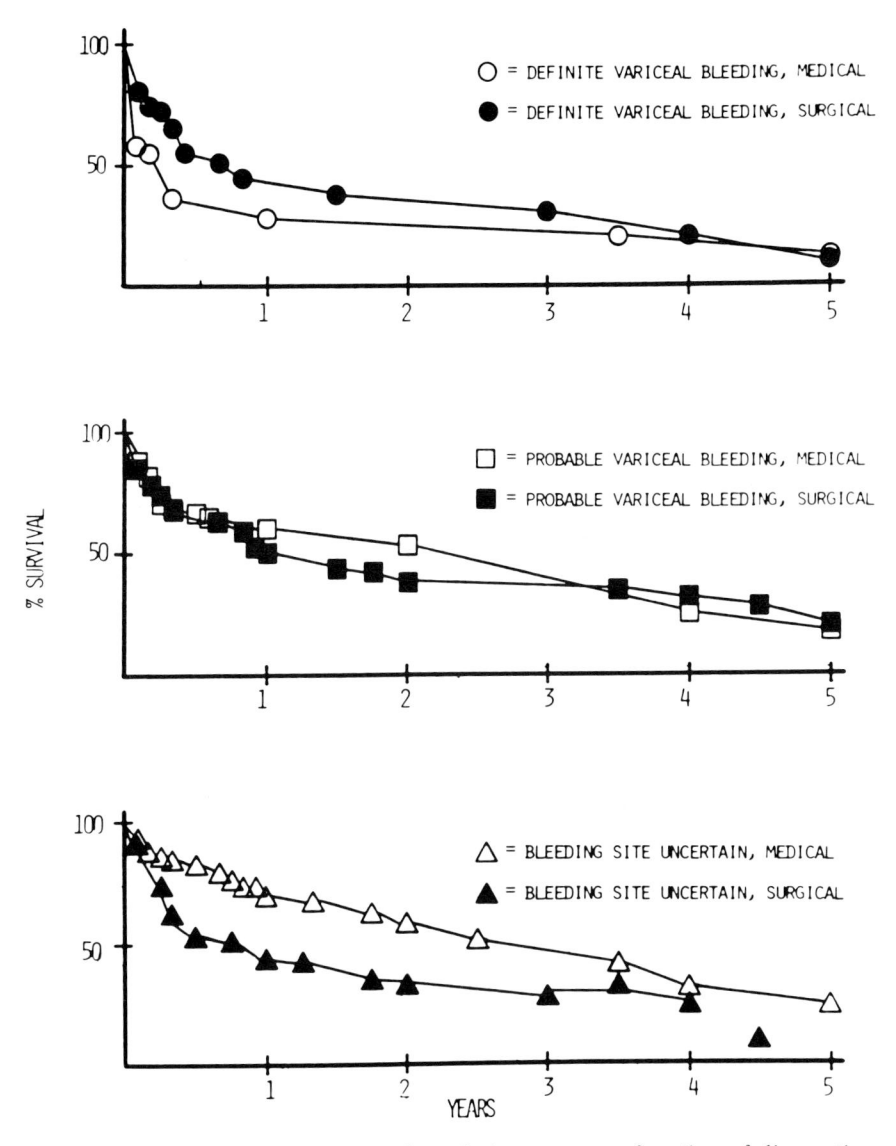

Fig. 1. Comparison of medical and surgical groups as a function of diagnostic criteria.

would be unfortunate if our suggestions were acted upon unless their validity has been rigorously proven.

The diagnosis of cirrhosis should be made by histopathological means; it cannot always be made with confidence otherwise. The etiology of cirrhosis and therefore its natural history is variable and many forms of cirrhosis, such as those of viral etiology, Wilson's disease and hemochromatosis are amenable to treatment. Patients must, therefore, be separated according to etiologies because the long held belief that cirrhosis represents an end stage of liver injury and is irreversible has been challenged [13].

Patients with a portahepatic pressure gradient of more than 12 mm Hg have larger sized varices and documented variceal bleeding was encountered only in that group [8, 15]. These studies require confirmation and some reexamination in terms of reproducibility and variability over periods of time. They did not prove that patients with a pressure gradient greater than 12 mm Hg will benefit from shunt therapy, but identified a group of patients who promise to be suitable for a prospective evaluation of such therapy.

If these patients are to be evaluated it is important to exclude those who present a prohibitive operative risk. This can be done judgmentally. Those who meet *all* of Child's C criteria are unlikely to survive long no matter what is done.

Other considerations of exclusion are based on hemodynamic measurements. Orloff has shown [11] that, if a clamp is placed across the portal vein, at operation patients whose pressure on the hepatic side of the clamp is greater than on the splenic side, i.e., patients who have significant collateral flow, will do poorly postoperatively. The apparent benefit of a Warren shunt, an operation which minimizes changes in hepatic flow, can be understood on that basis.

The existence of significant collateral flow can be assessed preoperatively. As pointed out by Cohn [4], in cirrhosis the splanchnic vascular bed can act as a huge arteriovenous fistula. Normally an indicator, injected as a pulse into the splanchnic vessels, can be recovered completely in the hepatic vein. In cirrhosis less is recovered and in 25% of cirrhotics, no indicator appears in the hepatic venous effluent. These patients ultimately may develop renal failure. For this reason, patients who show preoperative evidence of significant hepatofugal or collateral flow, as determined by the recovery of injected marker from the hepatic vein, are particularly at risk from early death regardless of treatment. They are best excluded from a trial seeking to establish the effectiveness of an elective operation intended to prolong life.

Finally, the function of the hepatocyte determines the fate of the patient. In alcoholic liver disease, there is a histopathological marker apparently associated with a higher surgical mortality, namely the Mallory body or alcoholic hyaline [10]. Studies by Eckhauser and his colleagues [5], have confirmed that abundant Mallory bodies are associated with poor long-term survival, regardless of other measurements. This observation has been verified only for patients with alcoholic liver disease. The significance of Mallory bodies seen in other conditions, such as primary biliary cirrhosis and Wilson's disease, remains to be assessed.

In summary, we suggest that the place of "elective" portal decompression operations be defined prospectively by the selection of patients who may benefit by the procedure. These patients should have evidence of hemorrhage from esophageal varices by direct observation and evidence of a portahepatic pressure gradient greater than 12 mm Hg. They should not demonstrate significant collateral flow of blood or have abundant Mallory bodies on liver biopsy (patients with alcoholic liver disease only).

REFERENCES

1. Atkinson M, Losowsky MS: Plasma colloid osmotic pressure in relation to the formation of ascites and edema in liver disease. Clin Sci 22:383, 1962
2. Brick IB, Palmer ED: One thousand cases of portal cirrhosis of the liver, implications of esophageal varices and their management. Arch Int Med 113:501, 1964
3. Child GC III, Turcotte JG: Surgery and portal hypertension. In Child CG III: The Liver and Portal Hypertension. Philadelphia, Saunders, 1964, p 1
4. Cohn JN: Renal hemodynamic alterations in liver disease. In Suki WN, Eknoyan G (eds): The Kidney and Systemic Disease. New York, Wiley, 1976, p 226
5. Eckhauser FE, Polley T Jr, Bloch D, et al: Hepatic pathology as a determinant of prognosis after portal decompression. Submitted for publication
6. Gray RS, Martin F, Amir-Ahmadi H, et al: Erroneous diagnosis of hemorrhage from esophageal varices. Am J Dig Dis 14:755, 1969
7. Jackson FC, Perrin EB, Felix R, et al: A clinical investigation of the portocaval shunt. V. Survival analysis of the therapeutic operation. Ann Surg 174:672, 1971
8. Joly JG, Marleau D, Lagare L, et al: Bleeding from esophageal varices in cirrhosis of the liver. Hemodynamic and radiological criteria for the selection of potential bleeders through hepatic and umbilicoportal catheterization studies. Canad Med Ass J 104:576, 1971
9. Malt RB, Malt RA: Tests and management affecting survival after portacaval and splenorenal shunts. Surg Gynecol Obstet 149:220, 1979
10. Mikkelsen WP: Therapeutic portacaval shunt. Preliminary data on controlled trial and morbid effects of acute hyaline necrosis. Arch Surg 108:302, 1974
11. Orloff MJ, Chandler JG, Charter AC III, et al: Emergency portacaval shunt treatment for bleeding esophageal varices. Arch Surg 108:293, 1974
12. Resnick RH, Iber FL, Ishahara RM, et al: A controlled study of the therapeutic portacaval shunt. Gastroenterology 67:843, 1974
13. Rojkind M, Dunn MA: Hepatic fibrosis. Gastroenterology 76:849, 1979

14. Turcotte JG, Wallin VW, Child CG III: End to side versus side to side portacaval shunt in patients with hepatic cirrhosis. Am J Surg 117:108, 1969
15. Viallet A, Marleau D, Huet M, et al: Hemodynamic evaluation of patients with intrahepatic portal hypertension. Relationship between bleeding varices and the portohepatic gradient. Gastroenterology 62:1297, 1975

Milton G. Mutchnick, M.D.

Vasopressin in the Management of Variceal Hemorrhage

ABSTRACT

The use of vasopressin to control variceal hemorrhage has enjoyed varying degrees of popularity over the past two decades. Although initial control of bleeding is obtained in a majority of patients, the high rate of recurrent hemorrhage, the frequent incidence of drug related complications and the dismal survival rate have slowed down the general clinical application of vasopressin. In practice, high-dose intravenous vasopressin is no longer used and low-dose intravenous administration of the drug appears to have supplanted the once acclaimed selective intraarterial route. It is now recognized that intraarterial vasopressin induces systemic hemodynamic effects and that low-dose intravenous vasopressin influences splanchnic hemodynamics to a degree comparable to that seen using the intraarterial route. Controlled studies comparing low-dose intravenous to intraarterial infusions strongly suggest that both are equally effective in stemming variceal bleeds. The use of vasopressin should be viewed as a temporizing measure preliminary to specific procedures designed to decompress the varices. It is recommended that low-dose intravenous vasopressin be utilized because of the technical ease of administration and the promptness of its application. If control of the hemorrhage is not attained within a few hours following initiation of vasopressin infusion, it is imperative that other modalities of treatment be instituted.

Bleeding esophageal varices constitute a major life threatening complication in patients with cirrhosis and portal hypertension. The mortality associated with this presentation may be catastrophic, with 40%-80% of patients succumbing during their initial hemorrhage [9]. Therapeutic efforts directed towards arresting variceal hemorrhage have included surgical and nonsurgical procedures.

Milton G. Mutchnick, M.D.: Assistant Professor of Internal Medicine, University of Michigan Medical Center, and Chief, Liver Disease Section, Veterans Administration Medical Center, Ann Arbor, Michigan.

These alternative approaches are associated with inherent hazards that in turn, may serve to seal the fate of the patient [14, 44].

The posterior pituitary extract, vasopressin, has been used for the past two decades in the management of variceal hemorrhage. Initially, it was suggested that vasopressin would provide a safe and effective means by which variceal hemorrhage could be controlled. Clinical experience however, has not validated these early expectations.

It is important to recognize that the use of vasopressin must be viewed as a temporizing measure. Vasopressin does not provide the definitive approach to the problem of variceal hemorrhage. It offers a pharmacologic means for temporarily controlling the bleeding so that the appropriate maneuver for ensuring permanent control can be instituted.

Three principal routes of vasopressin administration have been described: high and low dose intravenous, and selective intraarterial.

HIGH DOSE INTRAVENOUS

Kehne et al [30] are credited with the first attempt to control variceal hemorrhage using serial infusions of high dose intravenous vasopressin. These authors described 7 episodes of variceal bleeding in 2 patients which were controlled with either 10 or 20 units of vasopressin infused rapidly over a 10 minute period. They also described the first fatal complication associated with vasopressin use in patients with bleeding varices. This patient, who expired within 24 hours of vasopressin treatment, was found to have thrombosis of the entire extrahepatic portal venous system.

Data from clinical trials of high dose intravenous vasopressin administration for the control of bleeding varices reported initial success in 38%-88% of patients studied [10, 36, 50, 51]. However, bleeding recurred in most cases following discontinuation of therapy. In addition, significant complications were observed, notably coronary vasoconstriction, sinus bradycardia leading to sinus arrest, and small bowel infarction [10]. Despite what appeared to be a reasonable response with respect to control of hemorrhage, the mortality rate in these studies ranged from 62%-88% [10, 36, 51]. The frequency of adverse reactions and the disappointing survival rate associated with high dose intravenous vasopressin led to a waning of clinical interest in the use of this agent.

SELECTIVE INTRAARTERIAL INFUSION

In 1967, Nusbaum et al [41] described the consequences of selective infusions of low dose vasopressin into the superior mesenteric artery in dogs with surgically created portal hypertension. Vasopressin produced constriction of splanchnic arterial vessels with a resultant decrease in superior mesenteric venous flow and portal pressure. Continuous administration of small dosages

Table 1
Selective Intraarterial Vasopressin in Variceal Hemorrhage (Uncontrolled Studies)

Investigator	Year	Vasopressin Dosage Range (Units/min)	No. of Patients	Number of Discrete Episodes	Episodes With Initial Control Number	%	Episodes With Rebleed Number	%	Patient Mortality Number	%
Brant et al [7]	1972	0.10–0.30	11	11	7	64	4	57	7	64
Conn et al [11]	1972	0.10–0.40	13	19	15	79	9	60	10	77
Marubbio et al [34]	1973	0.15–0.30	8	8	8	100	5	63	4	50
Murray-Lyon et al [39]	1973	0.20–0.80	17	18	11	61	7	64	11	61
Nusbaum et al [43]	1974	0.20–0.40	41	41	40	98	NP	NP	25	61
Johnson et al [26]	1976	0.10–0.40	21	21	17	81	4	24	14	67
Kaufman et al [29]	1977	0.20–0.40	39	39	31	80	12	39	19	49
Sherman et al [52]	1978	0.20–0.40	25	28	20	71	5	25	12	48
Total			175	185	149	81	46*	42*	102	58

NP, not provided.
*Excluding data of Nusbaum et al [43].

(0.1 U/min) resulted in a rapid and sustained fall in portal pressure of 50% without apparent systemic side effects. The first clinical application of selective intraarterial vasopressin infusion was reported the following year [40]. Two patients received 0.1-0.4 U/min of vasopressin and subsequently stopped bleeding. There were no complications observed in either patient, but perhaps as a portent of findings to come, both subsequently rebled.

Reports from several uncontrolled studies of continuous intraarterial vasopressin infusion suggested that vasopressin might be effective in decreasing portal pressure and arresting variceal hemorrhage. Table 1 provides an overview of selected studies wherein 185 episodes of variceal bleeding in patients with portal hypertension are analyzed. While taking author's license to summate what may well be the equivalent of apples and oranges, the data suggest that vasopressin affords temporary control of bleeding in 4 of 5 patients. Bleeding recurred in nearly half of the patients studied. Observed patient mortality rates of 48%-77% were comparable to those seen prior to the era of vasopressin [9].

These data paralleled to a remarkable degree the results reported in the single prospective, controlled clinical study [13]. Conventional treatment was compared with conventional therapy plus intraarterial vasopressin in cirrhotic patients with variceal hemorrhage. Vasopressin was effective in controlling 71% of variceal hemorrhage as contrasted to the 31% control rate in conventionally treated patients. In addition, blood replacement requirements were less in the vasopressin treated group. Hemorrhage recurred in 45% of patients treated with vasopressin and in 33% of conventionally treated patients. Surprisingly, survival was not improved in the vasopressin treated group which had a 54% mortality rate as compared to the 56% mortality rate in the conventionally treated group. While the complication rate in patients receiving intraarterial vasopressin was 43%, none of these were considered life-threatening.

These discouraging results must be viewed in light of the inherent shortcomings noted in the study [13, 47]. Patients randomized for inclusion were critically ill and might not have been expected to survive even without enduring a massive gastrointestinal hemorrhage. Further, intravenous vasopressin was utilized in the conventionally treated group and patients who were designated as conventional therapy failures were given intraarterial vasopressin; if they survived, these patients were viewed for statistical purposes, as conventional treatment successes. Finally, a major modality of treatment, the Sengstaken-Blakemore tube, was not used at all in this study.

PHARMACOLOGIC ACTION OF VASOPRESSIN

Vasopressin exerts a direct effect on the smooth muscle of arteries resulting in vasoconstriction with reduced blood flow. This action is not antagonized by adrenergic blocking agents nor prevented by vascular denervation. Vasopressin decreases superior mesenteric arterial flow, particularly in the precapillary segment of the arterial tree [55]. This in turn decreases splanchnic venous return and portal flow resulting in lowered portal venous pressure. Other mechanisms postulated for vasopressin-induced lowering of portal pressure include: lowered hepatic resistance [35], increased hepatic flow [45] and closure of the submucosal gastroenteric arteriovenous shunts [18, 25].

Early experimental studies in normal dogs showed that intravenous vasopressin produced a 25% decrease in portal pressure [30]. Subsequent studies demonstrated that selective infusion of vasopressin into the superior mesenteric artery of dogs resulted in a 50% decrease in portal pressure in portal hypertensive dogs and a 20% decrease in normal dogs [41]. Similar studies in patients with bleeding varices demonstrated decreases of 51% in portal pressure and 60% in superior mesenteric artery flow following the intraarterial administration of 0.2 U/min of vasopressin [4].

Less impressive effects of vasopressin on portal venous pressure have been reported. Millete et al [37] noted that infusions of vasopressin into the superior mesenteric artery of nonbleeding cirrhotic patients produced only small decrements (10%) in portal venous pressure, at the same time decreasing portal venous pO_2, arterial blood pO_2 and cardiac output. Thus the predicated advantage of selective intraarterial as contrasted to systemic infusion of vasopressin to minimize systemic effects was not observed. Similar small decreases in portal venous pressure have been reported by other investigators using continuous peripheral or intraarterial vasopressin infusion in nonbleeding cirrhotic patients [3, 42, 56].

Nusbaum and Conn, in assessing the import of the apparent minimal effect of vasopressin on portal venous pressure, reviewed the data on cirrhotic patients from several studies [37, 42]. They noted that 10 of 12 nonbleeding patients (83%) infused with vasopressin showed a decrease in portal pressure while only 6 of 14 (43%) patients with variceal bleeding had a similar decrease. Moreover, patients exhibiting the greatest decrease in portal pressure evidenced minimal systemic effects while those having small decreases in portal pressure had the highest incidence of untoward systemic effects. These authors suggested several possible explanations for these findings. First, the decrease in portal pressure may represent a compromise between an initial large drop in pressure which is compensated in part by an increase in hepatic arterial flow. This hypothesis is supported by studies showing a compensatory increase in hepatic arterial flow with vasopressin-induced decreases in portal venous flow [19]. Second, pressure within the varices may not reflect actual portal pressure. Many of the patients studied did not have ascites or jaundice and were thus in a compensated state as contrasted to the usual cirrhotic patient experiencing a variceal hemorrhage. Finally, it was suggested that vasopressin may arrest hemorrhage by promoting contraction of esophageal smooth muscle with compression of the varices. Recent work however, appears to refute this mechanism of action [24].

It is not at all clear why variceal bleeding does not promptly recur with discontinuation of vasopressin. Perhaps the reduction in intravariceal pressure during treatment induces thrombosis within the vessel, or the time gained during therapy may allow for healing of the eroded mucosa overlying the bleeding site. It is apparent that a definitive conclusion is still lacking with respect to the mechanism by which vasopressin causes cessation of variceal hemorrhage.

Hepatic Arterial Flow

There has been alleviation of the initial concern that intraarterial vasopressin would decrease hepatic arterial flow and result in ischemic changes within the liver. A number of studies have adequately demonstrated that while there is an initial constriction of the hepatic artery with vasopressin infusion, the effects are transitory [12, 17, 20]. The hepatic artery response is characterized by a sustained autoregulatory escape mechanism which may in fact lead to a compensatory increase in hepatic arterial flow [12, 31, 54].

Complications Associated With Vasopressin Infusion

The initial expectation that administration of small amounts of intraarterial vasopressin would reduce the frequency of systemic complications seen with larger intravenous dosages has not been borne out by experience. Significant complications have been reported with both the catheterization procedure and with maintenance of the infusion [11, 13, 22, 26, 28, 29, 32, 34, 39, 43, 52]. There have also been reports of systemic side effects associated with intraarterial vasopressin that are similar to those reported in earlier studies of high dose intravenous vasopressin. The most frequent complications include bradycardia [11, 13, 21, 26, 43, 52] and elevated systemic blood pressure [11, 13, 26, 52]. Vasopressin may induce bradycardia by stimulating the vagus nerve through the cardioinhibitory center and by depressing the myocardium [21]. Blood pressure elevation appears to result from the peripheral vessel pressor effect and is usually associated with a decrease in pulse pressure [21]. Other significant side effects include water intoxication [33, 34], cardiac arrest [11, 13, 26], cardiac arrhythmia [5, 13, 26, 52], cardiac failure [26, 52], myocardial infarction [22], angina pectoris [11], intestinal ischemia and necrosis [6, 11, 22, 46, 49], reactive erythema [11], and pedal ischemia [38]. The frequency of complications associated with the use of intraarterial vasopressin is presented in Table 2 and while by no means complete, serves to indicate the significance of problems encountered with this technique. Clinical studies have shown that one third of patients given intraarterial vasopressin may be expected to suffer untoward side effects.

HEMODYNAMIC EFFECTS OF INTRAVENOUS VERSUS INTRAARTERIAL VASOPRESSIN

Numerous investigators have observed systemic effects with low-dose intraarterial vasopressin infusion. Since the biological half-life of vasopressin

Table 2
Frequency of Complications Associated With Intraarterial Vasopressin Therapy in Patients With Upper Gastrointestinal Hemorrhage

Investigator	Vasopressin Dosage Range (Units/min)	No. of Patients	Complications Associated With Catheterization Number	%	Complications Associated With Vasopressin Number	%	Total Number	%
Conn et al [13]	0.05–0.40	28	2	7	10	36	12	43
Conn et al [11]	0.10–0.40	34	NS	–	NS	–	12	35
Marubbio et al [34]	0.15–0.30	41	6	15	2	5	8	20
Geronilla et al [21]	0.20–0.40	17	1	6	4	24	5	29
MacKenzie et al [32]	0.20	24	5	21	0	0	5	21
Johnson et al [26]	0.10–0.40	74	4	5	6	8	10	14
Kaufman et al [29]	0.20–0.40	39	2	5	0	0	2	5
Johnson et al [27]	0.10–0.40	14	6	43	6	43	6*	43*
Sherman et al [52]	0.20–0.40	66	5	8	49	74	49*	74*
Murray–Lyon et al [39]	0.20–0.80	17	16	94	0	0	16	94
Chojkier et al [8]	0.10–0.50	12	3	25	2	17	5	42
Total		366	50†	15†	79†	24†	130	36

NS, not specified.
*Exact totals not provided; data given represent the minimum possible total.
†Excluding data of Conn et al [11].

ranges from 15 to 24 min, the difference between intraarterial versus intravenous infusions on hemodynamic events should be minimal [31]. Several studies in dogs have revealed little difference between the hemodynamic effects of intraarterial versus intravenous vasopressin infusion. Low-dose intravenous vasopressin (0.2 U/min in humans) resulted in 80 to 85% of the splanchnic effect obtained with doses comparable to 1 U/min in humans. Low dose vasopressin therapy caused fewer and milder systemic effects than the high dose regimen [3].

Comparable responses with respect to cardiac output, intestinal oxygen consumption, mesenteric arterial flow, and portal venous pressure have been obtained using either low dose intravenous or intraarterial infusions [2, 3, 15, 31, 53]. The similarity of systemic effects encountered using both routes of administration is not surprising as comparable levels of circulating vasopressin have been found irrespective of the route of infusion.

INTRAVENOUS VASOPRESSIN IN BLEEDING VARICES

Vasopressin administered through the intraarterial or intravenous route results in similar local and systemic hemodynamic responses. This observation coupled with the technical ease of the latter route of administration has led to clinical studies evaluating the efficacy of low-dose intravenous vasopressin. The first reports of success using low-dose (0.1-0.3 U/min) intravenous vasopressin [1, 48] to control variceal hemorrhage were followed by two additional controlled studies comparing intraarterial versus intravenous vasopressin infusion (Table 3) [8, 27]. No essential differences with respect to control of hemorrhage, recurrent bleed or mortality were noted with the intraarterial versus intravenous routes of administration. The complication rate in the West Haven series was 70% in the intravenous treated group and 42% in the intraarterial treated group [8]. The figures for the Boston series were 18% and 43%, respectively [41].

A disturbing observation noted in these studies was that although both intravenous and intraarterial vasopressin were equally efficacious in controlling variceal hemorrhage, the mortality rate was high with either route of administration (Table 3) and resembled, to a remarkable degree, the results of previous studies of intraarterial vasopressin (Table 1) as well as studies evaluating other conventional forms of therapy [9].

VASOPRESSIN IN THE TREATMENT OF VARICEAL BLEEDING

It does not appear that the administration of vasopressin by any route favorably influences survival even though bleeding may be controlled. Thus, the clinical justification for vasopressin has not been established.

Table 3
Comparison of Intraarterial Versus Intravenous Vasopressin in the Treatment of Variceal Bleeding

	Intraarterial									Intravenous								
	Dosage	No.	Initial				Patient			Dosage	No.	Initial				Patient		
	Range	of	Control		Rebleed		Mortality			Range	of	Control		Rebleed		Mortality		
Investigator	(Units/min)	Patients	No.	%	No.	%	No.	%		(Units/min)	Patients	No.	%	No.	%	No.	%
Johnson et al [27]	0.1–0.4	14	10	71	3	30	4	29		0.1–0.4	11	7	64	0	0	5	46
Chojkier et al [8]	0.1–0.5	12	6	50	3	50	9	75		0.3–1.5	10	5	50	2	40	7	70
Total		26	16	62	6	38	13	50			21	12	57	2	17	12	57

Perhaps vasopressin, while stemming acute hemorrhage, induces untoward hemodynamic effects which ultimately harm the patient. There is evidence to suggest that cirrhotic patients may enter a hyperdynamic state, particularly when stressed by an event such as bleeding, and develop high output cardiac failure [16]. The known effects of vasopressin in reducing cardiac output may provide the ultimate insult by accentuating cardiac failure and impairing effective tissue perfusion.

It has been suggested that inotropic agents should be administered with vasopressin to avert or ameliorate high output cardiac failure [16]. In a recent study in dogs concomitant infusion of nitroglycerin and vasopressin appeared to minimize the adverse cardiac effects exerted by vasopressin without adversely influencing the splanchnic hemodynamic effect of vasopressin [23].

It is reasonable to conclude that there may be a role for vasopressin in the control of variceal hemorrhage if we can identify better the candidate who would benefit most from its administration, while at the same time provide adequate protection against serious known and suspected systemic complications related to its use.

In keeping with the current state of the art, if vasopressin is to be used to control variceal bleeding, the continuous infusion of low dose intravenous vasopressin is recommended. If control is not achieved within a few hours, other therapeutic maneuvers should be considered.

REFERENCES

1. Athanasoulis CA, Waltman AC, Novelline RA, et al: Angiography. Its contribution to the emergency management of gastrointestinal hemorrhage. Radiol Clin North Am 14:265, 1976
2. Athanasoulis CA, Waltman AC, Simmons JT, et al: Effects of intravenous vasopressin on canine mesenteric arterial blood flow, bowel oxygen consumption, and cardiac output. Am J Roentgenol 130:1033, 1978
3. Barr JW, Lakin RC, Rösch J: Similarity of arterial and intravenous vasopressin on portal and systemic hemodynamics. Gastroenterology 69:13, 1975
4. Baum S, Nusbaum M: Control of gastrointestinal hemorrhage by selective mesenteric arterial infusion of vasopressin. Radiology 98:497, 1971
5. Beller BM, Trevino A, Urban E: Pitressin-induced myocardial injury and depression in a young woman. Am J Med 51:675, 1971
6. Berardi RS: Vascular complications of superior mesenteric artery infusion with pitressin in treatment of bleeding esophageal varices. Am J Surg 127:757, 1974
7. Brant B, Rösch J, Krippaehne WW: Experiences with angiography in diagnosis and treatment of acute gastrointestinal bleeding of various etiologies: Preliminary report. Am Surg 176:419, 1972

8. Chojkier M, Groszmann RJ, Atterbury CE, et al: A controlled comparison of continuous intraarterial and intravenous infusions of vasopressin in hemorrhage from esophageal varices. Gastroenterology 77:540, 1979
9. Conn HO: Cirrhosis. In Schiff L (ed): Diseases of the Liver, 4th Ed. Philadelphia, Lippincott, 1975, p 833
10. Conn HO, Dalessio DJ: Multiple infusions of posterior pituitary extract in the treatment of bleeding esophageal varices. Ann Int Med 57:804, 1962
11. Conn HO, Ramsby GR, Storer EH: Selective intraarterial vasopressin in the treatment of gastrointestinal hemorrhage. Gastroenterology 63:634, 1972
12. Conn HO, Ramsby GR, Storer EH: Hepatic arterial escape from vasopressin-induced vasoconstriction: an angiographic investigation. Am J Roentgenol Radium Ther Nucl Med 119:102, 1973
13. Conn HO, Ramsby GR, Storer EH, et al: Intraarterial vasopressin in the treatment of upper gastrointestinal hemorrhage: a prospective, controlled clinical trial. Gastroenterology 68:211, 1975
14. Conn HO, Simpson JA: Excessive mortality associated with balloon tamponade of bleeding varices. JAMA 202:587, 1967
15. Davis GB, Bookstein JJ, Hagan PL: The relative effects of selective intraarterial and intravenous vasopressin infusion. Radiology 120:537, 1976
16. Dicarlo V, Staudacher C, Chiesa R, et al: The role of cardiovascular hemodynamics and liver histology in evaluating bleeding cirrhotic patients. Ann Surg 190:218, 1979
17. Drapanas T, Crowe CP, Shim WK, et al: Effect of pitressin on cardiac output and coronary, hepatic, and intestinal blood flow. Surg Gynecol Obstet 113:484, 1961
18. Eiseman B, Silen W, Tyler P, et al: The portal hypotensive action of pituitrin. Surg Forum 10:286, 1960
19. Erwald R, Wiechel KL, Strandell T: Effect of vasopressin on regional splanchnic blood flows in conscious man. Acta Chir Scand 142:36, 1976
20. Fingeroth RJ, Storer EH, Ramsby GR: Effect of intra-arterial infusion of vasopressin on hepatic artery flow. Surg Forum 24:399, 1973
21. Geronilla DR, Sampliner JE, Lerner A: Gastrointestinal bleeding: treatment with intra-arterial vasopressin. Am Surg 41:321, 1975
22. Getzen LC, Brink RR, Wolfman EF: Survival following infusion of pitressin into the superior mesenteric artery to control bleeding esophageal varices in cirrhotic patients. Ann Surg 187:337, 1978
23. Groszmann RJ, Blei A, Gusberg R, et al: Hemodynamic effect of combined infusion of vasopressin (VP) and nitroglycerin (NG) in normal and cirrhotic dogs. Gastroenterology 77:A15, 1979
24. Häuptle B, Güller R: Effect of vasopressin on the lower esophageal sphincter. Study of the action mechanism of vasopressin in bleeding esophageal varices. Schweiz Med Wochenschr 108:1087, 1978
25. Johnson LL, Nelson HM Jr, Hardesty WH, et al: Enteric arteriovenous anastomoses and their contribution to portal hemodynamics. Surg Forum 11:272, 1960

26. Johnson WC, Widrich WC: Efficacy of selective splanchnic arteriography and vasopressin perfusion in diagnosis and treatment of gastrointestinal hemorrhage. Am J Surg 131:481, 1976
27. Johnson WC, Widrich WC, Ansell JE, et al: Control of bleeding varices by vasopressin: a prospective randomized study. Ann Surg 186:369, 1977
28. Kadir S, Athanasoulis CA: Catheter dislodgment: a cause of failure of intraarterial vasopressin infusions to control gastrointestinal bleeding. Cardiovasc Radiol 1:187, 1978
29. Kaufman SL, Harrington DP, Barth KH, et al: Control of variceal bleeding by superior mesenteric artery vasopressin infusion. Am J Roentgenol 128:567, 1977
30. Kehne JH, Hughes FA, Gompertz ML: The use of surgical pituitrin in the control of esophageal varix bleeding. An experimental study and report of two cases. Surgery 39:917, 1956
31. Kerr JC, Hobson RW II, Seelig RF, et al: Vasopressin: Route of administration and effects on canine hepatic and superior mesenteric arterial blood flows. Ann Surg 187:137, 1978
32. MacKenzie RL, Bury KD, Provan JL, et al: The failure of intraarterial pitressin infusion to control upper gastro-intestinal bleeding in cirrhotic patients. J Surg Res 20:505, 1976
33. Marubbio AT Jr: Anti-diuretic hormone effect of pitressin during continuous pitressin infusion. Gastroenterology 62:1103, 1972
34. Marubbio AT Jr, Lombardo RP, Holt PR: Control of variceal bleeding by superior mesentric artery pitressin perfusions – complication and indications. Am J Dig Dis 18:539, 1973
35. McMichael J: The portal circulation. I. The action of adrenaline and pituitary pressor extract. J Physiol 75:241, 1932
36. Merigan TC Jr, Plotkin GR, Davidson CS: Effect of intravenously administered posterior pituitary extract on hemorrhage from bleeding esophageal varices. A controlled evaluation. N Engl J Med 266:134, 1962
37. Millette B, Huet P-M, Lavoie P, et al: Portal and systemic effects of selective infusion of vasopressin into the superior mesenteric artery in cirrhotic patients. Gastroenterology 69:6, 1975
38. Motsay GJ, Sutherland DER, Simmons RL: Reversible pedal ischemia following intra-arterial infusion of vasopressin at a high dosage level required for control of massive bleeding from the small bowel: a case report. Ann Surg 178:648, 1973
39. Murray-Lyon IM, Pugh RNH, Nunnerley HB, et al: Treatment of bleeding oesophageal varices by infusion of vasopressin into the superior mesenteric artery. Gut 14:59, 1973
40. Nusbaum M, Baum S, Kuroda K, et al: Control of portal hypertension by selective mesenteric arterial drug infusion. Arch Surg 97:1005, 1968
41. Nusbaum M, Baum S, Sakiyalak P, et al: Pharmacologic control of portal hypertension. Surgery 62:299, 1967
42. Nusbaum M, Conn HO: Arterial vasopressin infusions: science or seance? Gastroenterology 69:263, 1975

43. Nusbaum M, Younis MT, Baum S, et al: Control of portal hypertension. Selective mesenteric arterial infusion of vasopressin. Arch Surg 108:342, 1974
44. Orloff MJ, Chandler JG, Charters AC, et al: Emergency portacaval shunt treatment for bleeding esophageal varices. Arch Surg 108:293, 1974
45. Orrego H, Mena I, Sepulveda G: Effects of pituitrin and vasopressin on hepatic circulation. Am J Dig Dis 9:109, 1964
46. Renert WA, Button KF, Fuld SL, et al: Mesenteric venous thrombosis and small-bowel infarction following infusion of vasopressin into the superior mesenteric artery. Diag Radiol 102:299, 1972
47. Resnick RH: Intraarterial vasopressin: A continuing challenge. Gastroenterology 68:411, 1975
48. Rigberg LA, Ufberg MH, Brooks CM: Continuous low dose peripheral vein pitressin infusion in the control of variceal bleeding. Am J Gastroenterol 68:481, 1977
49. Roberts C, Maddison FE: Partial mesenteric arterial occlusion with subsequent ischemic bowel damage due to pitressin infusion. Am J Roentgenol 126:829, 1976
50. Schwartz SI, Bales HW, Emerson GL, et al: The use of intravenous pituitrin in treatment of bleeding esophageal varices. Surgery 45:72, 1959
51. Shaldon S, Sherlock S: The use of vasopressin ('pitressin') in the control of bleeding from oesophageal varices. Lancet 2:222, 1960
52. Sherman LM, Shenoy SS, Cerra FB: Selective intra-arterial vasopressin. Ann Surg 189:298, 1979
53. Simmons JT, Baum S, Sheehan BA, et al: The effect of vasopressin on hepatic arterial blood flow. Radiology 124:637, 1977
54. Swan KG, Hobson RW II, Kerr JC: Experimental observations and clinical recommendations on vasopressin for control of gastrointestinal hemorrhage. Am Surg 43:545, 1977
55. Texter EC Jr, Chow CC, Merrill SL, et al: Direct effects of vasoactive agents on segmental resistance of the mesenteric and portal circulation. J Lab Clin Med 64:624, 1964
56. Thomford NR, Sirinek KR: Intravenous vasopressin in patients with portal hypertension: Advantages of continuous infusion. J Surg Res 18:113, 1975

Stephen R. Ramsburgh, M.D.
Jeremiah G. Turcotte, M.D.

Control of Gastroesophageal Variceal Bleeding With Balloon Tamponade

ABSTRACT

Gastroesophageal balloon tamponade is an effective method of temporarily managing patients hemorrhaging from varices. Gastric and esophageal balloon tubes are designed to compress these submucosal veins and thereby tamponade any bleeding site.

The Linton-Nachlas tube, the Boyce modification of the Sengstaken-Blakemore tube, and the Edlich (Minnesota) tube are the three most widely used tamponade balloon tubes in use today. A review of the literature reveals that bleeding varices can be controlled in about 90% of cases using a tamponade balloon tube. Complications include aspiration, airway obstruction and esophageal injury. They occur in about 10% of patients. The mortality rate directly attributable to the use of such a tube is 5%.

Balloon tamponade should only be used in the treatment of bleeding gastroesophageal varices when other less invasive treatment modalities have been tried without success. The risk of a life-threatening complication or death directly as a result of using such a tube must be weighed against the risk of death from exsanguination.

Approximately 30% of all patients with cirrhosis of the liver will hemorrhage at least once from gastroesophageal varices. The mortality of this complication ranges from 30% to 85% [19, 27, 36]. A variety of approaches, including balloon tamponade, Pitressin infusion, transhepatic coronary vein thrombosis, sclerotherapy, transesophageal varix ligation and emergency portosystemic shunting, have been employed to deal with these patients. Gastroesophageal balloon tamponade has proven to be a reliable and effective method of temporary management.

Stephen R. Ramsburgh, M.D.: Instructor, Department of Surgery, University of Michigan Medical Center; Jeremiah G. Turcotte, M.D.: Professor of Surgery and Chairman, Department of Surgery, University of Michigan Medical Center, Ann Arbor, Michigan.

HISTORICAL BACKGROUND

Westphal [37] in 1930 was the first to effectively control variceal bleeding with esophageal tamponade. Using an inflatable balloon on a length of whale bone (Gottstein's sound) he successfully abated gastroesophageal hemorrhage in 2 patients for 24 and 29 hours, respectively. He also described the use of an antiseptic gauze pack for tamponade in a patient bleeding at a higher level. Rowntree [32] in 1947 modified a standard Miller-Abbott tube by attaching a Latex bag to the distal end. After the tube was inserted the balloon was inflated and left in place for 4 days. This technique resulted in complete control of bleeding in 1 patient with esophageal varices.

Over the next several years sporadic reports describing various techniques for balloon tamponade of the esophagus appeared in the literature. The first double-balloon tube was developed by Bixby [6] in 1948, but was impractical because it lacked a lumen for the aspiration of gastric contents. A double-balloon, four-lumen tube, was introduced a year later by Patton and Johnston [29] which minimized gastric aspiration problems. This tube was the prototype of the more familiar Sengstaken-Blakemore, Linton-Nachlas, and Edlich tubes.

The tube originally described by Sengstaken and Blakemore [33] in 1950 had an esophageal and a gastric balloon attached to a tube with three channels. Two channels were for inflating the gastric and esophageal balloons, and the third was for aspiration of the stomach (Fig. 1). With widespread acceptance of balloon tamponade of the esophagus for control of variceal bleeding, it became apparent that aspiration of blood, pharyngeal secretions or both into the tracheobronchial tree was a significant and frequent complication. To deal with this problem of aspiration, Boyce [8] modified the Sengstaken-Blakemore tube by attaching a standard plastic nasogastric tube, the tip of which was secured in place with a silk ligature at a point just above the proximal end of the esophageal balloon (Fig. 2).

Edlich [16] noted that continuous aspiration of the esophagus using a nasogastric tube positioned above the inflated esophageal balloon of a Sengstaken-Blakemore tube was unsatisfactory because the additional tube was poorly tolerated by the patient and the constantly accumulating secretions were not reliably removed. In an attempt to more effectively deal with this problem, Edlich developed a double-balloon, four-lumen, esophagogastric tube similar to the one introduced in 1949 by Patton and Johnston. This new apparatus (marketed by Davol, Inc. as the Minnesota tube) is essentially a Sengstaken-Blakemore tube with a fourth channel. The proximal and distal balloons can be individually inflated through two separate channels within the wall of the tube. The remaining two channels, also incorporated within the tube, allow aspiration of the stomach distal to the gastric balloon and the esophagus proximal to the esophageal balloon (Fig. 3).

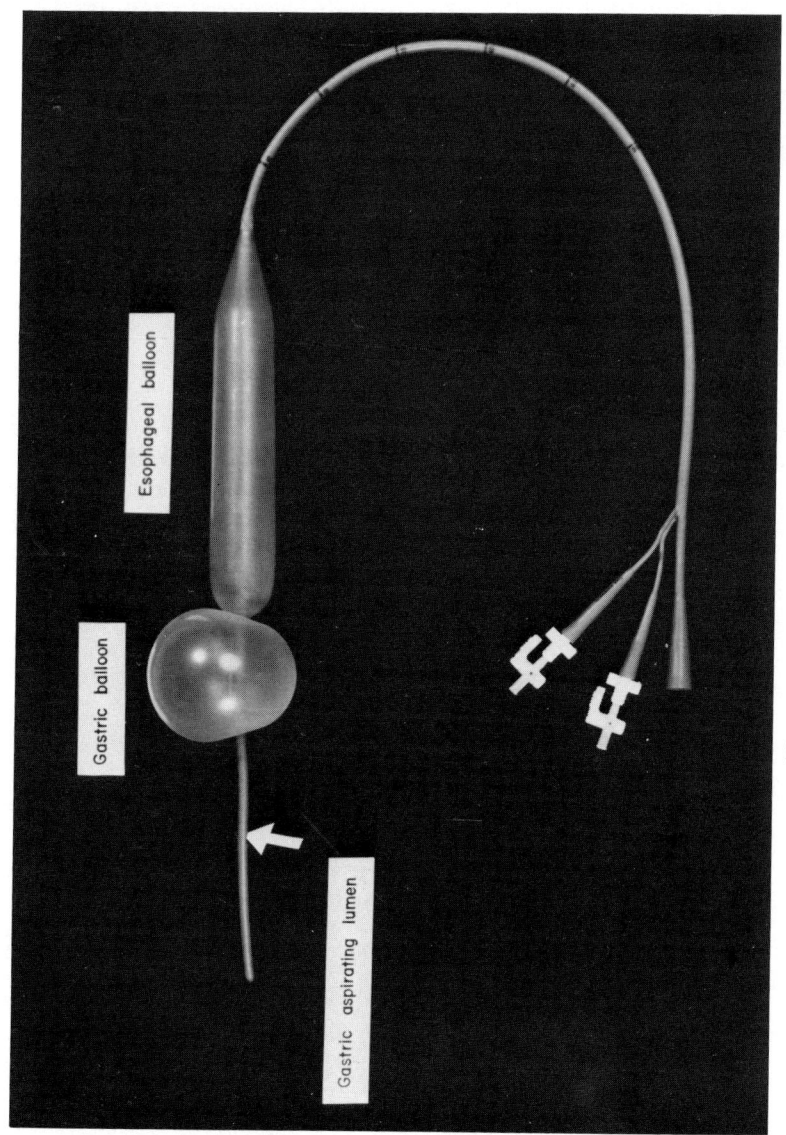

Fig. 1. Sengstaken-Blakemore tube.

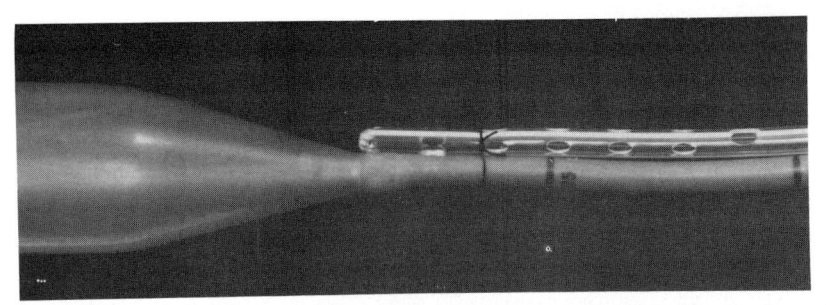

Fig. 2. Boyce modification of Sengstaken-Blakemore tube showing attachment of nasogastric tube to esophageal balloon.

Another esophageal tamponade tube in use today is the Linton-Nachlas tube. In 1953 Linton [23] designed and introduced a tube with only a gastric balloon and a distal aspirating lumen (Fig. 4). This balloon, unlike the gastric balloon in the Sengstaken-Blakemore tube, can be inflated to about 600 cc. The Linton tube was originally designed and used as a diagnostic instrument to determine whether gastroesophageal bleeding originated from above or below the cardia of the stomach. Soon after its introduction, however, it became apparent that this tube was also effective in controlling bleeding from gastric or esophageal varices. Once the effectiveness of the Linton tube had been clearly demonstrated, Nachlas [25, 26] introduced a modification by adding another channel to aspirate secretions in the esophagus and nasopharynx above the inflated gastric balloon (Fig. 5).

The Boyce modification of the Sengstaken-Blakemore tube, the Edlich or Minnesota tube and the Linton-Nachlas tube have been used extensively during the past ten years for balloon tamponade of bleeding esophageal varices. Recently, Idezuki [20] has described a new tamponade tube that is basically similar to the standard Sengstaken-Blakemore tube except for modifications which permit fiberoptic observation of the esophageal and gastric mucosa from within the main lumen of the core tube. The tube itself is made of transparent plastic; the core is polyvinyl chloride and the esophageal balloon is a polyurethane membrane. The inside diameter of the core tube is large enough to accommodate a small caliber fiberoptic endoscope. Proper use of this new tube ensures accurate placement in the stomach and allows direct visualization of the gastroesophageal varices as the balloons are inflated.

ANATOMY

Gastroesophageal varices develop as a compensatory response to elevated pressures within the portal venous system. The blood that courses through the esophageal varices of a patient with portal hypertension comes from two

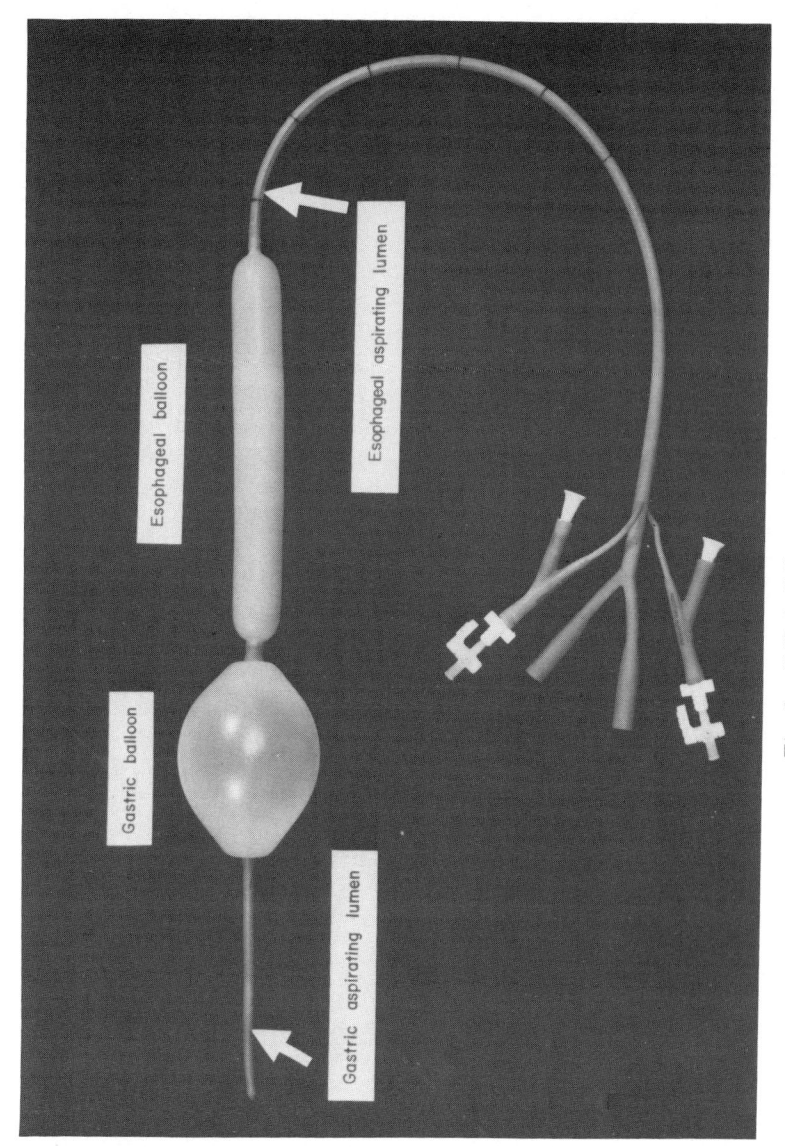

Fig. 3. Edlich (Minnesota) tube.

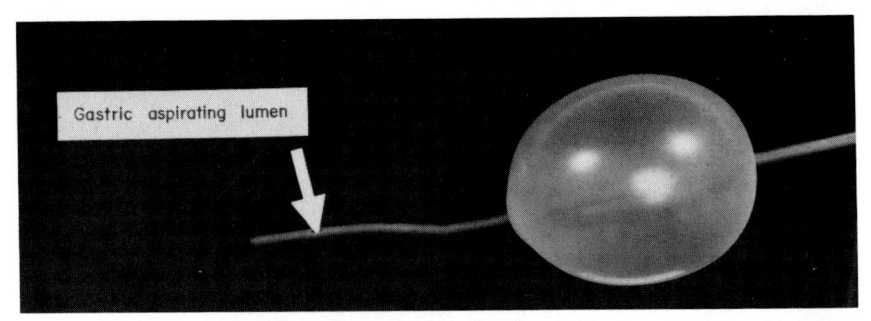

Fig. 4. Linton tube.

sources. Submucosal vessels of the stomach traverse the cardioesophageal junction to anastomose with esophageal submucosal veins and constitute the major source. Peri-esophageal veins with perforating branches ramifying through the wall of the esophagus to communicate with the submucosal varices provide the second source. These periesophageal veins also drain into the azygos, phrenic and intercostal veins, which normally have low or even negative pressures so that most of the extraesophageal blood flow drains toward the heart rather than through the muscular coats of the esophagus to the submucosal varices. Even though balloon tamponade at the cardioesophageal junction may not mechanically occlude the bleeding varices, it prevents the delivery of blood from the submucosal gastric varices to the submucosal esophageal varices [25, 26]. This is the anatomic explanation of why a single balloon tube, such as the Nachlas-Linton tube, is often successful in controlling esophageal hemorrhage.

The occasional failure of a single balloon tube to control esophageal bleeding necessitates the use of lateral esophageal compression and may be explained by the fact that infrequently the major contribution of blood to the esophageal varices is from the periesophageal veins through the large communicating veins that perforate the esophageal wall.

PHYSIOLOGY

The actual pathophysiologic mechanisms that initiate hemorrhage from gastroesophageal varices have never been clearly delineated. The importance of increased portal venous pressure is generally well accepted. The role of gastroesophageal reflux with resulting acid-peptic erosion of the esophageal mucosa has also been widely proposed as a possible etiologic factor. If peptic esophagitis causes varix rupture, gastroesophageal reflux must presumably be a common occurrence. Eckardt [15] undertook a study to determine the frequency of lower esophageal sphincter (LES) incompetency in patients with cirrhosis and variceal bleeding. Resting lower esophageal sphincter pressure measured in 35 patients with cirrhosis was similar to that found in 11

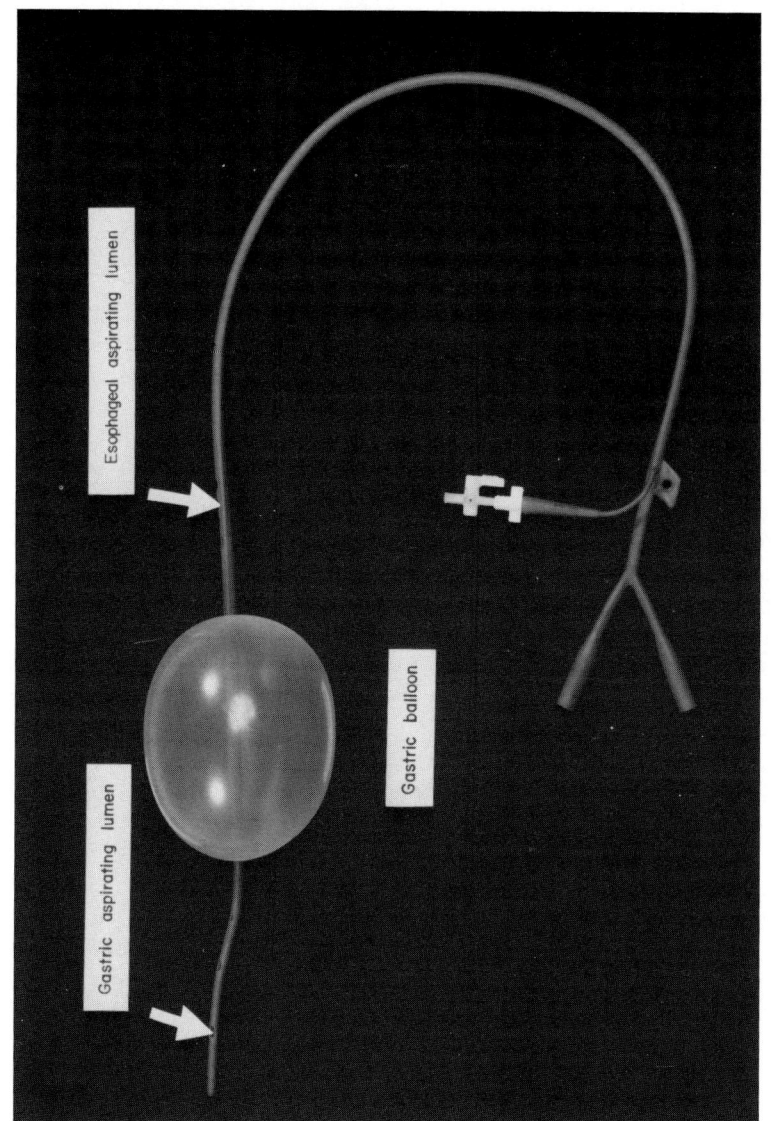

Fig. 5. Linton-Nachlas tube.

noncirrhotic, control patients. No differences were found among patients with variceal hemorrhage. Eckardt concluded that among individuals with cirrhosis of the liver and ruptured varices the occurrence of gastroesophageal reflux has no etiologic effect. Mucosal erosion over varices observed endoscopically in the distal esophagus or proximal stomach in patients who have suffered a recent variceal hemorrhage may reflect ischemic damage from impaired circulation and increased hydrostatic pressure within the varix, or it may be the effect of balloon compression during treatment of the bleeding.

One intriguing question associated with the use of balloon tamponade of bleeding esophageal varices is whether it is the pressure transmitted to the varices by the balloon that actually stops the hemorrhage [4]. Anderson [2] has clearly demonstrated that barium will freely pass both inflated balloons of a well positioned and properly employed Sengstaken-Blakemore tube.

Baxter [4] developed a method for measuring the transmitted pressure from the inflated esophageal balloon to the wall of the esophagus. The pressure within the balloon was measured by attaching the inflation arm of the tube to a manometer. By placing a fluid-filled, open-tipped catheter between the balloon and esophageal mucosa, 5 cm above the gastroesophageal junction, he found that transmitted (catheter) pressure at the esophageal wall was less than one-half the balloon pressure. This discrepancy between esophageal balloon pressure and the pressure transmitted to the esophageal wall has been confirmed by Agger and associates [1] who also measured the transmitted pressure in patients with verified bleeding esophageal varices. They observed that the inflation pressures required to obtain a transmitted esophageal pressure of 40 mm Hg (the recommended inflation pressure for the esophageal balloon of a standard Sengstaken-Blakemore tube) approached 100 mm Hg. At this inflation pressure all patients tested suffered severe retrosternal chest pain.

Agger also correlated the diameter of the esophageal balloon with transmitted pressure at increasing inflation pressures. The median diameter at 40 mm Hg was 27.3 mm, but further increases in inflation pressure caused only minor variations in diameter. At a median inflation pressure of 75 mm Hg (range 60-90 mm Hg) the balloon was noted to bulge at its proximal and distal ends, resulting in an actual fall in transmitted pressure at the midportion of the balloon to a median of 55 mm Hg (range 45-60 mm Hg) which was unaffected by further inflation.

Agger concluded from these measurements that the diameter of the esophageal balloon was probably not a significant hemostatic factor. This observation, coupled with the fact that actual transmitted pressure is often quite low, suggests that it is probably not necessary to equalize or exceed intravarix pressure to control bleeding.

In actuality, it is quite impossible to equalize or exceed intravarix pressure with an intraluminal pressure balloon. Transesophageal needling of a varix with a fine gauge needle has demonstrated that the venous pressure within a varix is very sensitive to slight changes in intrathoracic and intra-abdominal pressure. Even quiet respiration with such a needle in place causes a pressure fluctuation of as much as 7.5 mm Hg (rising during expiration). A sustained Valsalva effort can cause a rise in pressure of as much as 195 mm Hg [9] far greater than any that can be transmitted to the esophagus by an intraluminal balloon.

DIAGNOSIS

Rupture of gastroesophageal varices in cirrhotic patients accounts for less than half the total number of bleeding episodes [12, 28, 34]. Other sources of bleeding in these particular patients include gastroduodenal ulcer and acute erosive mucosal lesions; frequently these patients bleed from more than one lesion simultaneously. Prior to the widespread use of fiberoptic endoscopy to diagnose and localize upper gastrointestinal tract bleeding, esophageal tamponade tubes were used diagnostically. Nachlas [25] in 1955 used a single balloon tube to differentiate between bleeding from peptic ulcers and varices. The standard Sengstaken-Blakemore tube has also been used with intermittent success to localize upper gastrointestinal tract bleeding [24]. Unfortunately, bleeding from esophageal or gastric varices may persist despite tamponade by a properly employed tamponade balloon [13]. An erroneous diagnostic conclusion based on the use of a gastroesophageal tamponade tube may potentially be more serious than either recognized tube failure or a complication from improper use of the tube.

The enhanced accuracy of the fiberoptic endoscope in localizing sites of upper gastrointestinal tract bleeding mandates that varices be visualized as a source of bleeding before insertion and inflation of a tamponade balloon [28, 30]. The importance of accurately localizing bleeding to varices or some other site has obvious therapeutic implications. It is also important to localize the actual site of bleeding within a varix in relation to the cardioesophageal junction. Theoretically, bleeding from a gastric varix can be controlled without the use of an esophageal balloon [35].

INDICATIONS

The indications for the use of an esophageal balloon tamponade tube to control documented bleeding from gastroesophageal varices are not standardized. The use of such a tube must be weighed against possible complications, including death. The reported major complication rate secondary to esophageal tamponade ranges from 2% to 35%, with a mortality range of 3.7%-22% [3, 14, 18, 19, 30]. Nachlas [27], in a review of the life history of patients with cirrhosis of the liver and bleeding varices, noted that the use of esophageal tamponade has not significantly altered the prognosis of the patient with bleeding varices. Conn [14], who reported the highest incidence of both major complications and death directly related to the use of balloon tamponade, advises extreme caution in applying this technique for the control of variceal bleeding. More specifically, he believes that "good risk" patients with portal vein thrombosis, schistosomiasis or non-alcoholic cirrhosis of various types tend to survive both hemorrhage and operation and are therefore not candidates for balloon tamponade since the mortality from the use of the tube is greater than the risk of dying from the disease itself. The "poor risk" patients with bleeding varices who tend to die regardless of the type of treatment employed frequently fail to respond to less invasive measures and are more appropriate candidates for balloon tamponade. At the University of Michigan the primary indication for balloon tamponade is the failure to adequately control variceal bleeding with ice water lavage of the stomach and intravenous Pitressin infusion.

TECHNIQUE

The proper insertion and maintenance of gastroesophageal tamponade tubes contributes more directly to the success of treatment than any other single factor, including the severity of the underlying disease. Each time treatment is instituted a new tube should be used. We prefer the Boyce modification of the Sengstaken-Blakemore tube or the Edlich double-balloon, four-lumen tube. The balloons should be carefully checked for leaks and asymmetry and the channels tested for patency. The use of an adaptor and three-way stopcock at each inflation channel will help to prevent leaks once the tube in in place. The balloon inlets can be clamped with a rubber-shod hemostat to further prevent leakage. The stomach should be emptied by saline lavage prior to passing the tube to reduce the possibility of vomiting and aspiration during its insertion. A tracheal suction apparatus should be readily available at the bedside so that the trachea can be immediately suctioned if aspiration occurs during passage of the tube.

In our experience the majority of patients require endotracheal intubation prior to passage of a tamponade tube. Only those individuals who are alert and obviously capable of clearing their oropharyngeal secretions are not intubated. Unfortunately, the presence of an endotracheal tube makes passage of a tamponade tube extremely difficult. The tube is lubricated with xylocaine jelly and passed through the nose into the stomach. The gastric contents are aspirated again. Auscultation of the epigastrium while air is injected through the gastric channel should confirm the presence of the distal end of the tube in the stomach. The presence of the gastric balloon within the stomach is confirmed by roentgenogram or fluoroscopically. The gastric balloon is then slowly inflated to 250-275 cc of air and the tube withdrawn until firm resistance is encountered as the gastric balloon impacts at the cardioesophageal junction. The tube is then fixed to an overhead frame with one pound of traction. This method of securing the tube provides a more constant and reliable form of traction than can be obtained by fixing the tube to the face mask of a football helmet. The exact position of the inflated gastric balloon is immediately reconfirmed by another roentgenogram of the abdomen. After an hour, and periodically thereafter, the tautness of the tube is checked. Frequent readjustment, which may require withdrawal of as much as 5 cm, is necessary to compensate for diaphragmatic relaxation. Repeat abdominal x-rays should be obtained every 12-24 hours to assess correct positioning of the gastric balloon, as gradual relaxation of the diaphragmatic hiatus may allow the gastric balloon tube to displace upward into the esophagus. Constant or frequent intermittent gastric and esophageal suction is used to ensure that the stomach remains empty, to evaluate the rate of bleeding, and to remove all pharyngeal secretions.

Despite the fact that the failure of intravenous Pitressin to adequately control variceal bleeding has necessitated the use of balloon tamponade, Pitressin infusion is continued throughout the period of time the tube is in place. The initial rate of Pitressin infusion is 40 U/hr. After 24-48 hours, depending upon the patient's response, the dose is slowly tapered at a rate of 10 U/hr/day.

If, after the first hour, control of variceal bleeding has not been obtained, the esophageal balloon is inflated to 25-40 mm Hg as measured with a sphygmomanometer attached to the esophageal inflation tube. This pressure requires constant monitoring and readjustment. Roentgenograms are again used to detect malpositioning.

Unless the Boyce modification of the Sengstaken-Blakemore tube, the Linton-Nachlas tube, or the Edlich tube is employed, an oral pharyngeal aspiration tube should be positioned above the inflated esophageal balloon to collect secretions.

The patient is given nothing by mouth. Constant trained nursing attendance is mandatory. A pair of scissors is kept at the bedside with instructions that in the event of any sudden respiratory distress the tube is to be immediately cut across, below all the injection sidearms, and removed.

Periodic deflation of the esophageal balloon is recommended to prevent some of the adverse effects of prolonged pressure on the esophageal mucosa.

Once bleeding has been controlled for 24 hours the tube is removed through a series of timed maneuvers. Throughout this period the patient is carefully observed for any renewed gastroesophageal bleeding. With gastric and esophageal suction maintained throughout, the esophageal balloon is first deflated. The gastric balloon should remain inflated and traction maintained for an additional 12-24 hours. If hemorrhage does not recur, traction is removed and the gastric balloon is deflated. After deflation of both balloons, the tube should remain in place for yet another 12 hours and then be removed after transection to assure complete deflation of the balloons.

Gastroesophageal tamponade is generally well tolerated. Several authors [5, 36] have suggested an inflated tamponade balloon should not remain in place for more than 72 continuous hours. We have found that patient acceptance rarely extends beyond 48 hours, and 24 hours is the recommended maximum if esophageal ulceration is to be prevented.

RESULTS

The effectiveness of esophageal balloon tamponade in managing patients bleeding from gastroesophageal varices has remained remarkably consistent [3, 19, 21, 30, 31]. Initial hemorrhage was arrested in 170 of 191 patients (89%) reported since 1970 (Table 1). Among those patients in whom hemorrhage was initially controlled by tamponade, bleeding recurred soon after deflation of the balloons in 60 (35.4%). Permanent control of bleeding defined as hemostasis sufficient to allow appropriate resuscitation in anticipation of elective shunt surgery was obtained in 122 patients (71.2%). Unfortunately, a certain percentage of patients in whom hemostasis was obtained died of other causes while awaiting elective operation. These patients are included in the 71.2% permanent success figure, but it is difficult to determine with certainty how many of these would have rebled and thereby required emergency surgery. In a large number of patients bleeding was controlled to the point that shunt surgery could be performed, yet the tamponade balloons had to be in place and inflated until the operation was completed. These patients, although included in success estimates, are hardly comparable to those whose bleeding was controlled and the tube removed. Also included among the permanent successes are those patients who required two or more episodes of tamponade to obtain hemostasis. This is particularly significant because none of the authors comment as to how many times bleeding must recur after an initial success with balloon tamponade before urgent or emergent surgery is indicated.

Table 1
Survey of the Literature: Results With Balloon Tamponade for Bleeding Gastroesophageal Varices

Reference	No. of Patients	Primary Success with Tamponade (%)	Success With Recurrent Bleeding (%)	Permanent Hemostasis (%)
Hermann [19]	25	72	81	83.6
Pitcher [30]	50	92	62.5	78
Johansen [21]	91	88	82	45
Bauer [3]	25	84	67	80

Our current approach to this problem of rebleeding after initial success with esophageal balloon tamponade is that unless the patient with bleeding varices is a very poor risk, the first recurrence of bleeding after initial hemostasis indicates early surgical treatment. Early surgery is performed after reinflation of the tamponade balloons has controlled the bleeding and blood replacement is complete. The aim is to perform semielective rather than urgent or emergent surgery in the group of patients with rebleeding after cessation of balloon tamponade.

In summary, about one-third of patients with bleeding varices are controlled by balloon tamponade without rebleeding after removal of the tube. About one-third are controlled initially by tamponade but rebleed when the balloons are deflated and thereby require urgent or emergent operative portal decompression with the balloons in place and inflated. The remaining third are inconsistently controlled by tamponade or are not controlled at all and require emergent surgical intervention in the face of exsanguinating hemorrhage.

Two prospective, randomized clinical trials have been conducted to compare the Sengstaken-Blakemore tube to the Linton-Nachlas tube [10, 35]. In the first, 28 patients with 42 bleeding episodes were treated with balloon tamponade. Hemostasis was obtained in 74% of the patients treated with the Sengstaken-Blakemore tube and in 40% of those treated with the Linton-Nachlas tube. Unfortunately, the study was prematurely terminated when 2 patients in the Linton-Nachlas group suffered esophageal rupture secondary to inflation of the balloon in the esophagus.

In the second study, 79 patients with bleeding varices were prospectively randomized to treatment with Sengstaken-Blakemore or Linton-Nachlas tubes. Both tubes were initially effective in controlling hemorrhage (86%), but when bleeding arose from esophageal varices the Sengstaken Blakemore tube achieved permanent hemostasis in 52%, versus 30% when the Linton-Nachlas tube was used. When the bleeding originated from gastric varices the Sengstaken-Blakemore tube was much less effective than the Linton-Nachlas tube which achieved primary hemostasis in 50% of patients.

COMPLICATIONS

There are three major complications of esophageal balloon tamponade: respiratory obstruction, aspiration, and esophageal erosion, laceration or rupture. The major complication rates due to esophageal tamponade vary from a low of 2.2% to a high of 35% with an average of about 10%. Mortality rates range from 2.2% to 18% with an average of about 5% [3, 11, 14, 18, 19, 30].

The most frequent life-threatening complication is aspiration. The causes of aspiration include passage of the tube into a distended and unevacuated stomach, failure to control oral pharyngeal secretions and failure to control retching during passage of the tube [30].

Airway obstruction from an indwelling esophageal balloon usually results from migration upward into the hypopharynx. This migration is likely to occur if the gastric balloon is inadequately secured at the cardioesophageal junction [30], if it ruptures or is inflated with an insufficient volume of air (less than 200 cc), or if excessive traction is placed on the tube [5].

Erosion, lacerations and rupture of the esophagus tend to occur when the gastric balloon is inflated within the esophagus or if excessive, forceful traction is placed on the tube once it is in place. In addition, the gastric balloon may displace into the esophagus secondary to rupture, accidental deflation or insufficient insufflation. Improper passage of the tube or an endoscopy instrument, over-inflation of the esophageal balloon, and an excessively long period of tamponade with the esophageal balloon may all be contributory factors [7, 17, 30, 38].

There is one report in the literature describing occlusion of the innominate vein by an esophageal balloon. The patient's symptoms were limited to local edema of the area drained by the vein; diagnosis was confirmed by phlebography. Deflation of the balloon immediately corrected the problem [22].

SUMMARY

In summary, gastroesophageal balloon tamponade is an effective way to control hemorrhage from gastric or esophageal varices. The use and success of balloon tamponade is based on sound anatomic and physiologic principles. Both single-balloon and double-balloon tubes are acceptable, but neither should be used without the capacity to control oropharyngeal secretions. With meticulous attention to detail during insertion and maintenance of esophageal tamponade tubes, a primary success rate of about 90% can be expected with attendant complication and mortality rates not exceeding 10% and 5%, respectively.

The treatment of bleeding gastroesophageal varices by balloon tamponade should only be considered when other less invasive treatment modalities, such as gastric lavage and Pitressin infusion, have been unsuccessful. The risk of serious complication and death directly as a result of the tube must always be weighed against the risk of death from exsanguination.

REFERENCES

1. Agger P, Andersen JR, Burcharth F: Does the oesophageal balloon compress oesophageal varices? Scand J Gastroenterol 13:225, 1978
2. Andersen JR, Agger P: Passage of barium meal through esophagus in patients with balloon tamponade of esophageal varices. Scand J Gastroenterol 11:561, 1976
3. Bauer JJ, Kreel I, Kark AE: The use of the Sengstaken-Blakemore tube for immediate control of bleeding esophageal varices. Ann Surg 179:273, 1974

4. Baxter HK, Johnson AG, Kirk CJC, et al: Sense with Sengstakens. Lancet 1:1053, 1976
5. Bennett HD, Baker L, Baker LA: Complications in the use of esophageal compression balloons (Sengstaken tube). Arch Int Med 90:196, 1952
6. Bixby EW Jr: Correspondence. JAMA 138:908, 1948
7. Bouchier IAD: Impaction of the Sengstaken-Blakemore tube. Gastroenterology 45:274, 1963
8. Boyce HW Jr: Modification of the Sengstaken-Blakemore balloon tube. N Engl J Med 267:195, 1962
9. Brick IB, Palmer ED: One thousand cases of portal cirrhosis of the liver. Arch Int Med 113:501, 1964
10. Burcharth F, Malmstrom J: Experiences with the Linton-Nachlas and the Sengstaken-Blakemore tubes for bleeding esophageal varices. Surg Gynecol Obstet 142:529, 1976
11. Byrne WD, Samson PC, Dugan DJ: Complications associated with the use of esophageal compression balloons. Am J Surg 104:250, 1962
12. Cohn R, Mathewson C Jr: Observations on patients during the surgical treatment of acute massive hemorrhage from esophageal varices secondary to cirrhosis of the liver. Surgery 41:94, 1957
13. Conn HO: Hazards attending the use of esophageal tamponade. N Engl J Med 259:701, 1958
14. Conn HO, Simpson JA: Excessive mortality associated with balloon tamponade of bleeding varices: A critical appraisal. JAMA 202:135, 1967
15. Eckardt VF, Grace ND, Kantrowitz PA: Does lower esophageal sphincter incompetency contribute to esophageal variceal bleeding? Gastroenterology 71:185, 1976
16. Edlich RF, Landé AJ, Goodale RL, et al: Prevention of aspiration pneumonia by continuous esophageal aspiration during esophagogastric tamponade and gastric cooling. Surgery 64:405, 1968
17. Francis PN, Perkins KW, Pain, MCF: Rupture of the esophagus following use of the Sengstaken-Blakemore tube. Med J Aust 1:582, 1963
18. Hamilton JE: The management of bleeding esophageal varices associated with cirrhosis of the liver. Ann Surg 141:637, 1955
19. Hermann RE, Traul D: Experience with the Sengstaken-Blakemore tube for bleeding esophageal varices. Surg Gynecol Obstet 130:879, 1970
20. Idezuki Y, Hagiwara M, Watanabe H: Endoscopic balloon tamponade for emergency control of bleeding esophageal varices using a new transparent tamponade tube. Trans Am Soc Artif Intern Organs 23:646, 1977
21. Johansen TS, Baden H: Re-appraisal of the Sengstaken-Blakemore balloon tamponade for bleeding esophageal varices: Results in 91 patients. Scand J Gastroenterol 8:181, 1973
22. Juffé A, Tellez G, Eguaras MG, et al: Unusual complication of the Sengstaken-Blakemore tube. Gastroenterology 72:724, 1977
23. Linton RR, Ellis DS: Emergency and definitive treatment of bleeding esophageal varices. JAMA 160:1017, 1956
24. Lyons C, Patton TB: Bleeding esophageal varices. Surgery 39:540, 1956
25. Nachlas MM: A new triple-lumen tube for the diagnosis and treatment of upper gastrointestinal hemorrhage. N Engl J Med 252:720, 1955

26. Nachlas MM: The use of a triple-lumen single-balloon tube in the diagnosis and treatment of massive gastrointestinal hemorrhage. Surgery 38:667, 1955
27. Nachlas MM, O'Neil JE, Campbell AJA: The life history of patients with cirrhosis of the liver and bleeding esophageal varices. Ann Surg 141:10, 1955
28. Palmer ED: The vigorous diagnostic approach to upper-gastrointestinal tract hemorrhage: A 23-year prospective study of 1,400 patients. JAMA 207:1477, 1969
29. Patton TB, Johnston, CG: A method for control of bleeding from esophageal varices. Arch Surg 59:502, 1949
30. Pitcher JL: Safety and effectiveness of the modified Sengstaken-Blakemore tube: a prospective study. Gastroenterology 61:291, 1971
31. Read AE, Dawson AM, Kerr DNS, et al: Bleeding oesophageal varices treated by oesophageal compression tube. Br Med J 1:227, 1960
32. Rowntree LG, Zimmerman EF, Todd MH, et al: Intraesophageal venous tamponage. Its use in a case of variceal hemorrhage from the esophagus. JAMA 135:630, 1947
33. Sengstaken RW, Blakemore AH: Balloon tamponage for the control of hemorrhage from esophageal varices. Ann Surg 731:781, 1950
34. Terés J, Bordas JM, Bru C, et al: Upper gastrointestinal bleeding in cirrhosis: Clinical and endoscopic correlations. Gut 17:37, 1976
35. Terés J, Cecilia A, Bordas JM, et al: Esophageal tamponade for bleeding varices: Controlled trial between the Sengstaken-Blakemore tube and the Linton-Nachlas tube. Gastroenterology 75:566, 1978
36. Welch CS, Kiley JE, Reeve TS, et al: Treatment of bleeding from portal hypertension in patients with cirrhosis of the liver. N Engl J Med 254:493, 1956
37. Westphal K: Compression treatment in hemorrhage from esophageal varix. Deutsch Med Woschr 56:1135, 1930
38. Zeid SS, Young PC, Reeves JT: Rupture of the esophagus after introduction of the Sengstaken-Blakemore tube. Surgery 36:128, 1959

John G. Allison, M.D., M.B. Ch.B,
F.R.C.S. (Ed.), F.C.S. (S.A.)
Jeffrey W. Lewis, M.D.
Raphael S. Chung, M.D., F.A.C.S.

Esophageal Variceal Injection Using the Fiberoptic Endoscope

ABSTRACT

Injection sclerotherapy as a method for treating bleeding esophageal varices was first introduced in 1939. Initially a rigid esophagoscope was used to administer the sclerosant, but more recently, flexible esophagoscopes have been used. This paper describes a technique developed at the University of Iowa for injecting sclerosant, using a flexible endoscope.

Mounting dissatisfaction with portoazygos disconnection and portosystemic shunting in the management of actively bleeding esophageal varices and portosystemic shunting as an elective procedure to control subsequent hemorrhage has reawakened interest in the direct control of the bleeding source by injection sclerotherapy. The concept was introduced by Crafoord and Frenckner [1] in 1939 and there have been several recent reports in the literature attesting to the efficacy of injection sclerotherapy and the definite advantages to be gained in terms of morbidity and mortality. Sclerotherapy has been shown to control active hemorrhage and eradicate residual varices at subsequent elective injections. The risk of repeated bleeding from channels that remain patent and the problem of aggravating hepatocellular dysfunction that occurs after portosystemic shunting are almost entirely eliminated.

The use of a rigid Negus esophagoscope (or modification thereof) with the patient under general anesthesia has been reported by most authors using this modality of treatment. At The University of Iowa College of Medicine we have developed a technique of injection sclerotherapy for esophageal varices using a flexible fiberoptic endoscope. The advantages of the flexible endoscope are multiple and include ease of instrumentation, better visibility and greater

---

John G. Allison, M.D., M.B.Ch.B., F.R.C.S.(Ed.), F.C.S.(S.A.): Assistant Professor, Department of Surgery; Jeffrey W. Lewis, M.D.: Assistant Professor, Department of Surgery; Raphael S. Chung, M.D., F.A.C.S.: Associate Professor, Department of Surgery, University of Iowa College of Medicine, Iowa City, Iowa.

safety for the patient. A general anesthetic is not needed as topical application of a local anesthetic (0.5% Dyclone) and sedation with intravenous diazepam (Valium) are all that are required. A detailed description of our techniques and our early results has been published elsewhere [2]. The principle underlying our technique relies upon impaction of a balloon at the gastroesophageal junction during variceal injection. This serves to temporarily compress the varices and arrest the hemorrhage while the injection is being performed, as well as to prevent rapid washout of the sclerosant (sodium morrhuate, Lilly).

The balloon catheter (Fig. 1) is preinserted (retrograde) through one of the channels of a two-channel gastroscope, after which the endoscope and collapsed balloon are passed into the stomach. After withdrawal of the endoscope into the esophagus, the balloon is inflated and wedged into the gastroesophageal junction. Judicious use of irrigation and suction will clear the lower esophagus of clots and the varices can be easily identified. Brief relaxation of the tension on the balloon catheter permits identification of the source of the hemorrhage. The appropriate varix can then be injected with 2 ml of the sclerosant using a flexible injector (Olympus NMK-1) which has a retractable 5 mm 23 gauge needle. Bleeding usually ceases within two to five minutes, but a second injection may sometimes be necessary. Other nonbleeding varices may be injected at the same

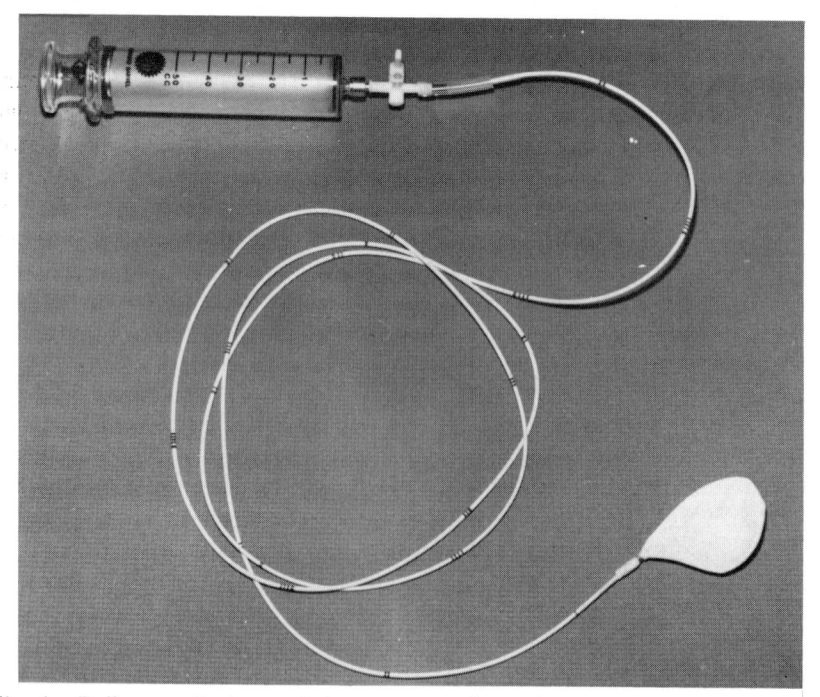

Fig. 1. Balloon catheter used to compress the varices at the gastroesophageal junction.

sitting and a loss of no more than 20 to 50 ml of blood can be expected from the injection site. The balloon is allowed to collapse after all bleeding has ceased and is withdrawn with the endoscope.

We are reluctant to inject bleeding varices in patients who have been managed with a Sengstaken-Blakemore tube as we feel the risk of lower esophageal necrosis is increased. A nasogastric tube is not used routinely in the postinjection period as this may contribute to erosions of the lower esophageal mucosa observed in some of our early patients.

Of the 9 patients who were actively bleeding from esophageal varices at the time of injection, immediate control was achieved in all. Subsequent variceal bleeding episodes in 2 of these of patients have been satisfactorily controlled with repeated injections. Three patients in this group have died, 1 from hepatic failure and 2 from unrelated causes. No patient has died as the result of uncontrollable or repeated variceal hemorrhage and all survivors have shown improvement in hepatocellular function.

Direct attack on the bleeding esophageal varices using injection sclerotherapy is a sensible and logical modality of treatment. Major surgery in critically ill patients is obviated and hepatopetal portal blood flow, which is often marginal, is not disturbed. The advent of the flexible fiberoptic endoscope has rendered esophagoscopy simple and safe, and injection of bleeding esophageal varices using this instrument is technically superior to the rigid esophagoscope though equally effective.

REFERENCES

1. Crafoord C, Frenckner P: New surgical treatment of varicous veins of the oesophagus. Acta Otolaryngol (Stockh) 27:422, 1939
2. Lewis JW, Chung RS, Allison JG: Sclerotherapy of esophageal varices. Arch Surg (in press)

Marshall J. Orloff, M.D.
Richard H. Bell, Jr., M.D.

Emergency Portacaval Shunt for Bleeding Esophageal Varices

Portosystemic shunt has been used under three circumstances in patients with esophageal varices: as *prophylactic* treatment, as *elective* therapy, and as *emergency* treatment. Each one of these circumstances is different and involves different patients, so that it is fallacious to compare them with each other or to lump them together in evaluating the results of treatment.

Prophylactic shunt is clearly of no value, as has been shown in three prospective studies [4, 12, 18]. I believe the results of these studies were predictable. The reason is that about two-thirds of patients with esophageal varices will never bleed from their varices. When a risky operation is performed to prevent a complication that would not occur in two-thirds of the patients if they did not have the operation, good results are unlikely. We have never performed a prophylactic shunt, either before or since these studies were reported. I cannot emphasize too strongly, however, that the results of prophylactic shunt have no bearing on what can be expected of therapeutic shunt.

Elective therapeutic shunt is still a matter of controversy. There is no question that by carefully selecting patients, elective shunt can be done with an operative mortality rate of less than 10%, with permanent prevention of varix rebleeding in over 90% of patients, and with a 5-year survival rate of 50%-60%. We have performed elective therapeutic portacaval shunt in 612 highly selected patients who were referred to us after having survived a bleeding episode at another hospital (Table 1). The operative mortality rate in our series was 2%, the 5-year survival rate has been 60%, and only 3 of the 612 patients have rebled from varices. Nevertheless, I must emphasize that elective treatment of bleeding varices is only a small part of the problem, and that our concentration on this

---

Marshall J. Orloff, M.D.: Professor and Chairman, Department of Surgery, University of California Medical Center; Richard H. Bell, Jr., M.D.: Assistant Professor of Surgery, Department of Surgery, University of California Medical Center, San Diego, California.

Table 1
Selected Patients With Cirrhosis Who Underwent Elective Therapeutic Portacaval Shunt for Bleeding Varicies

	Number of Patients	Percent of Group
Total group	612	100
Operative mortality	12	2
Five year survival	367	60
Varix rebleeding	3	0.5
Shunt patency	612	100
Encephalopathy at any time	127	21

aspect of portal hypertension during the past three decades has been seriously misplaced.

The cirrhotic patient entering the hospital with his first episode of variceal hemorrhage has had less than a 50-50 chance of leaving the hospital alive. Table 2 shows that the immediate mortality rate of the first bleeding episode has averaged about 70% during each of the past four decades. Moreover, only 10%-15% of bleeding cirrhotics have become eligible for elective therapy. In the prospective study of therapeutic portacaval shunt reported by the Boston Interhospital Liver Group [29], only 9% of 832 patients with bleeding varices

Table 2
Mortality Rate of First Variceal Hemorrhage in Patients With Cirrhosis

Authors	Year Reported	Type of Hospital	Number of Patients	Mortality (%)
Ratnoff and Patek [27]	1942	Five private-teaching	106	40
Higgins [11]	1947	City indigent	45	76
Atik and Simeone [1]	1954	City indigent	59	83
Nachlas, O'Neal, and Campbell [20]	1955	City indigent	102	59
Cohn and Blaisdell [6]	1958	City indigent	456	74
Taylor and Jontz [33]	1959	Veterans	102	45
Merigan, Hollister, Gryska, Starkey, and Davidson [17]	1960	City indigent	74	76
Orloff [22]	1962	City indigent	87	84
TOTAL			1,031	Mean 73

were subjected to elective portacaval shunt. Substantial evidence indicates that the traditional approach of using temporary, nonsurgical emergency measures in the hope of permitting deliberate, methodical preparation of patients for elective surgery has had little influence on the overall survival of the bleeding cirrhotic population.

As to emergency shunt, from these statistics it is apparent that emergency treatment of bleeding esophageal varices is unquestionably the single most important problem in the therapy of portal hypertension. The prompt and definitive control of the initial bleeding episode is where our efforts must be directed if the survival rate of patients with variceal hemorrhage is to be improved. For this compelling reason, we have focused our attention during the past 20 years on emergency therapy [23-25].

EMERGENCY DIAGNOSIS

In almost all patients, the diagnosis of bleeding esophageal varices can be made within 2-4 hours of admission to the hospital by means of an organized diagnostic plan that includes the following steps, in order of performance:

1. The importance of the history and physical examination requires no comment to those working in this field, other than to emphasize that confirmation of gastrointestinal bleeding by aspiration of the stomach and by gross and chemical examination of the stool is an essential part of the physical examination.
2. Blood studies include a complete blood count, a battery of liver function tests, and blood gas analysis. In our experience, the liver function test that is most consistently abnormal and of greatest value in cirrhosis is the excretion rate of a dye such as bromsulphalein or indocyanine green, if it is determined in the absence of jaundice, and after hypovolemic shock has been corrected.
3. Esophagogastroduodenoscopy with the flexible fiberoptic endoscope can be done in the emergency room in almost every patient shortly after admission and is the most valuable diagnostic procedure. Endoscopy is not a substitute for x-ray studies, but is an invaluable supplement.
4. Upper gastrointestinal series x-rays. We continue to obtain a barium contrast upper gastrointestinal series of x-rays in every patient as soon as shock has been corrected and the patient's condition stabilized. It is to be emphasized that x-ray studies are directed at determining the presence or absence not only of esophageal varices, but also of other lesions such as duodenal ulcer, gastric ulcer, or hiatus hernia. In our experience, emergency x-ray studies have accurately demonstrated esophageal varices at the time of bleeding in 95% of our patients.
5. Wedged hepatic vein pressure determinations by catheterization of the hepatic veins through a groin or arm approach are easy to perform and

require no more than 15-20 minutes. This procedure provides definitive evidence of the presence or absence of portal hypertension in alcoholic cirrhosis and, although it may not be essential in every patient, is extremely helpful when other findings are equivocal. We perform it routinely.

In our institution, the diagnosis of bleeding esophageal varices has been made accurately from information obtained in these first 5 steps in 99% of over 500 patients.

GENERAL MEASURES OF EMERGENCY THERAPY

Once the diagnosis of bleeding esophageal varices is made, there are six general principles of treatment that apply to all patients regardless of the specific therapeutic measures used to control the hemorrhage. These include:

1. Prompt restoration of the blood volume with as much fresh blood as can be obtained because of the coagulation defects associated with liver disease, compounded by those resulting from multiple transfusions of stored blood.
2. Prevention of hepatic coma by thorough and repeated cleansing of the intestine, both from above and below, and the instillation of intestinal antibiotics.
3. Support of the failing liver by the administration of concentrated glucose solutions and vitamins, parenterally.
4. Frequent monitoring of vital functions including the central venous pressure using a polyethylene catheter threaded through an arm cutdown into the superior vena cava.
5. Correction of the almost invariable hypokalemic, metabolic alkalosis, which we have found to exist preoperatively or immediately postoperatively, by infusion of large quantities of potassium chloride supplemented, occasionally, by parenteral administration of an acidifying agent such as ammonium chloride or arginine hydrochloride.
6. Treatment of the hyperdynamic state with digitalis and cardiotonic drugs.

SPECIFIC MEDICAL THERAPY TO STOP BLEEDING

A number of emergency nonsurgical measures are presently used specifically to stop variceal bleeding. The nonsurgical procedures include the use of esophageal balloon tamponade, systemic intravenous vasopressin, and selective mesenteric intraarterial vasopressin. Although each of these measures is capable of temporarily controlling bleeding, it has been our experience, as well as that of many others, that they have not significantly influenced the mortality rate of variceal hemorrhage in cirrhotic patients.

As shown in Table 3, there is no doubt that esophageal balloon tamponade has stopped variceal bleeding in many cirrhotic patients (45%-84%). The disheartening aspect of this form of management has been that many of the patients (50%-80%) have resumed bleeding when the balloons were deflated. Moreover, in our experience and that of others, tamponade has been associated with a high incidence of complications. In a two-year prospective study that we conducted several years ago, we observed 9 serious complications leading to death, including perforation of the esophagus, asphyxiation from regurgitation of the balloon into the pharynx, and aspiration pneumonia. Finally, and most importantly, balloon tamponade has failed to measurably influence the mortality rate of bleeding esophageal varices during a trial of three decades.

The second nonsurgical method of stopping variceal bleeding involves the use of systemic intravenous vasopressin. From our experience and that of others, it is apparent that systemic vasopressin promptly lowered portal pressure and stopped variceal bleeding in many patients. In our series of 218 patients, bleeding was controlled initially in 96% (Table 4). It is also apparent that most of the patients resumed bleeding (83% in our series), usually within several hours of receiving the drug. Therefore, vasopressin alone is not a definitive form of treatment but may be of value to "buy time" while other measures are being readied or the patient is being prepared for operation. Presently, all of our patients receive systemic intravenous vasopressin soon after admission in a rapid bolus dose of 20 units of Pituitrin, and this measure has largely replaced balloon tamponade as a means of obtaining immediate control of hemorrhage.

The third nonsurgical measure for controlling bleeding varices, selective mesenteric intraarterial vasopressin infused through an indwelling catheter, was introduced in 1967 [21]. Following this, a number of enthusiastic claims about the efficacy of intraarterial vasopressin were published, so that this modality has

Table 3
Results of Esophageal Balloon Tamponade in Cirrhotic Patients With Bleeding Esophageal Varices

Authors Year Reported	No. of Patients	Initial Control %	Ultimate Control %	Mortality %
Reynolds et al, 1952 [30]	32	66	50	47
Hamilton, 1955 [10]	20	45	–	75
Ludington, 1958 [15]	58	75	43	–
Conn, 1958 [7]	50	70	–	82
Read et al, 1960 [28]	38	84	24	74
Orloff, 1962 [22]	45	55.5	20	82

Table 4
Results of Systemic Intravenous Vasopressin
in Bleeding Esophageal Varices

Authors	Trials	Initial Success %	Rebled %	Mortality %
Schwartz et al [18]	25	88	"Frequent"	—
Merigan et al [19]	22	73	"Frequent"	93
Orloff	218	96	Immediate operation	—
	34	88	83	80

been used rather widely and, I might say, uncritically. However, within the last few years there have been at least five studies that have shown that mesenteric intraarterial vasopressin is no more effective than systemic intravenous vasopressin [2, 9, 13, 19]. Moreover, these prospective studies have shown that it is associated with similar systemic toxicity and a greatly increased incidence of local complications. Consequently, almost all workers have abandoned mesenteric intraarterial vasopressin therapy in the treatment of variceal hemorrhage. I might add that because of the cardiac effects of continuous infusion of vasopressin we have restricted the use of this agent to single bolus injection.

Recently, two additional nonsurgical measures have been introduced, namely, endoscopic sclerotherapy [14] and transhepatic embolization of varices [16]. Neither of these invasive techniques has been studied sufficiently to permit a conclusion about their efficacy.

SPECIFIC SURGICAL THERAPY

A number of surgical procedures have been employed to control bleeding esophageal varices, but, currently, emergency surgical treatment in the United States is largely confined to the use of two operations. These are transesophageal ligation of varices and the emergency portacaval shunt. Various devascularization procedures have been used in other countries, particularly in Japan, but the results are difficult to evaluate and may not be applicable to the cirrhotic population in the U.S.A.

Transesophageal Varix Ligation

Reported experience with transesophageal varix ligation is meager, and it has been difficult to assess the results. Because of this, and our dismal survival with medical therapy, we undertook a prospective evaluation of this procedure some years ago [22]. Every cirrhotic patient admitted to the hospital with variceal bleeding was included in the study, with no attempt at selection. The patients were assigned, by blindly drawing a card, to either a ligation or nonsurgical treatment group. The diagnosis in all patients was completed within six hours of admission to the hospital and operation through a transthoracic approach was performed within eight hours. The study group was made up entirely of chronic alcoholics with cirrhosis: 50% had ascites, 52% had jaundice, and 25% had hepatic encephalopathy at the time of admission.

The results of the study are shown in Table 5. The survival rate in the medical treatment group was only 14%, and esophageal balloon tamponade ultimately controlled the bleeding in only 29% of the patients. These results were almost identical to the survival rate of 18% obtained in a larger prestudy group of 45 bleeding cirrhotic patients, all of whom received identical modern medical therapy, so that the study and pre-study medical treatment groups were combined for analysis. In contrast, 54% of the 28 patients subjected to transesophageal varix ligation survived the operation. The bleeding in every patient in the surgical group was controlled by ligation, and the invariable cause of death was hepatic decompensation.

Experience has shown that transesophageal varix ligation is not a dependable procedure for the prolonged control of varix bleeding. Accordingly, all survivors were urged to undergo an elective portacaval shunt during the same period of hospitalization. All of the survivors who refused a second operation ultimately rebled and died. From our experience with varix ligation, we drew several conclusions. First, the procedure is uniformly effective in stopping the bleeding.

Table 5
Results of Emergency Transesophageal Varix Ligation and Medical Therapy in Patients With Alcoholic Cirrhosis

	Medical Treatment*	Varix Ligation*
Number of patients	59	28
Jaundice on admission	42%	57%
Ascites on admission	41%	50%
Encephalopathy on admission	25%	25%
Mean liver index	2.8	2.8
Admission hemoglobin 11 gm/100 ml or less	70%	71%
Varices demonstrated	95%	100%
Mean volume of blood transfused — liters	7.2	4.2
Early survival (30 days)	17%	54%
Ten-year survival	0	11%

*Followed by elective portacaval shunt when possible.

Second, it resulted in the immediate survival of 4 times as many patients as nonsurgical treatment. Third, as with medical therapy, it has the disadvantage of not being a definitive procedure, but must be considered the first of two stages in treatment, the second stage of which is a portacaval shunt. Therefore, operative mortality rate must include the mortality rate of the subsequent shunt. Finally, transesophageal varix ligation is just as large and traumatic an operation as portacaval shunt.

Emergency Portacaval Shunt

The other surgical procedure currently being used for treatment of bleeding esophageal varices is emergency portacaval shunt. The advantage of the venous shunt operation is that it is the definitive treatment for portal hypertension and esophageal varices. If it can be successfully accomplished during the bleeding episode, there is every reason to expect that it will permanently solve the problem of bleeding in the majority of patients. The question is: can cirrhotic patients tolerate an operation of this magnitude when it is performed as an emergency in the face of bleeding? To answer this question, we have been involved for the past 16 years in a prospective study of emergency shunts.

Important features of the study program are that it has been prospective in nature and has involved all persons with variceal bleeding, regardless of their condition. An extensive diagnostic workup was completed within seven hours of admission, operation was undertaken within eight hours, and a program of life-long follow-up was conducted in our Portal Hypertension Clinic so that the current status of 97% of the patients is known.

We have now performed emergency portacaval shunts in 255 unselected, consecutive patients. This report presents data on the 181 patients who were operated on up to June, 1978, and have had a minimum of 18 months of follow-up. All of them were chronic alcoholics and all had alcoholic cirrhosis on liver biopsy. On admission, 52% had ascites, 49% were clinically jaundiced, and 19% had frank encephalopathy or hepatic coma. Systemic intravenous Pituitrin temporarily controlled the varix bleeding in 95% of the patients and allowed sufficient time to complete the diagnostic workup. Emergency portacaval shunt promptly and permanently stopped variceal hemorrhage in 97% of the patients. The requirement for blood transfusion before and during operation averaged 5.1 liters.

Side-to-side portacaval shunt was performed in 151 patients, end-to-side shunt in 27, and another type of shunt in 3. There was no difference in survival rate between side-to-side and end-to-side anastomosis. The "skin-to-skin" operating time, which included various measurements of splanchnic pressures and blood flows, averaged 4.1 hours, and was less than 5 hours in 87% of the group. All patients had portal hypertension with corrected free portal pressures (obtained by subtracting the inferior vena cava pressure) that averaged 267 mm saline. The portacaval anastomosis reduced the portal pressure to normal in all but 1 patient.

One of the most important questions about portacaval shunt concerns the effect of portal diversion on liver function and, in turn, on survival and the development of encephalopathy. It has been proposed that patients with a large prograde portal blood flow will tolerate a portacaval shunt poorly, while those with a small prograde portal flow already have most of their portal blood diverted away from the liver and will not suffer ill effects from a shunt. Furthermore, it has been proposed that measurement of maximum perfusion pressure (MPP) is an accurate indicator of prograde portal blood flow. The uncertainty in this attractive hypothesis is related to the capacity of hepatic artery flow to compensate for diversion of portal flow, a critical factor that is unknown or difficult to predict. We examined the relationship of maximum perfusion pressure (MPP) to survival and encephalopathy in our series [5]. Contrary to the hypothesis, the patients with the lowest pre-shunt MPP had the lowest survival rate. In contrast, patients with the highest MPP, who might be expected to suffer serious consequences from portal diversion, had the highest survival rate and the lowest incidence of encephalopathy. It is clear that factors other than the maximum perfusion pressure or the magnitude of portal flow diversion play an important role in determining survival and the development of encephalopathy. Our results have been confirmed by the studies of three other groups [26, 32], and particularly by the detailed studies of Burchell, Moreno, and their colleagues [3] who clearly demonstrated no correlation between portal blood flow and the response to portacaval shunt.

Of the 181 unselected patients who entered the study, all comers included, 105 survived the emergency shunt operation, an early survival rate of 58% (Table 6). The survivors have been followed up for from 1½ to 16 years. The predicted

Table 6
Long-term Results of Emergency Portacaval Shunt in 181 Unselected Patients With Alcoholic Cirrhosis

		Percentage of Group	
Operative survival		58	
Predicted 10 year survival		30	
Encephalopathy in survivors at any time		34	
Patency of shunt		99	
Abstinence from alcohol in survivors		48	
		1 Yr	5 Yr
General Status:	Excellent or good	71	57
	Fair	24	33
	Poor	5	10
Working full time		46	57

5-year survival rate by the life-table method is 38% of the original group of 181, and the predicted 10-year survival rate is 30%. The early survival rate in the last 25 patients who have undergone emergency portacaval shunt is 80%.

Encephalopathy requiring dietary protein restriction at one time or another has occurred in 34% of the survivors. Long-term shunt patency has been demonstrated by yearly angiography in 99% of the patients. The 2 thrombosed shunts were of the end-to-side type. Forty-eight percent of the survivors have not consumed alcohol at any time during the follow-up period and an additional 24% have ingested alcohol only occasionally. The survival rate of the patients who consumed alcohol regularly was significantly lower than that of the abstainers. The general status of the survivors is excellent or good in 57%, fair in 33%, and poor in 10%, all but one of whom have resumed heavy alcoholism. Fifty-seven percent of the survivors are gainfully employed or doing full-time housework.

Beginning with the moment of admission and continuing through the life-long follow-up visits, detailed data on every patient were recorded on standard forms and continuously entered into a computer program. A total of 182 data categories were collected for each patient. The data have been analyzed statistically to identify the preoperative factors that influenced survival. Only four preoperative factors had a statistically significant adverse effect on survival (Table 7). One was the presence of ascites on admission (52% of patients). A past history of ascites was of no influence. The second was a SGOT level of 100 units or greater (34% of patients), which usually reflected acute liver damage by

Table 7
Preoperative Factors That Had a Statistically Significant Influence on Survival

Preoperative Factor	No. of Patients	Survival %	P Value
Ascites			
Present	95	46	<0.01
Absent	86	70	
SGOT			
≥100 units	56	43	<0.01
<100 units	110	69	
Last ingested alcohol			
≤7 days	119	52	<0.05
>7 days	48	71	
Blood transfusions			
≥5 liter	72	40	<0.001
<5 liter	109	70	

alcohol, and correlated with the presence of alcoholic hepatitis on operative liver biopsy. The third was ingestion of alcohol during the week preceding admission (75% of patients). The fourth was a requirement for five or more liters of blood transfusion, which reflected the magnitude of the variceal hemorrhage. Although all four of these factors significantly decreased survival, it should be emphasized that their presence was still associated with an acceptable survival rate of 40% or better and, therefore, they cannot be considered contraindicative to operation.

A large number of factors that have been alleged to be important in selecting patients for portacaval shunt had no statistically significant effect on survival. The notion that a patient who has survived several bleeding episodes is a better risk was not true in our study. Surprisingly, delirium tremens either on admission or in the past had no effect on survival. The presence of clinical jaundice did not affect the outcome. Nine patients had a serum bilirubin level greater than 10 mg/100 ml and 44% of these survived. The presence of encephalopathy on admission was associated with a higher mortality rate, but the increase was not statistically significant. The same was true of severe muscle wasting and a shrunken liver, i.e., the mortality rate was higher but not significantly higher. The liver function tests were of little help in predicting survival. Survival was decreased significantly only at the extremes of functional abnormality, namely, a liver index of greater than 3.4, which reflects terminal dysfunction and was found in less than 7% of patients.

A detailed hemodynamic evaluation was part of the emergency diagnostic workup. It provided no information of predictive value regarding survival. The corrected wedged hepatic vein pressure was about the same in survivors and nonsurvivors. The same was true of the portal pressure measured at operation. As we have reported previously, most of the patients had a hyperdynamic cardiovascular state. However, there was no significant difference in the degree of abnormality of cardiac output or systemic vascular resistance between those who lived and those who died. The maximum portal perfusion pressure, measured at operation, was essentially the same in survivors and nonsurvivors.

When combinations of commonly used selection criteria were analyzed, there was no statistically significant effect on survival. Thirty-six percent of patients who had ascites, jaundice, encephalopathy and severe muscle wasting at the time of admission survived the shunt operation compared to a 46% survival rate of patients with ascites alone (statistically not significantly different). However, as shown in Table 8, all 14 of these end-stage cirrhotics were dead within one year of operation, and it is now apparent that there is little to be gained in operating on such patients. Our analysis indicates that this constellation of admission findings, namely, ascites, jaundice, encephalopathy and severe muscle wasting, is the only contraindication to emergency portacaval shunt.

Table 9 compares the results of the three forms of emergency treatment of bleeding varices that we have evaluated prospectively during the past 20 years. Although the three groups of patients were not studied concurrently, they are

Table 8
Fate of Patients Undergoing Emergency Portacaval Shunt

	No. of Patients	Early Survival % P	One-Year Survival % P
Ascites alone	95	46	32
		N.S.	<0.01
Combined ascites, jaundice, encephalopathy, severe muscle wasting	14	36	0

quite similar from the standpoints of age, sex, liver function, incidence of jaundice, ascites and encephalopathy, and intensity of treatment. Early survival rates produced by the two forms of surgical therapy were about three times greater than those resulting from emergency medical treatment. Ten-year survival, both actual and predicted, was significantly greater following emergency shunt than after either of the two other types of emergency therapy. Figure 1 shows the cumulative survival curves resulting from the three types of emergency therapy. The differences between the groups are highly significant.

From our prospective studies in unselected patients, involving all comers, we have concluded that emergency portacaval shunt is the most effective treatment currently available for bleeding esophageal varices associated with alcoholic

Table 9
Types of Emergency Treatment of Bleeding Esophageal Varices in Patients With Alcoholic Cirrhosis

	Medical Treatment*	Varix Ligation*	Emergency Shunt
Number of patients	59	28	181
Jaundice on admission	42%	57%	49%
Ascites on admission	41%	50%	52%
Encephalopathy on admission	25%	25%	19%
Mean liver index	2.8	2.8	2.5
Admission hemoglobin 11 gm/100 ml or less	70%	71%	71%
Varices demonstrated	95%	100%	100%
Mean volume of blood transfused − liters	7.2	4.2	5.2
Early survival (30 days)	17%	54%	58%
Ten-year survival	0	11%	30%

*Followed by elective portacaval shunt when possible.

CUMULATIVE SURVIVAL

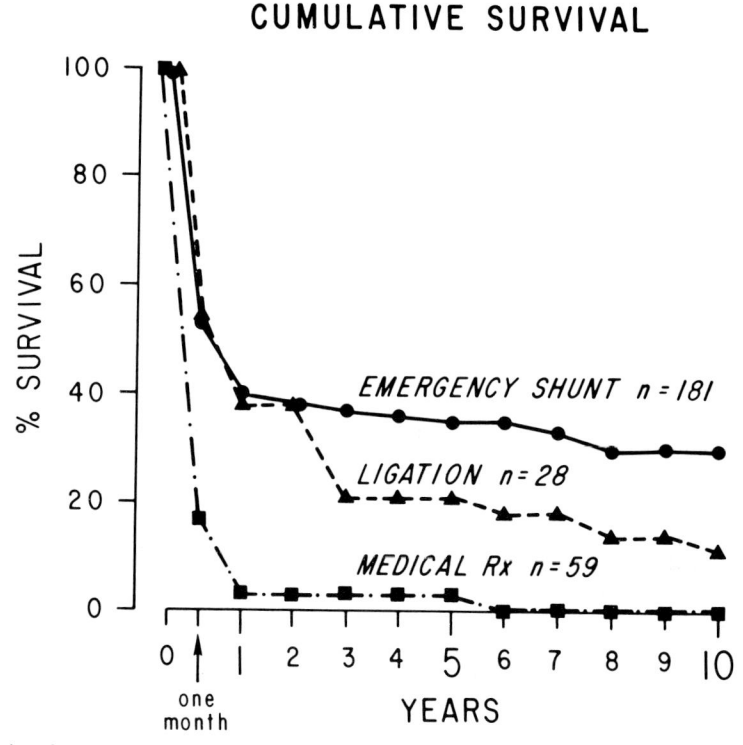

Fig. 1. Cumulative survival curves of patients with alcoholic cirrhosis who underwent three types of emergency therapy for bleeding esophageal varices.

cirrhosis. This conclusion should not be interpreted as advocacy of the use of emergency shunt in all bleeding cirrhotic patients. Rather, it should be emphasized that except in obviously terminal patients with concurrent ascites, jaundice, encephalopathy and severe muscle wasting, we do not yet have a sound basis for predicting which patients have no hope of survival, even with shunt therapy. Criteria for exclusion of those patients who are unlikely to benefit from shunt still remain to be defined.

SUMMARY

1. We have pointed out the extremely high mortality rate of bleeding esophageal varices in patients with cirrhosis and have emphasized the importance of concentrating our efforts on emergency treatment if we are to improve significantly the overall survival of patients with this disease.
2. We have discussed emergency diagnosis of bleeding varices and have indicated that, in the vast majority of patients, it is possible to arrive at the

correct diagnosis within 4-5 hours of admission to the hospital by means of the history and physical examination, liver function tests, esophagogastroduodenoscopy, upper gastrointestinal series x-rays, and wedged hepatic vein pressure measurements.
3. Regarding treatment, we have outlined some general measures which should be employed in all patients. These include: (a) prompt restoration of blood volume with fresh blood, (b) measures to prevent ammonia intoxication, (c) support of the liver with vitamins and glucose, (d) frequent monitoring of vital functions, (e) correction of metabolic alkalosis, and (f) treatment of the hyperdynamic state with digitalis and cardiotonic drugs.
4. As to specific measures to control bleeding, we have discussed nonsurgical methods, such as esophageal balloon tamponade, systemic intravenous vasopressin, and selective mesenteric intraarterial vasopressin, and have indicated that none of these consistently achieves hemostasis. We expressed our particular disappointment with balloon tamponade, a device that has failed to influence the high mortality rate and has been associated with many complications.
5. Regarding emergency surgical procedures, we indicated that our hopes have centered largely on two operations, transesophageal varix ligation, and the emergency portacaval shunt. Comparison of the results of medical treatment, varix ligation, and emergency shunt in a prospective study involving 268 unselected patients shows that 10-year survival is far better following operation and is best in patients treated by emergency shunt.
6. At present, the only contraindication to emergency shunt is concurrent ascites, jaundice, encephalopathy and severe muscle wasting at the time of admission.
7. It is concluded that emergency portacaval shunt is the therapy of choice in most cirrhotic patients who bleed from esophageal varices.

REFERENCES

1. Atik M, Simeone F: Massive gastrointestinal bleeding: a study of 296 patients at City Hospital of Cleveland. Arch Surg 69:355, 1954
2. Barr JW, Lakin RC, Rosch J: Similarity of arterial and intravenous vasopressin in portal and systemic hemodynamics. Gastroenterology 69:13, 1975
3. Burchell AR, Moreno AH, Panke WF, et al: Hemodynamic variables and prognosis following portacaval shunt. Surg Gynecol Obstet 138:359, 1974
4. Callow AD, Resnik RH, Chalmers TC, et al: Conclusions from a controlled trial of prophylactic portacaval shunt. Surgery 67:97, 1970
5. Charters AC, Brown BN, Sviokla SC, et al: The influence of portal perfusion on the response to portacaval shunt. Am J Surg 130:226, 1975
6. Cohn R, Blaisdell FW: The natural history of the patient with cirrhosis of the liver with esophageal varices following the first massive hemorrhage. Surg Gynecol Obstet 106:699, 1958

7. Conn HO: Hazards attending the use of esophageal tamponade. N Engl J Med 259:701, 1958
8. Conn HO, Lindenmuth WW: Prophylactic portacaval anastomosis in cirrhotic patients with esophageal varices. Interim results with suggestions for subsequent investigations. N Engl J Med 279:725, 1968
9. Conn HO, Ramsby GR, Storer EH, et al: Intra-arterial vasopressin in the treatment of upper gastrointestinal hemorrhage. A prospective, controlled clinical trial. Gastroenterology 68:211, 1975
10. Hamilton JE: Management of bleeding esophageal varices associated with cirrhosis of liver. Ann Surg 141:637, 1955
11. Higgins HW Jr: The esophageal varix: A report of one hundred and fifteen cases. Am J Med Sci 214:436, 1947
12. Jackson FC, Perrin EB, Smith AG, et al: A clinical investigation of the portacaval shunt. II. Survival analysis of the prophylactic operation. Am J Surg 115:22, 1967
13. Johnson WC, Widrich WC, Ansell JE, et al: Control of bleeding varices by vasopressin: A prospective randomized study. Ann Surg 186:369, 1977
14. Johnston GW, Rodgers HW: A review of 15 years' experience in the use of sclerotherapy in the control of acute haemorrhage from oesophageal varices. Br J Surg 60:797, 1973
15. Ludington AG: A study of 158 cases of esophageal varices. Surg Gynecol Obstet 106:519, 1958
16. Lunderquist A, Vang J: Transhepatic catheterization and obliteration of the coronary vein in patients with portal hypertension and esophageal varices. N Engl J Med 291:646, 1974
17. Merigan TC Jr, Hollister RM, Gryska PF, et al: Gastrointestinal bleeding with cirrhosis: study of 172 episodes in 158 patients. N Engl J Med 263:579, 1960
18. Merigan TC, Plotkin GR, Davidson CS: Effect of intravenously administered posterior pituitary extract on hemorrhage from bleeding varices. N Engl J Med 266:134, 1962
19. Millette B, Huet P-M, Lavoie P, et al: Portal and systemic effects of selective infusion of vasopressin into the superior mesenteric artery in cirrhotic patients. Gastroenterology 69:6, 1975
20. Nachlas MM, O'Neil JE, Campbell AJA: The life history of patients with cirrhosis of the liver and esophageal varices. Ann Surg 141:10, 1955
21. Nusbaum M, Younis MT, Baum S, et al: Control of portal hypertension. Selective mesenteric arterial infusion of vasopressin. Arch Surg 108:342, 1974
22. Orloff MJ: A comparative study of emergency transesophageal ligation and nonsurgical treatment of bleeding esophageal varices in unselected patients with cirrhosis. Surgery 52:103, 1962
23. Orloff MJ: Emergency portacaval shunt: a comparative study of shunt, varix ligation and nonsurgical treatment of bleeding esophageal varices in unselected patients with cirrhosis. Ann Surg 166:456, 1967
24. Orloff MJ, Chandler JG, Charters AC, et al: Emergency portacaval shunt for bleeding esophageal varices. Prospective study in unselected patients with alcoholic cirrhosis. Arch Surg 108:293, 1974

25. Orloff MJ, Charters AC, Chandler JG, et al: Portacaval shunt as emergency procedure in unselected patients with alcoholic cirrhosis. Surg Gynecol Obstet 141:59, 1975
26. Price JB Jr, Britton RC, Voorhees AB Jr: The significance and limitations of operative hemodynamics in portal hypertension. Arch Surg 95:843, 1967
27. Ratnoff OD, Patek AJ Jr: Natural history of Laennec's cirrhosis of the liver: analysis of 386 cases. Medicine 21:207, 1942
28. Read AE, Dawson AM, Kerr DNS, et al: Bleeding oesophageal varices treated by oesophageal compression tube. Br Med J 1:227, 1960
29. Resnik RH, Iber FL, Ishihara AM, et al: A controlled study of the therapeutic portacaval shunt. Gastroenterology 67:843, 1974
30. Reynolds TB, Freedman T, Winsor W: Results of the treatment of bleeding esophageal varices with balloon tamponade. Am J Med Sci 224:500, 1952
31. Schwartz SI, Bales HW, Emerson GL, et al: Use of intravenous Pituitrin in treatment of bleeding esophageal varices. Surgery 45:72, 1959
32. Smith GW: Use of hemodynamic selection criteria in the management of cirrhotic patients with portal hypertension. Ann Surg 179:782, 1974
33. Taylor FW, Jontz GJ: Cirrhosis with hemorrhage. Arch Surg 78:786, 1959

Jeremiah G. Turcotte, M.D.
Frederic E. Eckhauser, M.D.

Elective Portosystemic Shunts

ABSTRACT

Fundamental experimental and clinical observations have guided the development of portosystemic shunts since Eck described his classic anastomosis in 1877. Prophylactic portacaval shunts are not indicated, but the weight of evidence is that therapeutic portacaval shunts do prolong survival as well as improve the quality of life. In a recent study we have noted the presence of many Mallory bodies to be contraindicative to shunt surgery. In the last few years, investigators have demonstrated that there is a great variability in the amount of blood diverted around the liver with all types of side-to-side portosystemic shunts. Even the Warren distal splenorenal shunt is probably partially diverting, especially with the passage of time. Unless there are physiological or anatomical contraindications, we would prefer a Warren shunt, since it seems to be the least diverting. The recent series indicate that in patients with reasonable hepatic reserve, all types of shunts can be constructed with a low operative mortality and with good prospects for long term survival in more than half of the patients.

HISTORY

The development of operative therapy to achieve portal decompression has been based on a series of fundamental physiological and anatomical observations. The work of Nicolai Eck, the Russian military surgeon who first described the portacaval shunt in the dog, was really an extension of the observations of Lautenbach of Philadelphia. Lautenbach had reported in 1877 that dogs die rapidly after ligation of the portal vein; he mistakenly concluded, however, that

---

Jeremiah G. Turcotte, M.D.: Professor of Surgery and Chairman, Department of Surgery, University of Michigan Medical Center; Frederic E. Eckhauser, M.D.: Assistant Professor of Surgery, Department of Surgery, University of Michigan Medical Center, and Assistant Chief, Surgical Service, Ann Arbor Veterans Administration Medical Center, Ann Arbor, Michigan.

death was caused by depriving the liver of portal blood flow. Eck's fistula experiment demonstrated that survival was possible despite diversion of portal blood around the liver. Eck's report stated, "This preliminary communication was stimulated by the work of Lautenbach, 'On A New Function of the Liver,' which I read in the 'Journal Review' in the Military Medical Journal of July of this year." Eck, somewhat over optimistically, foresaw the future with the comment, "I consider the main reason to doubt that such an operation can be carried out on human beings has been removed because it was established that the blood of the portal vein, without any danger to the body, could be diverted into the general circulation and this by means of a perfectly safe operation." Only 1 of Eck's 8 experimental dogs was a long-term survivor. It is doubtful that such a report would ever have survived the editorial review of one of today's surgical journals.

Other early efforts to achieve portal diversion were centered primarily on attempts to study and relieve ascites formation. Omentopexy as first described independently by Drummond and Morison and by Talma was the first operation applied with some success in humans. The concept of the time was that collateral vessels would form, portal blood would be diverted and that the stimulus for the production of ascites would be eliminated. Shortly thereafter, Tansine, an Italian, described a technique of "termino-lateral" portacaval shunt in the dog and the next year, 1903, Vidal presented to the 16th Congress of French Surgeons a detailed case report in which such a shunt was constructed in a human for the treatment of both ascites and hemorrhage. Through a series of experimental and clinical observations, surgeons, physiologists and anatomists had, at this point, not only developed a technique of portacaval anastomosis, but had demonstrated that humans and animals could survive such an operation and that ascites and hemorrhage might be relieved by a direct portosystemic shunt. The early history of portosystemic shunt development is outlined in Table 1.

Direct anastomosis of the portal vein to the vena cava soon fell into disrepute as an acceptable technique for relieving either ascites or hemorrhage. Several European surgeons attempted the procedure, but no patient survived. McIndoe of the Mayo Foundation in his classic report of 1928 rekindled interest in the concept of a direct portosystemic anastomosis for the relief of portal hypertension. From postmortem dissections he accurately described the major collateral venous channels which formed subsequent to cirrhosis and portal hypertension and suggested "considering that the whole tendency of portal cirrhosis is to divert the stream of portal blood away from the liver, leaving the arterial blood to provide for the parenchymal requirements, the most logical and effective method of dealing radically with the embarrassed portal circulation would doubtless be to perform a simple Eck fistula."

The scene then shifted to the State of New York. Dr. George Whipple, Dean of the School of Medicine at Rochester and a Nobel laureate, had found that an inbred strain of dogs he was using for studies of protein metabolism could

Table 1
Early History of the Development of Portosystemic Shunts

	Year	Investigator
Death after ligation of portal vein in dog	1877	Lautenbach
Portacaval shunt in the dog	1877	Eck
Omentopexy for ascites	1896	Drummond & Morison
Omentopexy for ascites	1898	Talma
End-to-side portacaval shunt in the dog	1902	Tansini
End-to-side portacaval shunt in the human	1903	Vidal
Side-to-side portacaval shunt	1912	Rosenstein
	1912	Franke

survive after construction of a portacaval shunt. Encouraged by this information, Dr. Allen Whipple, Chairman of the Department of Surgery at Columbia Presbyterian Hospital in New York City, began constructing splenorenal shunts in his patients seen in the "Spleen Clinic" at that hospital. With experience and under the direction of Blakemore, Lord and Rousselot the technique was modified and the end-to-side portacaval shunt was adopted as reported in 1945. Since that time multiple technical variations have been described. Table 2 summarizes the history of the introduction of the major types of shunts which have wide clinical application today. Current interest centers on proper selection

Table 2
Modern History of the Development of Portosystemic Shunts

	Year	Investigator
Vascular anatomy of cirrhosis	1928 •	McIndoe
Splenorenal and portacaval shunt for clinical use	1945	Whipple
	1945	Blakemore & Lord
	1947	Linton
Side-to-end mesocaval shunt	1953	Clatworthy
	1953	Marion
Interposition mesocaval shunt	1951	Reynolds & Southwick
Side-to-end portorenal shunt	1963	Simeone
	1964	Erlik
Distal splenorenal shunt	1967	Warren

of patients and development of shunts which will minimize postoperative complications, especially encephalopathy, and enhance long-term survival.

INDICATIONS FOR ELECTIVE PORTOSYSTEMIC SHUNTS

The classic indications for recommending an elective portosystemic shunt are (1) demonstration of gastroesophageal varices, (2) occurrence of a major hemorrhage from ruptured varices, and (3) a patient who is a reasonable operative risk.

Varices are best demonstrated by fiberoptic endoscopy. Small or localized varices are not always easily visualized. A 33% variance in the interpretation of findings from one endoscopist to another has been documented [22]. At times, repeated studies by an experienced endoscopist are needed to verify the presence of varices. An important aspect of the endoscopic study is to rule out the presence of other lesions such as peptic ulcer or gastritis which might be the source of hemorrhage. Only about one-third of patients with varices ever experience a variceal hemorrhage and 25%-50% of patients with hepatic cirrhosis have lesions other than varices as a source of hemorrhage. In our experience, however, if the patient has had a typical episode of variceal hemorrhage and no other lesion is demonstrated by endoscopy and upper gastrointestinal x-rays, the bleeding is almost always from varices. We do not recommend actually visualizing hemorrhage or a clot on the varix, since to do so may prove to be impossible and may destine the patient to repeated hemorrhages before surgical intervention is recommended.

The Child risk classification system based on an estimate of hepatic reserve has proved to be useful in predicting operative mortality and long-term prognosis [33]. Operation is recommended for Class A and B patients and selected Class C patients. The comatose patient with gross ascites or markedly elevated serum bilirubin is not a candidate for operation. Other clinical observations helpful in estimating hepatic reserve are the patient's tolerance of a major hemorrhage and the size of the liver. Surviving a major hemorrhage without becoming comatose or encephalopathic and without the development of marked jaundice is good evidence of a patient with reasonable hepatic reserve. Although we are not aware of any firm substantiating data, long-term survival seems to be poorer for patients with small shrunken livers. Malt and Malt have recently published an excellent paper in which they point out that serum bilirubin is the best predictor of operative mortality and serum albumin is the best predictor of long-term prognosis [27]. This subject is discussed in more depth in other chapters.

In 1974 Mikkelson reported that the presence of Mallory bodies in liver biopsy specimens was associated with poor long-term survival and an operative mortality rate of 65% if a portosystemic shunt was constructed [28, 40]. These intracytoplasmic inclusion bodies were first described by F. B. Mallory in 1911. Presumably they are the result of hydropic degeneration of hepatocytes and are most often seen in alcoholic cirrhosis, especially when acute alcoholic hepatitis is present. We recently reported our experience based on 124 perioperative liver biopsies [23]. When "many" Mallory bodies were present the one year survival after shunt surgery was less than 10%. A few patients with Mallory bodies had been categorized as Child Class A and these patients also did poorly. Thus, the presence of Mallory bodies is associated with a high mortality independent of Child classification. We now recommend that liver biopsies be obtained preoperatively whenever possible. We would consider the presence of many Mallory bodies to be a contraindication to shunt surgery. The presence of Mallory bodies seem to augur an even poorer prognosis if a shunt has to be constructed with urgency.

Prophylactic portacaval shunt surgery is not recommended. Results of prospective randomized trials in which shunts were performed before hemorrhage had occurred, uniformly showed no benefit [48]. Four prospective randomized studies of the therapeutic portacaval shunt did not demonstrate a statistically significant improvement in survival in any single study [37, 40, 43, 44]. The three studies conducted in the United States, however, did demonstrate a trend toward improved survival of at least 20% at 3 and 5 years following construction of the shunt (Table 3). Since all three studies demonstrate a trend in the same direction, the weight of evidence would seem to be that shunts may improve survival. These three studies analyze quite small cohorts of patients and one would not expect statistically significant differences unless truly dramatic differences in survival between the groups occurred. Moreover, most agree that there is less hemorrhage, easier control of ascites, and less hospitalization after construction of a shunt. The incidence of encephalopathy is about the same in medical and surgical groups, but the authors of these studies do note that encephalopathy tends to be more severe in the shunted group when it occurs. These studies are largely concerned with the portacaval shunt and conclusions should not be applied to hemodynamically dissimilar shunts such as the distal splenorenal shunt of Warren. For a more complete critique of these studies see Turcotte and Erlandson [48].

A fourth study by Rueff et al from Clichy, France demonstrated a statistically nonsignificant improvement in survival for controlled versus shunted patients [44]. Only a brief report with a three year followup of this study has been published. None of the studies stratify patients by hepatic reserve and the distribution of this major variable could significantly alter results. Table 3 summarizes these important clinical trials, and together with Table 4 provides a good estimate of results which may be achieved today following portacaval shunt surgery in the cirrhotic patient. Some of the patients originally randomized in the medical group in Table 3 had subsequent shunts.

Table 3
Prospective Therapeutic Portacaval Shunt Studies

	Number	30 Day Mortality%	Actuarial Survival (%) 3 Year	5 Year	Encephalopathy (%)
Jackson-VA [17]					
Medical-NS + S	77	—	42	31	44
Surgical-S	67	8	61	52	34
Resnick-BILG [43]					
Medical-NS + S	25	17	40	40	35
End-to-side	25	20	65	65	16
Side-to-side	21	5	40	30	24
Mikkelsen-Los Angeles [40]					
Medical-NS + S	38	—	37	10	—
Surgical-S + NS	37	5.4	70	60	—
Rueff-Clichy, France [44]					
Medical-NS + S	49	—	56	—	44
Surgical-S	31	19.4	47	—	32

S, shunt; NS, no shunt. In some instances actuarial survival figures are estimates from published graphs.

Table 4
Results of Recent Series of Elective Portacaval Shunts

Series	n	Operative Mortality	Months Followup	Late Deaths	Encephalopathy (%)
Bristol 1975 [49]					
Portacaval	57	7% (4)	15 yrs	44% (25)	38
MGH 1976 [38]					
Portacaval	35	20% (7)	60	70% dead (actuarial)	46
Michigan 1976 [48]					
Portacaval	119	14% (17)	60	59% (66)	—
Class A	43	5% (2)		49% (20)	
Class B	56	13% (7)		78% (38)	
Class C	20	40% (8)		67% (8)	
Alabama 1979 [41]					
Portacaval	56	11% (6)	84	56% (28)	67
UCLA 1979 [34]	17	24% (4)	Mean 57	54% (7)	85

PHYSIOLOGICAL CONSIDERATIONS
IN THE SELECTION OF SHUNTS

There are 2 major physiological considerations which may guide the surgeon in his selection of a specific type of portosystemic shunt. The first is the presence of ascites and the potential effect of the shunt on salt and water homeostasis. The second is the potential harmful effects of diversion of portal blood around the liver.

Patients with hepatic cirrhosis are known to have significant impairment of their ability to excrete sodium and free water [24]. There is little information available comparing the direct effects of various types of portosystemic shunts on sodium metabolism. Side-to-side portacaval shunts are known to regularly improve salt and water excretion and relieve ascites [30]. End-to-side portocaval shunts may also improve salt and water excretion, but the effect is inconsistent, and at times may actually increase ascites formation. The presence of significant ascites is a contraindication to construction of a distal splenorenal shunt. Tense ascites may appear after this operation and can be a serious clinical problem. On 3 occasions we have had to insert a Leveen peritoneojugular shunt to relieve ascites following construction of a distal splenorenal shunt. Two of these were inserted in the early postoperative period and one was inserted after ascites appeared one year after construction of shunt. Generally we will not select a distal splenorenal shunt unless ascites is absent or easily controlled, that is, with a 40 mEq sodium diet and no more than 25 mg of spironolactone qid. When ascites is significant we prefer a side-to-side portacaval shunt or a hemodynamically similar shunt such as portorenal or interposition mesocaval shunt.

There is substantial evidence indicating that diversion of portal blood around a *normal* liver can lead to hepatic atrophy, hepatic insufficiency, encephalopathy and even death. Because portal hemodynamics are altered and hepatofugal flow of portal blood may even be present, the construction of a diverting shunt may have a variable effect on patients with hepatic cirrrhosis as compared to patients without portal hypertension and liver disease. Many patients have survived for long periods of time without any demonstrable ill effects after a totally diverting end-to-side portacaval shunt. Nevertheless, it would seem prudent to avoid diverting shunts whenever possible, especially when the liver is histologically normal as occurs in idiopathic portal hypertension. Patients with hepatic schistosomiasis, a presinusoidal intrahepatic block, also seem to tolerate diverting shunts poorly. The end-to-side portacaval shunt is necessarily completely diverting and also restricts outflow from the liver since the hepatic limb of the portal vein is ligated in this operation. We recommend avoiding end-to-side shunts wherever possible, especially in the presence of a normal liver or hepatofugal flow.

Debate continues, supported by a limited amount of data only, concerning the hemodynamic consequences of side-to-side shunts. In this group are included

Table 5
Hemodynamic Categorization of Portosystemic Shunts

Shunt	Hemodynamic Characteristics	Indications	Contra-indications
Distal spleno-renal shunt	Minimal portal diversion; permits hepatic portal outflow	Shunt of choice when feasible; schistosomiasis	Ascites; hepatofugal flow
Side-to-side portacaval; portorenal; interposition; mesocaval; central splenorenal	Variable portal diversion; permits hepatic portal outflow	When distal splenorenal shunt not possible or contra-indicated; ascites; hepatofugal flow	
End-to-side portacaval shunt	Total portal diversion; hepatic portal vein outflow prevented	As emergent shunt when other is not simple to construct	Normal liver; Budd-Chiari or hepatofugal flow; replaces hepatic artery

side-to-side portacaval, portorenal, interposition and Marion-Clatworthy mesocaval, and central splenorenal shunts. There is also debate as to whether the distal splenorenal shunt of Warren truly separates the right-sided portal-mesenteric flow from left-sided splenogastric venous flow and whether it is nondiverting or partially diverting. Burchell measured portal flow following construction of side-to-side portacaval shunts [21]. He found that 46% of patients maintain some antegrade portal flow averaging 377 ml/min. Reichle and Owen studied awake, stable patients with cirrhosis by observation of radiopaque water soluble droplets before and after construction of either an interposition mesocaval or distal splenorenal shunt [31]. These investigators found that there was no significant change in portal venous flow after a distal splenorenal shunt. After interposition shunt portal vein flow changed from 772±177 ml/min hepatopetal to −1021±310 ml/min hepatofugal. Six of their 7 patients had reversal of portal flow after mesocaval shunt. Nabseth utilized percutaneous transhepatic portal venography to establish direction of portal flow and measure pressure [29]. Three of five patients after nonselective splenorenal shunts were found to have prograde flow in the portal vein. A "watershed" area in the region of the distal splenic vein with bidirectional flow was demonstrated. In 5 patients with modified distal splenorenal shunts prograde flow was maintained in the portal vein in four, and in 1 portal flow was static. Maillard et al demonstrated with mesenteric angiography that in only 2 of 18 patients was there complete separation of the portal-mesenteric from the gastrosplenic venous beds following a distal splenorenal shunt [26]. In the others, collateral could be visualized between the two beds which seemed to increase with time. Thus, all types of side-to-side anastomosis seem to be partially diverting in many patients, especially with the passage of time. Most diversion occurs after side-to-side portacaval and interposition mesocaval and the least after central or distal splenorenal. Table 5 provides a hemodynamic classification of shunts together with our current recommendations.

ANATOMIC AND TECHNICAL CONSIDERATIONS

Certain anatomic and technical considerations are paramount in shunt selection. Since the theoretical hemodynamic advantages of one type of shunt versus another are not well established, in no case would we recommend a specific type of shunt if it is not technically feasible and safe. Thrombosis of the portal, splenic or superior mesenteric vein is an obvious contraindication to utilizing these veins for a shunt. Although thrombectomy is sometimes possible, the rate of shunt failure will be unacceptable if such a vein is used. In 18% of patients, a replaced right hepatic artery occurs [48]. This artery courses within the inferior edge of the hepatic trinity. If any type of portacaval shunt is fashioned, the portal vein may be kinked as it courses over the origin of the replaced artery from the superior mesenteric or celiac arteries. At times the portal vein may be transposed beneath the origin of the replaced hepatic artery, but the safest course is to select another type of shunt.

The "surgical trunk" of the superior mesenteric vein is also quite variable. Holyoke et al found the superior mesenteric vein in 26 of 36 cadaveric dissections to be quite suitable for a mesocaval shunt [25]. In 8 others anatomic variations, usually a short or bifurcated surgical trunk or unusual locations of mesenteric arteries would have presented technical problems. In two cases the authors judged that a mesocaval shunt would not have been possible. A splenic vein of less than 1.5 cm in diameter or a very short, double or retroaortic renal vein may preclude construction of a splenorenal shunt [20]. Knowledge of all these variations and study of the preoperative angiogram is helpful in guiding dissection or influencing choice of shunt [32].

At times one may need to alter his choice of shunt based on intraoperative findings. If in attempting to construct a side-to-side portacaval shunt it is found that the portal vein and vena cava will not easily approximate, then selection of a portorenal shunt is a feasible alternative. A portorenal shunt is hemodynamically similar to a lateral portacaval anastomosis. The renal vein can be exposed from the right side of the abdomen beneath the duodenum. With portal hypertension the renal vein can be divided safely near the hilum of the kidney and the adrenal and gonadal veins may also be divided to gain additional length. Only a temporary reduction in renal function of the left kidney will occur. A feasible alternative after beginning the dissection for a distal splenorenal shunt is a mesocaval shunt. Usually the superior mesenteric vein has already been partially dissected and it is a relatively simple dissection to locate the cava caudal to the third portion of the duodenum and pancreas through the same general dissection site as used for the distal splenorenal shunt. Other alternatives may need to be selected in the individual case and the surgeon should be quite familiar with performing all major types of portosystemic shunts.

RESULTS OF ELECTIVE PORTOSYSTEMIC SHUNT SURGERY

Portacaval Shunts

The prospective trials of the therapeutic portacaval shunt provide some of the most accurate data available regarding postoperative morbidity and mortality. Postoperative mortality varied from 5%-18% in these studies. Three year actuarial survival varied from 40%-70%. The most favorable three year actuarial survival of 70% was reported from Los Angeles. These patients were all Child Class A patients. The rate of postoperative encephalopathy did not differ from that of medically treated patients. However, the authors of these studies do note that encephalopathy tended to be more severe in shunted patients and in some studies more chronic encephalopathy occurred in shunted patients.

Other large and recent series of results with the portacaval anastomosis are summarized in Table 4. Unfortunately, most series are not reported in terms of actuarial survival, so that we have converted the followup to actual numbers and percentages of late deaths. These studies, together with the prospective therapeutic shunt studies confirm that portacaval shunts can be constructed with a relatively low operative mortality in good risk patients. The operative mortality in both the Michigan and the Los Angeles Child Class A patient was 5%. Three year actuarial survival for the Mikkelsen-Los Angeles study was 70% and for Child Class A patients in the Michigan study was 71.5%. In contrast, three year survival in the Michigan series of elective portacaval shunt for Child Class C patients was only 20%. Thus, good risk patients, even when utilizing a portacaval anastomosis which is not our shunt of choice at present, have a reasonable prognosis.

In Table 4, in the Alabama series 8 shunts were emergent and in the UCLA series 2 shunts were urgent; all others were elective. In the Bristol series the etiology of cirrhosis was cryptogenic in 38 patients. Late deaths are those occurring after the postoperative period, that is, deaths attributed to operative mortality are not included. The numbers in parentheses are the actual numbers of patients. The percentages under encephalopathy express the percent of patients who survived operation and who subsequently experienced hepatic encephalopathy.

Mesocaval Shunts

Table 6 illustrates that operative mortality is directly related to hepatic reserve with mesocaval shunts also. Both elective and urgent/emergent shunts are included. In the Arkansas series 19 patients had interposition shunts using jugular vein grafts between the portal vein and inferior vena cava. The remaining 36 patients underwent interposition mesocaval shunts. See Table 4 for additional explanation. An operative mortality of 0%-6% occurred with Class A patients and of 18%-58% with Class C patients. The Tulane series updates the experience at that institution from their report of 80 patients in 1974 by Dr. Drapanas. Unfortunately, long-term results are not stratified by Child risk class. In the experience from Tulane 22 of 137 shunts (16%) were known to be clotted either by angiography or at autopsy. The report from Johns Hopkins includes emergent and semiemergent shunts. There were no operative deaths with patients undergoing elective shunts. Predicted actuarial survival for the entire Johns Hopkins' experience is 30% at five years. Four of their shunts were known to have clotted. In the Temple series 14 mesocaval shunts were elective and 14 were emergent. Only one of the patients undergoing elective shunt died postopera-

Table 6
Results with Mesocaval Shunts

Series	n	Operative Mortality	Months Followup	Late Deaths	Encephalopathy (%)
Arkansas 1977 [46, 47]					
Mesocaval	54	11% (6)	108	22% (12)	10
Class A	0				
Class B	10				
Class C	44				
Johns Hopkins 1976 [35]					
Mesocaval	44	23% (10)	60	44% (15)	9
Class A	16	6% (1)			
Class B	16	13% (2)			
Class C	22	58% (7)			
Temple 1978 [42]					
Mesocaval	28	18% (5)	72	22% (5)	—
Class A	4	0			
Class B	13	23% (3)			
Class C	11	18% (2)			
Tulane 1979 [36]					
Mesocaval	137	10% (14)	120	7% (8)	19
Class A	20	0			
Class B	54	4% (2)			
Class C	63	19% (12)			

tively and four of the 14 patients undergoing emergency shunts died. Two of the 28 mesocaval shunts are known to have thrombosed.

Distal Splenorenal Shunt of Warren

Table 7 summarizes results with the distal splenorenal shunt. The series from Emory and Temple are prospective studies of the distal splenorenal shunt as compared to randomized controls. The series from UCLA is compared with matched retrospective controls. Unfortunately, none of the studies has entered enough patients so that results may be stratified and reported in terms of Child risk class. Zeppa reported only 1 operative death in his entire series of elective distal splenorenal shunts despite the fact that some of the patients were Child

Table 7
Results With Distal Splenorenal Shunts

Series	n	Operative Mortality	Months Followup	Late Deaths	Encephalopathy (%)
Miami 1977 [50]					
DSR	91	1% (1)	72	20% (18)	—
Alcoholic	52				
Nonalcoholic	39				
Emory 1978 [45]					
DSR	26	12% (3)	72	44% (10)	12%
Control	29	10% (3)	72	31% (8)	52%
(nonselective)					
OSU 1978 [39]					
DSR	50	10% (5)	24	16% (7)	18%
Class A	12				
Class B	32				
Class C	6				
Temple 1978 [42]					
DSR	13	8% (1)	72	25% (3)	
Control	14	7% (1)	72	23% (3)	Higher
(elective mesocaval)					
Michigan 1979					
DSR	55	16% (9)	60	18% (8)	—
UCLA 1979 [34]					
DSR	17	12% (2)	Mean 28	13% (2)	8%
Class A	7				
Class B	7				
Class C	3				

DSR, distal splenorenal; PCS, portacaval shunt.

Class C. He found a much poorer late survival in the alcoholic patient, but results were not compared in terms of preoperative hepatic reserve. In Warren's series from Emory, the nonselective shunts were comprised of interposition shunts between the superior mesenteric and left renal veins in 18 patients, interposition shunts between the superior mesenteric vein and inferior vena cava in 6 patients, 4 splenorenal, and only 1 end-to-side portacaval shunt. Five nonselective and 2 selective shunts had occluded. In none of the controlled series is there a significant difference in operative mortality or actuarial survival. Encephalopathy is significantly lower in the patients undergoing distal splenorenal shunt in the Emory series and is noted to be much lower in the Temple series of patients with Warren shunts. The Michigan series reports an operative mortality of 16%. This includes our entire experience in all risk classes; our operative mortality has decreased since performance of the first shunt in 1972.

Perusal of the results from all these series suggests that operative mortality and long-term survival is more dependent upon hepatic reserve than on any specific type of shunt. Some of the lowest operative mortalities have been reported with the mesocaval or distal splenorenal shunt, but these are also the series performed most recently. There is good evidence that all of these types of shunts can be constructed with low operative mortality in the better risk patients. The mesocaval shunt seems to be associated with a higher rate of thrombosis of the graft. The longer these patients are followed the greater the frequency of graft thrombosis. Distal splenorenal shunts do not seem to offer any advantage in either lower operative mortality or improved long-term survival. However, the controlled studies do report a decreased incidence of hepatic encephalopathy. This advantage of distal splenorenal shunt may disappear with time as hepatic cirrhosis progresses and as collateral forms between the right and left side of the splanchnic bed, thus diverting more portal blood away from the liver [26]. At the present time, we would recommend that distal splenorenal shunts be performed when feasible, since they can be constructed with a low mortality and since they hold the best promise of minimizing hepatic encephalopathy.

REFERENCES

History

1. Blakemore AH, Lord JW: The technique of using vitallium tubes in establishing portacaval shunts for portal hypertension. Ann Surg 122:476, 1945
2. Child CG III: Eck's fistula. Surg Gynecol Obstet 96:375, 1953
3. Donovan AJ, Covey PC: Early history of the portacaval shunt in humans. Surg Gynecol Obstet 147:423, 1978
4. Drummond D, Morison R: A case of ascites due to cirrhosis of the liver, cured by operation. Br Med J 2:728, 1896

5. Erlik D, Barzilai A, Shramak A: Porto-renal shunt. Ann Surg 158:72, 1964
6. Franke: The side-to-side anastomosis of the portal vein in the inferior vena cava as a substitute for the Eck fistula. Zischr I biol Tschnik u Methodik. 2:262, 1912
7. Lautenbach BF: On a new function of the liver. Phila Med Times 7:387, 1877
8. Linton RR, Jones CM, Wolwiler W: Portal hypertension: The treatment by splenectomy and splenorenal anastomosis with preservation of the kidney. Surg Clin N Am 27:1162, 1947
9. Marion P: Les obstructions portales. Sem Hop Paris 29:2781, 1953
10. McIndoe AH: Vascular lesions of portal cirrhosis. Arch Path Lab Med 5:23, 1928
11. Reynolds JT, Southwick HW: Portal hypertension: use of venous grafts when side-to-side anastomosis is impossible. Arch Surg 62:79, 1951
12. Rosenstein P: Ueber Die Behandlung Der Leberchirrhose Durch Anlegung Einer Eck'Schen Fistel. Arch Klin Chir 98:1082, 1912
13. Simeone FA: Personal communication, 1963
14. Talma S: Surgical opening of a new channel for the blood of the vena porta. Berl Klin Wuchsler 35:833, 1898
15. Tansini J: Diversion of the portal blood by direct anastomosis of the portal vein with the vena cava. Zentralbl Chir Leipz 29:937, 1902
16. Vidal M: Traitement chirurgical des ascites dans les cirrhoses du foie. 16th Cong Fran de Chir 16:294, 1903
17. Warren WD, Zeppa R, Fomon JJ: Selective transsplenic decompression of gastroesophageal varices by distal splenorenal shunt. Ann Surg 166:437, 1967
18. Whipple AO: Problems of portal hypertension in relation to hepatosplenopathies. Ann Surg 122:449, 1945
19. Whipple GH: Personal communication to AO Whipple. Ann Surg 122:149, 1945

Indications

20. Anson BJ, Kurth LE: Common variations in the renal blood supply. Surg Gynecol Obstet 100:157, 1955
21. Burchell AR, Moreno AH, Panke WF, et al: Hemodynamic variables and prognosis following portacaval shunts. Surg Gynecol Obstet 138:359, 1974
22. Conn HO, Smith HW, Brodoff M: Observer variation in endoscopic diagnosis of esophageal varices. N Engl J Med 272:830, 1965
23. Eckhauser FE, Polley T Jr, Bloch D, et al: Hepatic pathology as a determinant of prognosis after portal decompression. Am J Surg (in press)
24. Epstein M: Deranged sodium homeostasis in cirrhosis. Gastroenterology 76:622, 1979
25. Holyoke EA, Davis WC, Harry RD: Surgical anatomy of the mesocaval shunt. Surgery 78:526, 1975
26. Maillard J, Flamant YM, Hay JM, et al: Selectivity of the distal splenorenal shunt. Surgery 86:663, 1979

27. Malt RB, Malt RA: Tests and management effecting survival after portacaval and splenorenal shunts. Surg Gynecol Obstet 149:220, 1979
28. Mikkelson WP, Kern WH: The influence of acute hyaline necrosis on survival after emergency and elective portacaval shunt. In Child CG III (Ed): Portal Hypertension. Philadelphia, Saunders, 1974, p 233
29. Nabseth DC, Widrich WC, O'Hara ET, et al: Flow and pressure characteristics of the portal system before and after splenorenal shunts. Surgery 78:739, 1975
30. Orloff MJ: Effect of side-to-side portacaval shunt on intractable ascites, sodium excretion, and aldosterone metabolism in man. Am J Surg 112:287, 1966
31. Reichle FA, Owen OE: Hemodynamic patterns in human hepatic cirrhosis: a prospective randomized study of the hemodynamic sequelae of distal splenorenal (Warren) and mesocaval shunts. Ann Surg 190:523, 1979
32. Stevens JC, Morton D, McElwee R, et al: Preduodenal portal vein: two cases with differing presentation. Arch Surg 113:311, 1978
33. Turcotte JG: Portal hypertension as I see it. In Child, CG III (ed): Portal Hypertension. Philadelphia, Saunders, 1974, p 78

Results

34. Busuttil RW, Brin B, Tomkins RK: Matched control study of distal splenorenal and portacaval shunts in the treatment of bleeding esophageal varices. Am J Surg 138:62, 1979
35. Cameron JL, Zuidema GD, Smith GW, et al: Mesocaval shunts for the control of bleeding esophageal varices. Surgery 85:257, 1979
36. Dowling J: Ten years' experience with mesocaval grafts. Surg Gynecol Obstet 149:520, 1979
37. Jackson FC, Perrin EB, Felix WR, et al: A clinical investigation of the portacaval shunt: V. Survival analysis of the therapeutic operation. Ann Surg 174:672, 1971
38. Malt RA, Szczerban J, Malt RB: Risks in therapeutic portacaval and splenorenal shunts. Ann Surg 184:279, 1976
39. Martin EW, Molnar J, Cooperman M, et al: Observations on fifty distal splenorenal shunts. Surgery 84:379, 1978
40. Mikkelsen WP: Therapeutic portacaval shunt. Preliminary data on controlled trial and morbid effects of acute hyaline necrosis. Arch Surg 108:302, 1974
41. Ravelo HR, Aldrete JS: Comparative group study between patients surviving five or more years after portacaval shunt procedure and those surviving less than one year. Am J Surg 133:169, 1977
42. Reichle FA, Fahmy WF, Golsorkhi MG: Prospective comparative clinical trial with distal splenorenal and mesocaval shunts. Am J Surg 137:13, 1979
43. Resnick RH, Iber FL, Isihara AM, et al: Liver physiology and disease. A controlled study of the therapeutic portacaval shunt. Gastroenterology 67:843, 1974

44. Rueff B, Degos F, Degos JD, et al: A controlled study of therapeutic portacaval shunt in alcoholic cirrhosis. Lancet 655, 1976
45. Rikkers LF, Rudman D, Galambos JT, et al: A randomized, controlled trial of the distal splenorenal shunt. Ann Surg 138:271, 1978
46. Thompson BW, Casali RE, Read RC, et al: Results of interposition "H" grafts for portal hypertension. Ann Surg 187:515, 1978
47. Thompson BW, Read RC, Casali RE: Interposition grafting for portal hypertension. Am J Surg 130:733, 1975
48. Turcotte JG, Erlandson EE: Portacaval shunts. Indications, techniques and results. In Rutherford RB (Ed): Vascular Surgery. Philadelphia, Saunders, 1977, p 891
49. Windle R, Peacock JH: Prognosis after portocaval anastomosis: a 15-year follow-up. Br J Surg 62:701, 1975
50. Zeppa R, Hensley GT, Levi JU, et al: The comparative survivals of alcoholics versus nonalcoholics after distal splenorenal shunt. Ann Surg 187:510, 1978

Miscellaneous Causes of Gastrointestinal Bleeding

Duane T. Freier, M.D.

Gastrointestinal Hemorrhage in the Immunosuppressed Patient

ABSTRACT

Gastrointestinal hemorrhage in patients receiving immunosuppressive drugs is a relatively uncommon occurrence with a highly fatal outcome. The etiologies in patients undergoing treatment for transplantation, cancer, or other diseases requiring steroids include peptic ulcers, superficial erosions, cecal ulcerations, diverticulosis, tumor implants, platelet deficiencies and other unusual causes. The incidence of gastrointestinal hemorrhage is 3%-17% in transplant series and is similar in the other immunosuppressed groups. Fatality from this complication is high, 30% or greater overall, 50% if an operation is required, and 90% if an emergency operation is performed. Prophylactic operative management in transplantation is recommended for documented peptic ulcer disease and diverticulosis in elderly patients. Therapeutic management should be aggressive with early endoscopy and arteriography. Brief nonoperative treatment should be followed by operation when necessary. Early cessation of immunosuppression and sacrifice of the graft is important.

The immunosuppressed patient, a compromised host, is at special risk with gastrointestinal hemorrhage. The serious nature of the reason for the immunosuppressive treatment portends a dire outcome when complications result. The patients to be discussed all suffered from severe, often end stage systemic diseases. Fortunately, gastrointestinal hemorrhage is not a common complication and can be self-limited. However, it must always be considered life-threatening because massive hemorrhage is unpredictable and has an extremely high mortality. No site in the alimentary tract is spared from bleeding complications. The oropharynx, esophagus, stomach, small bowel, colon and anorectum are all at risk.

Duane T. Freier, M.D.: Chief, Surgical Service, Veterans Administration Medical Center, and Associate Professor of Surgery, University of Michigan Medical Center, Ann Arbor, Michigan.

This discussion is limited to the intentional primary or secondary immunosuppression of drug therapy as seen in renal transplantation, cancer chemotherapy, rheumatoid arthritis and other systemic maladies. The term "immunosuppressed patient" refers to one receiving an immunosuppressive agent. Etiology, incidence, mortality, diagnosis and treatment of gastrointestinal bleeding in these patients are presented.

ETIOLOGY

The etiology of gastrointestinal hemorrhage in immunosuppressed patients is similar to that of other patients but with notable and bizarre additions. Underlying platelet abnormalities and other coagulopathies of uremia, rejection, myelosuppression and infections change apparently mild hemorrhage into life-threatening bleeding.

In the field of renal transplantation many studies review gastrointestinal complications in general, but few carefully analyze the specific causes of gastrointestinal bleeding. Meyers et al [17] reported a large series of 81 hemorrhagic complications of the gastrointestinal tract in 367 renal grafts. Twenty-five occurred from peptic ulcer disease of the stomach and duodenum, 20 from superficial gastric erosion, and 19 from other sources, 11 of which were not determined. They also cite various sources of lower gastrointestinal bleeding in 17 patients, which included hemorrhoids, pseudomembranous colitis, generalized submucosal hemorrhage, cecal ulcers, a cecal polyp and other undetermined locations. Owens, et al [22] report 18 patients with posttransplant hemorrhage from a known site in a series of 109 transplant patients. Fourteen had peptic ulcerations and 4 had superficial erosive lesions of the esophagus, stomach and duodenum. These two studies substantiate the concept that posttransplant patients bleed from the gastrointestinal tract from causes similar to other patients with a preponderance of peptic ulcer disease and erosive superficial gastritis.

Peptic ulcer disease documented prior to transplant is a strong predictive factor that posttransplant hemorrhage will occur. Meyers et al [17] reported that 11 of 14 recipients with previous peptic ulcer disease had at least one bleeding episode following transplantation. Owens et al [22] noted that in 11 patients with previous peptic ulcer disease, 7 had a posttransplant recurrence. In contrast, 10 of 96 patients without previous ulcer disease had a posttransplant peptic ulcer complication. Spanos et al [29], reporting the extensive Minnesota experience, found that 30 of 377 patients had a pretransplant peptic ulcer history. Nineteen had a prophylactic vagotomy and pyloroplasty or antrectomy pretransplant, with a resulting recurrence of ulcers in 3 patients. Eleven patients did not receive a prophylactic operation and 9 had ulcer recurrence just prior to or after transplantation. Despite the above findings, it is important to remember the report of Palmer [23] which showed that in 1,400 cases of general diseases, 40% of the patients known to have a pre-existing lesion were bleeding from a different site. Also, Morrissey [20] found that in 110 patients examined after bleeding stopped, 15% had two lesions capable of being the cause of hemorrhage.

Oropharyngeal and esophageal ulcerations are common in posttransplantation patients, usually in association with candidiasis. Two cases of small bowel intussusception secondary to an intramural hematoma have been reported by Carr et al [4] in end stage renal failure patients. Cytomegalovirus has been implicated as a cause of ulceration and hemorrhage in the esophagus, stomach, and colon in the post transplantation state [1, 8, 25, 32]. All authors agree, however, that to consider cytomegalovirus as the etiology of the ulcers is highly speculative. Their presence may be incidental only.

The direct contribution to gastrointestinal hemorrhage of the drugs commonly used in transplantation is unknown but accepted as being significant. No report on posttransplant hemorrhage fails to mention steroids as a contributing agent. The pros and cons of this controversial subject will be fully discussed later. Suffice it to say, transplant surgeons are attuned to the possibility that steroids somehow contribute to esophageal, gastroduodenal, jejunal and colonic ulcerations and hemorrhage and that cytomegalovirus organisms are occasionally found in the ulcers.

Azathioprine (Imuran) is the second universal drug used in transplantation immunosuppression. Its myelosuppressive side effects are well known. These most often include leukopenia but occasionally thrombocytopenia occurs with its subsequent threat of secondary hemorrhage. Antilymphocytic globulin, used regularly in many transplant centers, can be thrombocytopenic. It is a biological product, being produced by the immune system of an animal such as a horse, rabbit, or goat. Each batch differs in its potential properties depending upon the antigenic source, the animal used to make the antibody, the state of response of the specific animal, and the process of purification. The antilymphocytic globulin product may be specifically thrombocytopenic to the point of requiring prophylactic splenectomy.

In cancer patients the causes of complicating gastrointestinal hemorrhage are usually from a nonmalignant source. Multiple studies done at Memorial Sloan-Kettering Cancer Center show hemorrhagic gastritis to be the most common source of gastrointestinal bleeding in their patient population [14, 16]. Tumor was present in 72% of their patients [16]. Half of these ulcerating lesions were postulated to be from stress and half from exogenous gastric irritants which include aspirin, steroids, ethanol, chemotherapeutic agents, radiotherapy, indomethacin, and phenylbutazone. Peptic ulcers were second most common as cause of gastrointestinal hemorrhage, equally distributed between stomach and duodenum. Hemorrhage from the tumor itself occurred in only 12% of the patients overall. If the tumor was in the stomach this percentage increased to

50% and if it was a primary gastric adenocarcinoma or lymphoma, 75%. Esophagitis, often in association with candidiasis, was present in 10% of the bleeding patients. The authors do not report what proportion of their overall cancer population was on chemotherapy when hemorrhaging.

Leukemic infiltration of the gastrointestinal tract is not uncommon and as a source of hemorrhage occurred in 27 of 148 (18%) patients reported by Prolla and Kirsner [24]. This complication is augmented by the platelet abnormalities and leukostasis of leukemia as well as the thrombocytopenia induced by the chemotherapeutic agents. Metastases to the gastrointestinal tract are common in breast cancer, melanoma and testicular tumors [28]. Direct invasion of the stomach or duodenum by pancreatic carcinoma can result in massive hemorrhage. Steroids appear to be associated with a high frequency of gastroduodenal metastases in breast carcinoma. In a report by Hartmann and Sherlock [11], gastroduodenal metastases were 6 times more frequent in the patients with breast cancer who received steroids than in those who did not. Furthermore, the steroid treated group who developed gastrointestinal lesions had a 54% chance of bleeding from them and a 38% chance of dying from the hemorrhage if it occurred.

A review by Belt et al [2] reported hemorrhage during chemotherapy in a group of 718 patients with solid tumors. The causes of bleeding were categorized into those secondary to thrombocytopenia, direct extension or invasion by the tumor, disseminated intravascular coagulopathy and causes unrelated to the malignancy. Seventy-five (10%) patients had bleeding during the course of chemotherapy, 37 of which were secondary to thrombocytopenia. Only 2 of the thrombocytopenic patients bled from the gastrointestinal tract and 11 of the 37 (30%) had a preceding fever or verified infection associated with the hemorrhage. Tumor invasion accounted for 25 episodes of bleeding, 7 secondary to gastrointestinal lesions. Seven patients had disseminated intravascular coagulopathy and 6 bled from causes unrelated to malignancy or chemotherapy. Other causes included 3 benign peptic ulcers and a single gastric erosion occurring in a patient on steroids. Thus of the entire series of 718 patients on chemotherapy, only 4 (0.6%) bled from the commonest causes noted in other cancer studies and the general population.

Drugs used for and during chemotherapy have direct hemorrhagic effects in addition to the indirect one of thrombocytopenia. Pain medications containing salicylates are well known for their irritation of the gastrointestinal tract in addition to their effect on platelet function. Antifolic compounds (e.g., methotrexate) and the fluorinated pyramidines (e.g., 5-fluorouracil) cause increased mitotic counts in small bowel epithelial cells and interfere with epithelial cell proliferation in the colon [28]. Gastrointestinal ulceration has been associated with these drugs and rarely hemorrhage can result. Arterial infusion of 5-fluoro-2'-deoxyuridine into the celiac artery has been reported to lead to acute gastritis which mimicked carcinoma of the antrum in one case [27].

The controversial issue of steroids and their relationship to gastrointestinal ulceration and hemorrhage has been mentioned previously. Diethelm [7], in an excellent review of steroid complications states, "The complications best known to the general surgeon and least well documented by statistical analysis relate to the effect of corticosteroids upon the gastrointestinal tract." Clinical evidence, reported in the early experience with the drug, was biased in favor of there being a causal relationship. Kammerer, et al [13] showed by routine x-ray studies that 31% of 117 patients on steroids for rheumatoid arthritis had ulcers in the stomach and duodenum. Most were clinically silent. Glenn and Grafe [9] retrospectively studied 53 patients on steroids for inflammatory, allergic, collagen, granulomatous, malignant, and other miscellaneous diseases. These 53 patients had no less than 109 complications, 42 having single and 11 multiple adverse effects. A total of 53 ulcerations occurred from the esophagus to the colon. Forty episodes of hemorrhage and 11 perforations were documented in the gastrointestinal tract. Lewicki et al [15] attempted to characterize roentgenographic features of hemorrhaging transplant patients with peptic ulcers to show a steroid induced origin. They cited occurrence while steroid dosage was highest, high incidence of multiple ulcerations, and a reversal of the gastroduodenal ratio of ulcers as evidence of steroid influence. Meyers et al [17] reported 11 of 32 HLA-identical transplant recipients developed gastrointestinal disease while on stable maintenance of steroids, and only 1 of 13 HLA-identical recipients not on maintenance steroids developed a similar problem.

Despite these reported retrospective findings and many other similar reports, exhaustive reviews of this question fail to statistically prove a clear association of steroids to gastrointestinal ulcerations and hemorrhage [3, 5, 6, 7]. Conn and Blitzer [5] reviewed 26 prospective double blind investigations, including 3550 patients, and 16 prospective nondouble blind studies, including 1773 more patients. The combined results showed that ulcer frequency was slightly higher in the steroid treated patients but the difference was not statistically significant (2.1% vs 1.8%). Most surgeons, however, continue to accept the relationship on strong clinical retrospective evidence and treat their patients accordingly. Studies such as that of Conn and Blitzer, by their own admission, will probably not change that prejudice.

INCIDENCE AND MORTALITY

The very nature of the use of immunosuppression for end stage and other severe systemic diseases augers poor results when complications occur. Gastrointestinal hemorrhage is no exception. Early reports of post transplantation hemorrhage by Starzl and his group [30] and Moore and Hume [19], showed an extremely high mortality. Moore and Hume in 1969 stated, "Emergency operations for gastrointestinal bleeding has proved to be the most lethal complication in our transplant experience. Seven of our patients have been operated upon in emergency circumstances for gastrointestinal bleeding and all have died" [19]. Hadjiyannakis et al [10] in 1971 reported a gastrointestinal hemorrhage complication rate of 12% in 139 patients and a resulting mortality of over 50%. Aldrete et al [1], reporting on 126 transplant patients in 1975 noted a 3% incidence of hemorrhage from peptic ulcer disease culminating in a 50% mortality in the immediate postoperative period. Owens et al [22] reported their own series of 109 transplants in 1976 with a 13% incidence of peptic ulcer hemorrhage. Three were operated upon of whom 2 died, and 6 were treated nonoperatively with 3 resulting deaths for an overall posthemorrhage mortality of 36%. Four of their patients had erosive gastritis; 3 of these died. Owens et al [21] reviewed reports from 12 transplant centers which included 1852 patients. Fifty recipients had hemorrhage from peptic ulcer disease and of 21 patients, bleeding severely enough to require emergency operations, 19 died. Meyers et al [17], in 1979, reported 367 transplant recipients who had 64 upper gastrointestinal hemorrhages (17% incidence) which resulted in a 29% mortality.

Gastrointestinal hemorrhage in leukemia is likewise an ominous complication. Prolla and Kirsner [24] outlined the gastrointestinal lesions and complications in 148 patients with leukemia. Twenty-five percent had leukemic infiltrates in the gastrointestinal tract, 18% had gastrointestinal hemorrhage and

Table 1
Incidence and Mortality in Transplantation

Authors	Transplant Patients at Risk	Number of Patients at Risk Who Hemorrhaged	Patient Mortality From Hemorrhage
Moore & Hume, 1969	113	14 (12%)	100%*
Hadjiyannakis et al, 1971	139	16 (12%)	50%†
Aldrete et al, 1975	126	4 (3%)	50%†
Owens et al, 1976	109	14 (13%)	36%†
Owens et al, 1977	1,853	50 (3%)	75%†
Meyers et al, 1979	367	64 (17%)	90%*
Summary	>2,000	Range 3%-17%	95%* 44%†

*Emergency operations only.
†Overall.

30% of those who hemorrhaged died of that complication. Hersh, et al [12] showed that 52% of deaths from leukemia in their series were from complications of hemorrhage.

The mortality of chronic steroid therapy for nontransplantation disease states as reported by Glenn and Strafe [9] was significant. Fifteen of their 53 patients were operated upon for hemorrhage or perforation with a postoperative mortality of 33%. The 718 patients on chemotherapy with solid tumors reported by Belt et al [2] had an overall death rate of 1.5% from hemorrhage alone. Of those 75 who bled, 11 died to give a mortality of 15% in this group. Upper gastrointestinal bleeding occurred in only 19 patients, an incidence of 3%. The mortality from upper gastrointestinal bleeding is not given.

Table 1 summarizes the results of thousands of transplant patients reported. The incidence of upper gastrointestinal hemorrhage ranges from 3%-17% with an overall mortality of about 30%. Fifty percent or more of the patients undergoing an operation for upper gastrointestinal bleeding died. If the operation was emergent, 90%-100% of the patients died. Table 2 summarizes the results of groups of patients immunosuppressed for reasons other than transplantation. The overall mortality of hemorrhage in these groups is also bleak.

Table 2
Incidence and Mortality in Nontransplant Immunosuppression

Authors	Patients at Risk	Number of Patients at Risk Who Hemorrhaged	Patient Mortality From Hemorrhage
Prolla & Kirsner, 1964	148*	27 (18%)§	30% of those who hemorrhaged
Hersh et al, 1965	414*	215 (52%)‖	100%, hemorrhage was considered cause of death
Glenn & Grafe, 1967	53†	40§	33%, postoperative for hemorrhage and perforation
Belt et al, 1978	718‡	19 (3%)§	Unknown
		75 (10%)‖	15% of those who hemorrhaged

*Leukemia.
†Miscellaneous benign diseases and cancer.
‡Solid tumors on chemotherapy.
§UGI only.
‖All hemorrhage sites.

DIAGNOSIS AND TREATMENT

The diagnosis and treatment of gastrointestinal hemorrhage in immunosuppressed patients warrants an aggressive approach by virtue of the incidence and mortality. Numbers of patients are small. The incidence of hemorrhage is relatively low and so a constant high degree of suspicion must be maintained. Gastrointestinal hemorrhage in steroid treated patients often is asymptomatic and frequently occurs during another attention-holding crisis such as infection or rejection. The hematocrit must be constantly monitored and the platelet count routinely obtained in all immunosuppressed patients. When gastrointestinal hemorrhage is apparent the urgency is great. An aggressive endoscopic approach should be utilized. A high proportion of gastric erosions will probably be found [16]. Approximately 90% of the source of hemorrhage should be found by endoscopy alone [28]. Upper gastrointestinal roentgenography will show obvious peptic ulcers, but will usually miss the more prevalent erosions. Arteriography is especially helpful in diagnosing more distal lesions and has been used for treatment of small and large bowel ulcers through infusion of Pitressin and other drugs [31].

Prophylactic management of peptic ulcer disease in transplantation is standard. A pretransplant history of peptic ulcer disease, especially if hemorrhage is documented, justifies a pretransplant ulcer operation [17, 21, 22, 29]. Vagotomy and antrectomy appears to have a better outcome compared to vagotomy and pyloroplasty in recurrence of posttransplant hemorrhage [29]. A prior history of significant diverticular disease is also justification for surgical correction before transplantation [17, 26]. Misra et al [18] recommend a pretransplant barium enema in all patients over 50 years of age. Transplantation affects diagnosis of colonic disease in numerous ways. Steroids mask the symptoms of pain, postgrafting local irradiation may initiate inflammation of the colon, the position of the graft in the iliac fossa allows graft rejection symptoms to mimic colonic disease, and routine use of antacids to prevent ulceration promotes constipation. Cimetidine has been advocated as a prophylactic drug after transplantation, especially in patients with high gastric acidity. However, Zammit and Toledo-Pereyra [33] have reported evidence that rejection may be augmented by the use of this drug in dogs. More needs to be known about the immunological effects of cimetidine before it can be routinely used in transplantation, however, selective use may be justified in the light of high postoperative mortality from upper gastrointestinal hemorrhage.

Therapeutic management of gastrointestinal hemorrhage in immunosuppressed patients should follow similar guidelines to treatment of other patients, but with added urgency. After diagnosis, brief attempts at nonoperative treatment (lavage, infusion of drugs intraarterially, cimetidine, endoscopic electrocoagulation, etc.) should be promptly followed by operative intervention if they are unsuccessful. Only early operative intervention will improve the formidable postoperative mortality. Attempts to save a graft should be abandoned early in the course of posttransplant hemorrhage.

REFERENCES

1. Aldrete JS, Sterling WA, Hathaway BM: Gastrointestinal and hepatic complications affecting patients with renal allografts. Am J Surg 120:115, 1975
2. Belt FJ, Leite C, Haas CD, et al: Incidence of hemorrhagic complications in patients with cancer. JAMA 239:2571, 1978
3. Bowen R, Mayne JG, Cain JC, et al: Peptic ulcer in rheumatoid arthritis and relationship to steroid treatment. Proc Mayo Clin 35:537, 1960
4. Carr BJ, Luft FC, Hamburger RJ, et al: Intussusception in chronic renal failure. Arch Surg 111:866, 1976
5. Conn HO, Blitzer BL: Nonassociation of adrenocorticosteroid therapy and peptic ulcer. N Engl J Med 294:473, 1976
6. Cushman P: Glucocorticoids and the gastrointestinal tract. Gut 11:534, 1970
7. Diethelm AG: Surgical management of complications of steroid therapy. Ann Surg 185:251, 1977
8. Diethelm AG, Gore I, Chien LT: Gastrointestinal hemorrhage secondary to cytomegalovirus after renal transplantation. Am J Surg 131:371, 1976
9. Glenn F, Grafe WR: Surgical complications of adrenal steroid therapy. Ann Surg 165:1023, 1967
10. Hadjiyannakis EJ, Evans DB, Smellie WAB, et al: Gastrointestinal complications with renal transplantation. Lancet 2:781, 1971
11. Hartmann WH, Sherlock P: Gastroduodenal metastases from carcinoma of the breast. An adrenal steroid-induced phenomenon. Cancer 14:426, 1961
12. Hersh EM, Bodey GP, Nies BA, et al: Causes of death in acute leukemia: a 10 year study of 414 patients from 1954-1963. JAMA 193:105, 1965
13. Kammerer WH, Freiberger RH, Rwelis AL: Peptic ulcer in rheumatoid patients on corticosteroid therapy. Arthr Rheum 1:122, 1958
14. Klein MS, Ennis F, Sherlock P, et al: Stress erosions. A major cause of gastrointestinal hemorrhage in patients with malignant disease. Am J Dig Dis 18:167, 1973
15. Lewicki AM, Saito S, Merrill JP: Gastrointestinal bleeding in the renal transplantation patient. Radiology 102:533, 1972
16. Lightdale CJ: Cancer and upper gastrointestinal tract hemorrhage. Benign causes of bleeding demonstrated by endoscopy. JAMA 226:139, 1973
17. Meyers WC, Harris N, Stein S, et al: Alimentary tract complications after renal transplantation. Ann Surg 190:535, 1979
18. Misra MK, Pinkus GS, Birtch AG, et al: Major colonic diseases complicating renal transplantation. Surgery 73:942, 1973
19. Moore TC, Hume DM: The period and nature of hazard in clinical renal transplantation. Ann Surg 170:1, 1969
20. Morrissey JF: Gastrointestinal endoscopy. Gastroenterology 62:1241, 1972

21. Owens ML, Passaro E, Wilson SE, et al: Treatment of peptic ulcer disease in the renal transplantation recipient. Ann Surg 186:17, 1977
22. Owens ML, Wilson SE, Saltzman R, et al: Gastrointestinal complications after renal transplantation. Arch Surg 111:467, 1976
23. Palmer ED: The vigorous diagnostic approach to upper gastrointestinal hemorrhage. JAMA 207:1477, 1969
24. Prolla JC, Kirsner JB: The gastrointestinal lesions and complications of the leukemias. Ann Int Med 61:1084, 1964
25. Rosen P, Armstrong D, Rice N: Gastrointestinal cytomegalovirus infection. Arch Int Med 132:274, 1973
26. Sawyer OI, Garvin PJ, Codd JE, et al: Colorectal complications of renal allograft transplantation. Arch Surg 113:84, 1978
27. Sherlock P: Acute gastritis resulting from regional infusion of an antimetabolite. Bull Gastrointest Endosc 9:16, 1963
28. Sherlock P, Winawer SJ: Differential diagnosis of upper gastrointestinal bleeding and cancer. Cancer J Clin 28:7, 1978
29. Spanos PK, Simmons RJ, Rattazi TC: Peptic ulcer disease in the transplant recipient. Arch Surg 109:193, 1974
30. Starzl TE: Experience in renal transplantation. In Starzl TE (ed): Gastrointestinal Hemorrhage. Philadelphia, Saunders, 1964
31. Sutherland D, Frech RS, Weil R, et al: The bleeding cecal ulcer: pathogenesis, angiographic diagnosis and nonoperative control. Surgery 71:290, 1972
32. Wolfe BM, Cherry JD: Hemorrhage from cecal ulcers in cytomegalovirus infection. Ann Surg 177:490, 1973
33. Zammit M, Toledo-Pereyra LH: Cimetidine for kidney transplantation: experimental observations. Surgery 86:611, 1979

S. Martin Lindenauer, M.D.

Hemobilia

ABSTRACT

Hemobilia is an uncommon variety of gastrointestinal hemorrhage and has diverse causes. The triad of gastrointestinal hemorrhage, biliary colic and jaundice should suggest the diagnosis and lead to precise anatomical delineation of the lesion by arteriography. Most commonly, hemobilia follows blunt hepatic trauma appearing 4-8 weeks after injury. The safety and important role of hepatic artery ligation has been clarified.

The subject of hemobilia is appropriately associated with the contributions of the Swedish surgeon, Philip Sandblom, who described his first case in 1948 [14]. Sandblom is credited with assigning the name hemobilia to the phenomenon of blood loss from the liver into the intestinal tract through the common bile duct and for clarification of numerous aspects of this phenomenon. However the possibility of hemorrhage through the biliary tract was discussed almost 300 years earlier in the first detailed description of the anatomy of the liver in 1654 by Francis Glisson [6]. Glisson observed and described the first case of hemobilia in the literature when a young nobleman was pierced by a sword while fighting a duel and bled to death through the biliary tract. Sandblom [13] notes that by the nineteenth century, there had been numerous reports of hemobilia and that every known kind of hemobilia had been described. In 1871, Quincke [10] described the pathognomonic symptom triad of gastrointestinal hemorrhage, biliary colic and jaundice.

The number of reported cases has increased rapidly since 1950, due to improved diagnostic skills and the increasing number of traffic accidents resulting in traumatic hemobilia.

S. Martin Lindenauer, M.D.: Professor of Surgery, Department of Surgery, University of Michigan Medical Center, and Chief of Staff, Veterans Administration Medical Center, Ann Arbor, Michigan.

CLINICAL MANIFESTATIONS

Sandblom in 1972 [13] collected 545 cases of gross hemobilia from the world literature and analyzed 355 "fully described cases." Sandblom [13] pointed out that hemobilia is less often recognized than hematuria when the rate of bleeding is small. The clinical manifestations of hemobilia depend to a large degree upon the rate of bleeding. A slow ooze of blood into the biliary tract is not distinguishable from any other form of gastrointestinal hemorrhage. However, more copious amounts of bleeding will form clots in the biliary tree and cause biliary colic and jaundice. Sandblom [13] estimates that the concentration of blood in the bile has to reach 70% before it will begin to clot. The symptoms of hemobilia therefore, are directly related to the rate of bleeding. Slow bleeding will at first be occult, then present as melena and if prolonged, manifest itself as blood loss anemia. Profuse arterial hemorrhage will distend the biliary ductal system and cause severe biliary colic and even hypovolemic shock. Massive hemorrhage can also present as hematemesis.

More often, the bleeding is intermittent because of the limited capacity of the biliary tree and the resistance of the sphincter of Oddi which slows the rate of bleeding and allows clots to form. Blood clots in the biliary tree act like stones, obstructing the flow of bile causing biliary colic and jaundice. The obstructed biliary tree will also result in liver swelling and tenderness. If infection is present, fever will be encountered. Because of the fibrinolytic activity of bile, clots that have formed may loosen and pass into the duodenum with relief of symptoms [16]. Occasionally a clot may remain in the common bile duct causing recurring attacks of pain, jaundice, and even pancreatitis. Clots in the gallbladder also act like stones and can cause symptoms of cholecystitis. Hemobilia secondary to an aneurysm may result in a thrill and bruit. In Sandblom's experience [13], melena was present in 90% of instances, while colicky pain, anemia, hematemesis, jaundice and shock were present in 60%-70%.

ETIOLOGY

The source of bleeding was noted by Sandblom [13] to arise from the liver in 53% of cases and from the gallbladder, bile ducts and pancreas in 47%. The cause was due to trauma in 55% of cases, gallstones and inflammation in 28%, vascular disorders in 11% and tumor in 6%. While trauma was the predominant cause in the United States and Western Europe, inflammatory etiologies are far more prevalent in Asia [1, 17]. Among the traumatic causes of hemobilia, traffic accidents account for 70% while surgical trauma was responsible in 30%. Blunt trauma to the liver due to automobile accidents is the single most common cause of hemobilia [9]. Surgical trauma is more often penetrating. It is due to suture ligatures, biopsy and cholangiogram needle punctures.

Blunt trauma to the liver resulting in capsular rupture or subcapsular hematoma seldom causes hemobilia. Trauma resulting in central hepatic rupture disrupts blood vessels and bile ducts, forming a cavity filled with blood and bile and is the setting in which hemobilia can occur. Penetrating trauma may also cause a central cavity or may simply result in an arteriobiliary fistula with little evidence of injury. There is no correlation between the size of the cavity and the degree of hemobilia. Sandblom [13] cites an incidence of hemobilia following hepatic trauma of 2.5% and an incidence of occult hemobilia of 3% to 10% following liver puncture. Rarely, hemobilia may be associated with a traumatic arteriovenous fistula and secondary portal hypertension. Central hepatic rupture causes hepatic necrosis, heals poorly and frequently becomes infected. Following hepatic injury, hemobilia seldom is noted immediately. There usually is a variable silent interval (average 4-8 weeks; median 2 weeks [13]) before hemobilia is clinically evident [9]. It is presumed that, during this interval, necrosis and autolysis of intervening walls of ducts and arteries occurs, allowing direct connection between these structures. It is also possible that occult hemobilia is present during this time. The formation of clots and their subsequent lysis accounts for the intermittent signs and symptoms. Isolated blunt trauma to the gallbladder or extrahepatic ducts is rarely a cause of hemobilia and is more often associated with hepatic parenchymal injury.

An important cause of hemobilia, comprising 17% of Sandblom's cases [13], is surgical injury to the liver and bile ducts. Injury to the structures of the porta hepatis may occur with attempts to control bleeding during a difficult cholecystectomy. A suture ligature may cause an arteriobiliary fistula or a false aneurysm which may then erode into a bile duct. Iatrogenic hemorrhage may occur after operation upon the common bile duct. The most common cause is probably injury to hepatic parenchyma with resultant hepatic necrosis, superinfection and abscess, or direct injury to intrahepatic vessels. Erosion due to indwelling drainage tubes has also been implicated. Puncture of the liver for diagnostic purposes can cause hemobilia [4]. This is more common when thick needles are used for this purpose [11].

Inflammatory disorders were the primary cause of hemobilia in 13% of Sandblom's cases [13] involving the liver and the extrahepatic biliary structures with equal frequency. Hepatic injury due to anesthetics, drugs, viral hepatitis, parasites, and pyogenic infection have all been described. Pancreatic inflammatory disease involving the head of the pancreas will result in hemobilia on occasion.

Gallstones are a common cause of occult biliary bleeding. Prior to the advent of cholecystography, the presence of occult blood in the stool was an important finding supporting the diagnosis of biliary lithiasis. Sandblom [13] cites an incidence of occult hemobilia in 25% of patients with cholelithiasis and in 37% of those with choledocholithiasis. In contrast, major hemorrhage due to gallstones is uncommon. Nevertheless, hemobilia due to gallstones accounted for 13% of cases in Sandblom's [13] collected series and was associated with a 55%

mortality, often due to exsanguinating hemorrhage. Gallstones can cause pressure necrosis and erosion into an adjacent hollow organ with resultant bleeding into both the biliary and intestinal tracts.

Vascular disorders were the cause of hemobilia in 11% of cases in Sandblom's experience [13]. Arterial aneurysms, true, false or mycotic, all may erode an adjacent bile duct and result in hemobilia. They may be intrahepatic or extrahepatic. Rupture of an aneurysm into the biliary tract is often associated with the sudden onset of severe pain. Portal hypertension on rare occasions is associated with rupture of a varix into the biliary tree.

Tumors causing hemobilia were least common in Sandblom's experience comprising 6% of his collected cases [13]. Such neoplasms may be benign or malignant and occur in the liver or biliary tree with almost equal frequency. Liver tumors rarely cause hemobilia which is in sharp contrast to urinary tumors which almost always are associated with hematuria. Metastatic liver neoplasms account for the bulk of liver tumors and almost never are associated with hemobilia. Primary hepatic neoplasms also seldom cause hemorrhage into the biliary system. The rare tumor that causes hemobilia infiltrates large bile ducts and becomes necrotic leading to hemorrhage.

DIAGNOSIS

The characteristic signs and symptoms of hemobilia — gastrointestinal hemorrhage, jaundice and biliary colic — should make the diagnosis relatively easy. However, the relative rarity of the condition sometimes makes it difficult. Furthermore, Sandblom estimates that in 10% of cases there are biliary symptoms without major gastrointestinal hemorrhage [15]. He has termed these instances "minor hemobilia" and has pointed out its importance. A small amount of hemorrhage can cause clots in the biliary tree but they rarely acquire clinical significance because they usually are promptly dissolved by the fibrinolytic action of bile. Interference with this mechanism by the diversion or obstruction of bile flow will allow such clots to persist. When biliary colic with obstructive jaundice is present and no cause is found, it is generally assumed that it was due to a small stone that has passed. In some instances this no doubt is due to obstruction by a blood clot. It is possible that some "retained stones" that are removed by various perfusion techniques represent the dissolution of clots rather than the dissolution of biliary calculi [15]. One should also think of hemobilia when there is gastrointestinal bleeding for which a cause cannot be found, especially if there are symptoms of biliary disease. Arteriography at present is the most important tool to localize the source of bleeding. Selective celiac as well as superior mesenteric angiography is required since the hepatic blood supply may be derived from the superior mesenteric circulation in 20% of instances. Arteriography may show a central hepatic cavity, aneurysm, tumor vessels or displacement of normal vessels which is of great help in localizing the site of hemorrhage even if the study is done when the patient is not actively bleeding. Portal venography, in contrast, is seldom useful. Cholangiography may visualize a clot in the biliary tree and a liver scan may reveal a filling defect due to a necrotic cavity, hematoma, abscess or tumor. The use of the duodenoscope may be extremely helpful in ruling out more common causes of gastrointestinal hemorrhage and may allow identification of active hemorrhage from the papilla.

TREATMENT

Hemobilia is a symptom or an expression of a primary pathologic entity; while generally, it is not good practice to treat only a symptom there are certainly exceptions to this generalization. Additionally, hemobilia is an entity that may itself require specific attention because of its life threatening potential. The treatment of hemobilia depends on the nature of the lesion associated with cause of hemorrhage and has to be individualized. Procedures commonly utilized include: hepatic artery ligation, hepatic debridement and drainage, hepatic resection, and cholecystectomy.

Hepatic artery ligation was previously thought to be almost universally associated with hepatic necrosis. Recent evidence suggests, however, that hepatic necrosis is uncommon if there is an intact portal circulation with no underlying hepatic parenchymal disease, if measures are taken to ensure adequate hepatic oxygenation (correction of hypovolemia, hypotension and hypoxia), and if hepatic metabolic requirements are decreased (treatment of pyrexia, maintenance of blood glucose levels). It is clear that the portal circulation can sustain the hepatic parenchyma under proper circumstance and that the collateral arterial supply to the liver is extensive, making hepatic artery ligation entirely feasible [2, 3, 5, 7, 8, 12]. Hepatic artery ligation is useful to control bleeding due to hepatic trauma, both blunt and penetrating, bleeding due to tumor and abscess, arteriobiliary fistula and arterial aneurysm [2, 8, 9]. Hemobilia due to blunt trauma may also be treated by debridement and drainage or hepatic resection, depending on the location and nature of the injury [8, 9, 13]. Debridement or resection is most appropriate for peripheral lesions, whereas hepatic artery ligation may be better to control hemorrhage from large central traumatic cavities. The use of packing and the superficial suture of deep central lesions is contraindicated and associated with rebleeding and abscess and an unacceptable incidence of complications and death. Hemobilia originating in the gallbladder is easily controlled by cholecystectomy. The accurate delineation of the site of bleeding will avoid the futility of the so-called "blind resection."

REFERENCES

1. Amberson JR and Ferguson IA: Traumatic hemobilia. Surgery 54:729, 1963

2. Ariyan S, Cahow CE, Greene FL, et al: Successful treatment of hepatic artery aneurysm with erosion in the common duct. Ann Surg 182:169, 1975
3. Brittain RS, Marchioro TL, Hermann G, et al: Accidental hepatic artery ligation in humans. Am J Surg 107:822, 1964
4. Cahow CE, Burrell M, Greco R: Hemobilia following percutaneous transhepatic cholangiography. Ann Surg 185:235, 1977
5. Gelin LE, Lewis DH, Nilsson LAV: Liver blood flow in man during abdominal surgery. II. Effect of hepatic artery ligation on the blood flow through metastatic tumor nodules. Acta Hepatosplen 15:21, 1968
6. Glisson F: Anatomia Hepatis, 1654
7. Madding GF, Kennedy PA, Sogemeier F: Hepatic artery ligation for metastatic tumor in the liver. Am J Surg 120:95, 1970
8. Mays ET: Lobar dearterialization for exsanguinating wounds of the liver. J. Trauma 12:397, 1972
9. McGehee RN, Townsend CM, Thompson JC, Fish JC: Traumatic hemobilia. Ann Surg 179:311, 1974
10. Quincke H: Ein fall von aneurysma der leberarterie. Berl Klin Wschr 8:349, 1871
11. Redecker AG, Karvountzis GG, Richman RH, et al: Percutaneous transhepatic cholangiography: An improved technique. JAMA 231:386, 1975
12. Redman HC, Reuter SR: Arterial collaterals in the liver hilus. Radiology 94:575, 1970
13. Sandblom P: Hemobilia. Springfield, IL, Charles C. Thomas, 1972
14. Sandblom P: Hemorrhage into the biliary tract following trauma — "traumatic hemobilia." Surgery 24:571, 1948
15. Sandblom P, Mirkovitch V: Minor hemobilia, clinical significance and pathophysiological background. Ann Surg 190:254, 1979
16. Sandblom P, Mirkovitch V, Saegesser F: Formation and fate of fibrin clots in the biliary tract. Ann Surg 185:356, 1977
17. Steichen FM and Scheiner NM: Traumatic intrahepatic hemobilia. Arch Surg 92:838, 1963

James C. Stanley, M.D.
Walter M. Whitehouse, Jr., M.D.
Linda M. Graham, M.D.

Splanchnic Artery Aneurysms and Gastrointestinal Hemorrhage

ABSTRACT

Splanchnic artery aneurysms are an uncommon cause of gastrointestinal hemorrhage. Aneurysms of the splanchnic circulation include lesions of the celiac (4%), gastric (4.5%), gastroepiploic (0.5%), gastroduodenal (1.5%), hepatic (19%), jejunal-ileal-colic (3.5%), pancreaticoduodenal-pancreatic (3%), splenic (56%), and superior mesenteric (8%) arteries. Etiologies are varied, as are the natural histories of these aneurysms. Bleeding into the intestinal tract is most often associated with aneurysms developing as a consequence of periarterial inflammation. Diagnosis and treatment of gastrointestinal hemorrhage due to splanchnic artery aneurysms must be undertaken with an understanding of distinguishing clinical characteristics of individual lesions.

Visceral artery aneurysms affecting splanchnic vessels have been discovered with increasing regularity as a consequence of more common arteriographic studies of both vascular and nonvascular disease. More than 1600 splanchnic arterial aneurysms have been described in the literature. Many of these lesions are initially recognized as a cause of major gastrointestinal hemorrhage. Others are often silent, being diagnosed during studies or treatment for unrelated disease. Splanchnic artery aneurysms are best addressed separately because of the marked variability in their biological character, especially in regard to intestinal bleeding.

James C. Stanley, M.D.: Associate Professor of Surgery, Head, Division of Peripheral Vascular Surgery, Department of Surgery, University of Michigan Medical Center; Walter M. Whitehouse, Jr., M.D.: Assistant Professor of Surgery, Division of Peripheral Vascular Surgery, Department of Surgery, University of Michigan Medical Center; Linda M. Graham, M.D.: Research Fellow in Vascular Surgery, Resident in General Surgery, Department of Surgery, University of Michigan Medical Center, Ann Arbor, Michigan.

CELIAC ARTERY ANEURYSMS

Aneurysms of the celiac artery are a rare cause of gastrointestinal hemorrhage. They account for 4% of all splanchnic aneurysms. During the past 40 years males and females have been equally affected. Medial degeneration appears to be the most common pathologic finding in these lesions. Arteriosclerotic changes are common, but are considered a secondary event, rather than a primary etiologic factor in most aneurysms. Traumatic, mycotic, and luetic aneurysms were more commonly cited in early reviews, but have been unusual in recent reports.

Celiac artery aneurysms are usually asymptomatic. Vague epigastric discomfort is common when symptoms do occur. Although rare, intense pain radiating to the back, with nausea and vomiting, has been attributed to expanding aneurysms. Pulsatile masses rarely are evident on physical exam. Rupture is the most serious clinical complication of celiac artery aneurysms. Although nearly 80% of early reported aneurysms ruptured, most recent experience suggests a rupture rate less than 10%. Intraperitoneal hemorrhage is more likely with rupture than bleeding into the intestinal tract. Gastrointestinal hemorrhage is in fact an exceedingly uncommon complication of celiac artery aneurysms, having been reported by only a few authors during the past four decades [19, 24]. Direct bleeding into the stomach and duodenum, as well as indirect communication through the pancreatic ductal system have been encountered.

Recognition of celiac artery aneurysms with angiography or abdominal operation for unrelated disease has been the most common means of diagnosing these lesions in recent times [17]. Aneurysmal wall calcification is uncommon. Displacement of contiguous gastrointestinal structures is a frequent radiographic finding of larger aneurysms. Although antemortem recognition is increasing, preoperative diagnosis, as recently as a decade ago, had been made only 7 times [39].

Operative intervention is advocated for all celiac artery aneurysms [12, 36]. More than 90% of surgically treated cases during the past two decades have had a successful outcome. Aneurysmectomy constitutes appropriate treatment of most celiac artery aneurysms. Use of autologous vein or prosthetic graft reconstruction is preferred over aortic implantation of the celiac artery in these circumstances. Aneurysmorrhaphy, because of the inherent weakness of the dilated vessel wall, is not recommended in managing these lesions. Simple ligation of the celiac artery may be adequate therapy if hepatic blood flow is not severely compromised.

GASTRIC AND GASTROEPIPLOIC ARTERY ANEURYSMS

Aneurysms of gastric and gastroepiploic arteries may occasionally be confused with gastric ulcers or malignancies as a cause of upper gastrointestinal

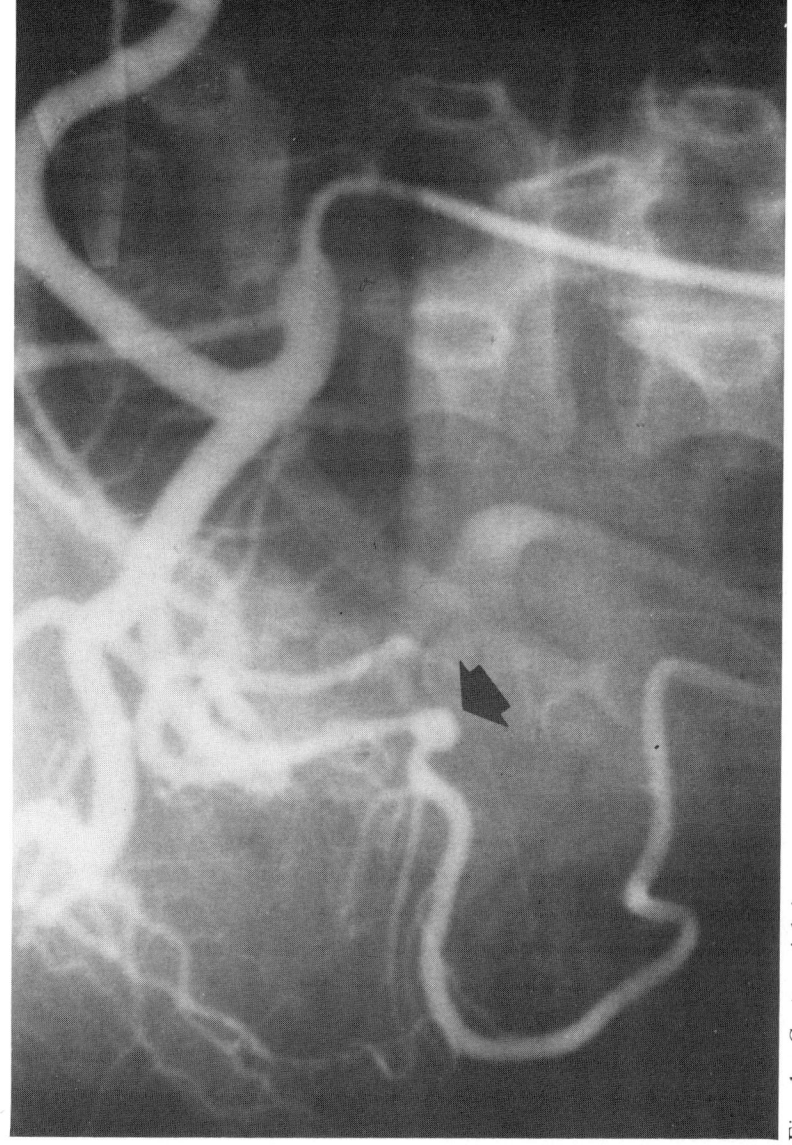

Fig. 1. Gastroepiploic artery aneurysm associated with traumatic pancreatic pseudocyst and massive gastrointestinal hemorrhage.

bleeding. These lesions account for approximately 5% of splanchnic aneurysmal disease. Gastric artery aneurysms occur 9 times more often than gastroepiploic artery aneurysms. Most lesions are solitary. The male:female ratio of patients with these aneurysms is 3:1. Arteriosclerotic changes as seen in many aneurysms are unlikely representatives of a primary process. In most of these aneurysms medial generation or periarterial inflammation, such as that accompanying gastric ulcer disease, may predispose to secondary arteriosclerosis.

Most reported gastric or gastroepiploic artery aneurysms have ruptured at the time of diagnosis. Rupture was associated with serious gastrointestinal bleeding manifested by hematemesis in 70% of patients [23, 25, 39]. Chronic gastrointestinal bleeding occurs less often. A few patients experience antecedent dyspeptic epigastric discomfort but most have no abdominal pain prior to aneurysmal rupture. Intraperitoneal bleeding is less common, occurring in approximately 30% of cases [40].

Antemortem diagnosis usually is established with urgent operations for gastrointestinal or intraperitoneal bleeding. More recently, arteriographic studies for unexplained gastrointestinal bleeding have provided preoperative recognition of these lesions (Fig. 1). Mucosal changes with these aneurysms are nondiagnostic, causing endoscopic recognition to be exceedingly difficult.

Approximately 70% of patients with gastric or gastroepiploic artery aneurysms reported before 1970 died following rupture [39]. Intramural lesions, especially when associated with gastrointestinal tract hemorrhage, are best excised with adjacent gastric tissue [3, 23]. Ligation, with or without excision of the lesion is often possible in treating extraintestinal aneurysms.

GASTRODUODENAL, PANCREATICODUODENAL, AND PANCREATIC ARTERY ANEURYSMS

These aneurysms are uncommon, but among splanchnic aneurysms are one of the more frequent causes of gastrointestinal hemorrhage. Gastroduodenal artery aneurysms account for 1.5% of these lesions, with pancreaticoduodenal and pancreatic artery aneurysms accounting for 3% of all splanchnic aneurysms. Men are affected 4 times more often than women. Periarterial inflammation associated with acute or chronic pancreatitis, often with pseudocyst formation, appears responsible for most of these aneurysms [13, 37]. Arteriosclerosis, when present, is often a secondary event.

Gastroduodenal, pancreaticoduodenal, or pancreatic artery aneurysms are usually symptomatic when recognized. Pain associated with these lesions is often difficult to distinguish from that of pancreatitis. Approximately 65% of reported aneurysms have ruptured into the intestinal tract. Bleeding directly into the stomach or duodenum is most common, although indirect communcations through biliary or pancreatic ducts have been reported [16, 44]. Hemoperi-

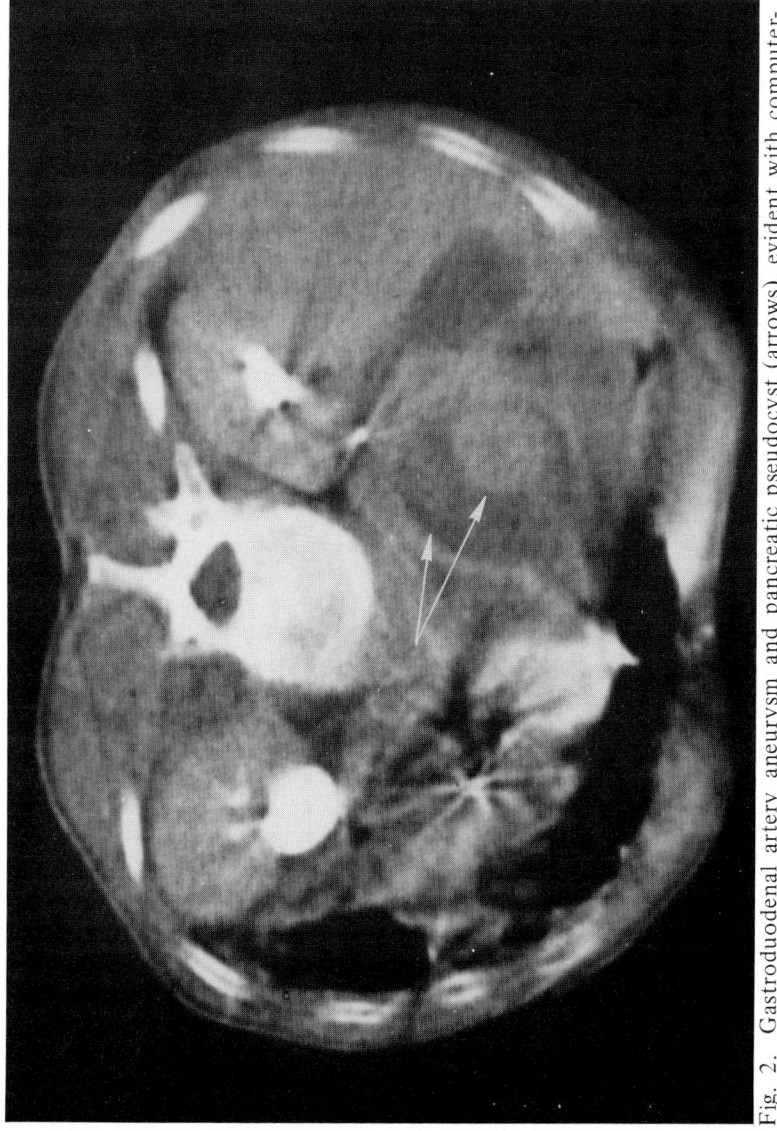

Fig. 2. Gastroduodenal artery aneurysm and pancreatic pseudocyst (arrows), evident with computerized axial tomography, as a cause of massive gastrointestinal hemorrhage following pseudocyst penetration into the duodenum.

toneum is unusual. Arteriography is very important in establishing a preoperative or antemortem diagnosis of these aneurysms. Endoscopic recognition of these lesions with bleeding from the papilla of Vater has been reported [4]. Occasionally computerized axial tomography will be diagnostic (Fig. 2).

A mortality of 50% follows rupture of gastroduodenal or pancreaticoduodenal artery aneurysms. Urgent operative intervention is justified in all but the poorest risk patients [9, 41]. Gastroduodenal artery aneurysmectomy can usually be performed electively without great risk. Aneurysmal ligation within the sac is more appropriate than excision if it has ruptured into a viscus or is embedded within the pancreas [9]. Treatment of pancreaticoduodenal and pancreatic artery aneurysms is more difficult [35, 44]. Multiple vessels communicating with these aneurysms limit the efficacy of simple ligature. Pancreatic resections, including pancreaticoduodenectomy, may become necessary treatment. Occasional transangiocatheter embolic occlusion of these lesions has proved successful, although rebleeding and rupture occur too frequently for this to become standard therapy [21, 30].

HEPATIC ARTERY ANEURYSMS

Hepatic artery aneurysms are a recognized cause of gastrointestinal bleeding in the form of hemobilia. These lesions comprise 19% of aneurysms affecting splanchnic vessels. Etiologic factors include arteriosclerosis (32%), medial degeneration (24%), trauma (22%) and infection (10%). Mycotic lesions associated with endocarditis were more prevalent in the past. Infection from illicit drug abuse may reverse this trend. True aneurysms and pseudoaneurysms following blunt abdominal trauma are occurring with increasing frequency. Periarterial inflammation with cholecystitis or pancreatitis are less common causes of hepatic artery macroaneurysms.

Hepatic artery aneurysms greater than 2 cm in size tend to be solitary and saccular. Approximately 80% involve the extrahepatic vessels, with 20% occurring within the liver parenchyma [11]. A review of 163 aneurysms documented the following locations: common hepatic (63%), right hepatic (28%), left hepatic (5%) and both right and left hepatic arteries (4%) [39].

Aneurysmal calcifications or displacement of contiguous structures noted during barium contrast studies or cholecystocholangiography may raise a suspicion of hepatic aneurysms. Arteriographic studies have resulted in increased recognition of these lesions. Certainly, preoperative arteriographic studies are essential in planning optimal surgical management of hepatic artery aneurysms [43]. Ultrasonography and computerized axial tomography in select cases have provided a noninvasive means of diagnosing and following these lesions. Symptomatic intact aneurysms may be associated with discomfort suggesting cholecystitis. Expanding hepatic artery aneurysms often produce serere abdominal pain with radiation to the back. Pulsatile masses are not commonly observed with these aneurysms.

Rupture of hepatic artery aneurysms occurs with equal frequency into the hepatobiliary tract and the peritoneal cavity. The former may present with characteristic findings of hemobilia. Intermittent pain similar to biliary colic, gastrointestinal bleeding with periodic hematemesis, and jaundice are hallmarks of this complication. Many patients in this group are febrile. Bright red rectal bleeding or melena are less common manifestations of hemobilia [32]. Direct rupture into the stomach or duodenum is very uncommon. Intraperitoneal bleeding may accompany extrahepatic aneurysmal rupture, but occurs much less frequently than hemorrhage into the gastrointestinal tract. Rupture affected 44% of hepatic artery aneurysms reported from 1960 to 1970, although the true risk of this event may be much less [39]. Mortality with reported ruptures has been approximately 35%.

Aneurysmectomy or aneurysm exclusion by proximal and distal ligation, without reconstruction of the involved vessel has been the most common means of treating hepatic aneurysms. These procedures are most appropriate for aneurysms occurring proximal to the gastroduodenal and right gastric vessels. Diseases compromising hepatic blood flow make ligation of the proximal hepatic artery unacceptable. Aneurysmorrhaphy or arterial reconstructions are preferable in such situations, as well as in management of proper hepatic artery aneurysms. Complicated intrahepatic aneurysms often require hepatic territory resection. In occasional patients, bleeding intrahepatic aneurysms may be controlled by simple ligation of the proximal artery. This may be preferable to undertaking major liver resections, although it is not universally successful [14]. In select cases percutaneous transangiocatheter embolization may be a satisfactory form of therapy [10].

JEJUNAL, ILEAL, AND COLIC ARTERY ANEURYSMS

Jejunal, ileal, and colic artery aneurysms are often insidious as a cause of intestinal bleeding. They account for approximately 3.5% of all splanchnic aneurysms. Men and women are affected with equal frequency. Most mesenteric branch aneurysms appear to originate from congenital or acquired medial defects [20, 29]. Arteriosclerosis when present is probably a secondary event. Most clinically important lesions have been solitary.

Intact symptomatic aneurysms are rare, with most being recognized after rupture into the intestinal lumen. Massive rectal bleeding as well as chronic melena may follow such an event. Rupture into the mesentery or peritoneal cavity occurs less often. Rarely, a tender mass with contained rupture has been the initial manifestation of these lesions. Bland mesenteric branch aneurysms are becoming recognized more often during arteriographic studies for unrelated disease including gastrointestinal hemorrhage [33]. Treatment of intestinal artery branch aneurysms usually entails ligation, aneurysmectomy or bowel resection for intramural lesions. Aneurysms of the inferior mesenteric artery and its branches are exceedingly rare [8]. Their causes, natural history and optimal treatment remain to be defined.

SPLENIC ARTERY ANEURYSMS

Splenic artery aneurysms are the most common splanchnic aneurysms associated with gastrointestinal hemorrhage, and account for 56% of all splanchnic aneurysms. The incidence of these aneurysms has been reported to range from 0.098% in a collection of nearly 195,000 necropsies to 10.4% in a select autopsy study of elderly patients [1, 26]. Incidental arteriographic demonstration of these aneurysms in 0.78% of cases studied at one institution may reflect their true frequency in the general population [38]. Females are affected with these aneurysms 4 times more often than males. Splenic aneurysms are usually saccular, occur at arterial bifurcations, and are multiple in 20% of cases.

Three distinct conditions associated with medial degeneration have been related to the evolution of these lesions. First, 4% of patients with renal artery medial fibrodysplasia exhibit splenic artery aneurysms [38]. Second, portal hypertension with splenomegaly may also be a contributory factor in certain cases [2, 29, 34]. Seven percent of portal hypertensives in one report exhibited splenic artery macroaneurysms [38]. Vascular effects of repeated pregnancy are a third factor related to splenic aneurysms. Forty percent of women in a recent series, without other etiologic factors present, had completed 6 or more pregnancies [38]. Gestational vessel wall alterations due to hormonal and local hemodynamic events may enhance the development of these aneurysms.

Frequent localization of calcific arteriosclerotic changes to aneurysms, without involvement of adjacent vessels, suggests that arteriosclerosis often is a secondary process, rather than a primary etiologic event. Occasional aneurysms may be due to primary arteriosclerotic weakening of the splenic vessel wall. Inflammatory processes affecting tissues adjacent to the splenic artery, particularly pancreatitis with pseudocysts [37], are an important cause of aneurysms associated with intestinal hemorrhage (Fig. 3).

Most splenic artery aneurysms are asymptomatic and their clinical importance is the subject of considerable controversy [18, 38]. Vague abdominal discomfort is the most common complaint in those 20% of patients alleged to be symptomatic. Abdominal bruits were more often associated with turbulent blood flow through tortuous splanchnic vessels than aneurysmal disease. Splenic artery aneurysms, being usually less than 2 cm in size, are rarely palpable.

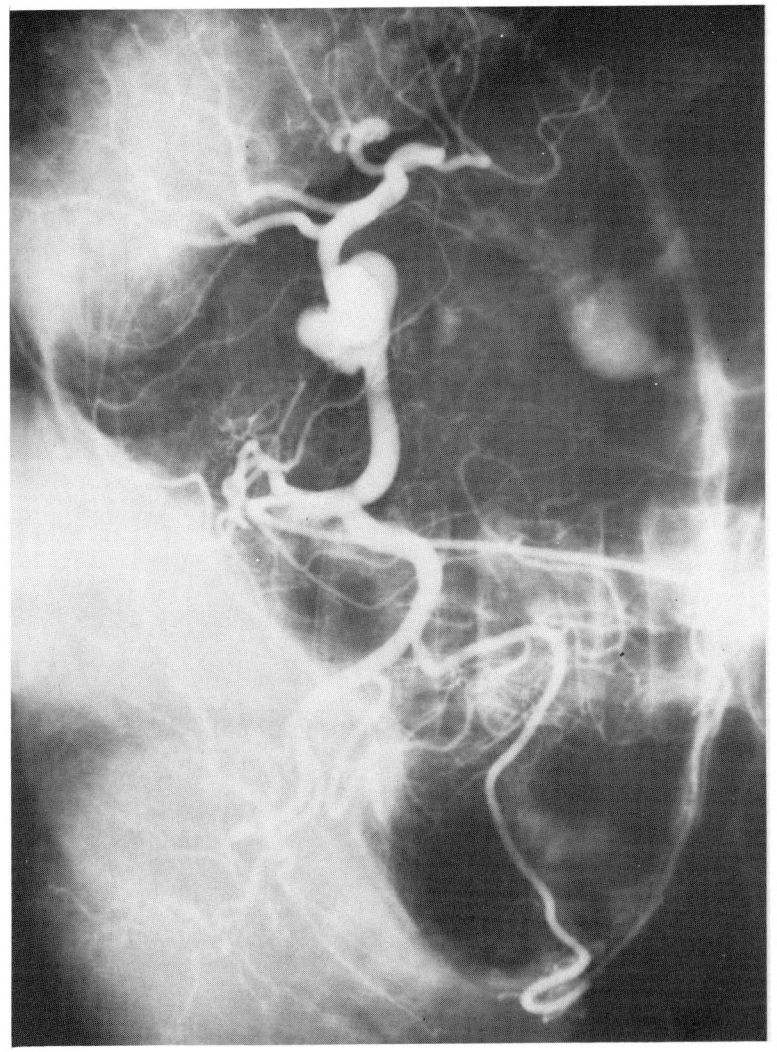

Fig. 3. Splenic artery aneurysm as a consequence of chronic pancreatitis and pseudocyst extension about the midsplenic vessel. Massive gastrointestinal hemorrhage followed pseudocyst erosion into the stomach.

Splenic artery aneurysms are most often incidental findings of arteriographic studies. These lesions may be suspected when curvilinear, signet ring-like calcifications are observed within the left upper quadrant on abdominal radiographs. Ultrasonography and computerized axial tomography may prove useful noninvasive means of diagnosing these aneurysms.

Aneurysmal rupture represents the most serious complications of splenic artery aneurysms. Intermittent gastrointestinal hemorrhage reflects an occult form of rupture. Presentation of bleeding stomach masses in such instances often leads to an erroneous clinical diagnosis of leiomyoma or leiomyosarcoma [5, 15]. Hemorrhage into the gastrointestinal tract may be indirect through the pancreatic ducts or by way of a pancreatic pseudocyst that erodes into the lumen of adjacent bowel. Rupture with splenic arteriovenous fistula formation and portal hypertension is a rare but recognized complication of these aneurysms.

Intraperitoneal bleeding is more common than gastrointestinal hemorrhage. Some patients bleed massively, whereas others bleed slowly into the retrogastric area. Catastrophic intraperitoneal bleeding often results when the lesser sac containment is lost. This double rupture phenomenon may allow treatment before fatal hemorrhage develops.

Life-threatening splenic artery aneurysm rupture occurs in fewer than 2% of cases [38]. Death following operation for aneurysmal rupture in nonpregnant patients occurs in fewer than 25% of cases [39]. Thus surgical therapy for most splenic artery aneurysms appears justified only when the risk of operation approaches 0.5%. Aneurysmal rupture with pregnancy is common [22, 28]. More than 95% of reported splenic artery aneurysms have ruptured in such a setting. Splenic aneurysms in pregnancy are considered emergencies with the mortality of aneurysmal rupture during pregnancy being greater than 65%.

Operative management of splenic artery aneurysms usually entails splenectomy. Exclusion of certain bland proximal splenic aneurysms may be preferred to excision. However, proximal aneurysms embedded in pancreatic tissue, that are associated with bleeding into the ductal system, are best treated by pancreatectomy. Aneurysms associated with hemorrhagic gastric erosions nearly always require excision of the involved stomach wall. Proximal splenic artery aneurysms have often been treated by aneurysmectomy and ligation, with avoidance of splenectomy. Operative mortality following elective aneurysmectomy for bland lesions has not been reported in the recent literature. The role of transangiocatheter embolization for certain of these lesions may prove important as preservation of splenic tissue assumes greater clinical significance [31].

SUPERIOR MESENTERIC ARTERY ANEURYSMS

Superior mesenteric artery aneurysms are an extremely rare cause of gastrointestinal hemorrhage. These lesions comprise 8% of splanchnic artery aneurysms. The sexes are equally affected. Mycotic aneurysms are the most common lesion, being frequently associated with endocarditis due to non-hemolytic streptococcus. Medial degeneration, arteriosclerosis and trauma are less common causes of superior mesenteric artery aneurysms.

Abdominal discomfort that becomes persistent, severe, epigastric pain is often the first manifestation of a superior mesenteric artery aneurysm. Early manifestations of these lesions often represent intestinal angina due to reduced midgut blood flow with propagation of intraluminal thrombus beyond the inferior pancreaticoduodenal middle colic vessels. Tender, mobile, pulsatile abdominal masses are occasionally seen with expanding lesions. Rupture of these lesions, especially into the gastrointestinal tract is very unusual. Bleeding, when it has been noted, was associated with aneurysm thrombosis and intestinal ischemia [6].

The first successful surgical treatment of superior mesenteric artery aneurysm was reported more than three decades ago [7]. The most common treatment has been ligation. Aneurysmal ligation without arterial reconstruction has proved a successful means of treatment. Preexisting collaterals due to coexisting occlusive disease often make this direct approach feasible. Aneurysmorrhaphy has also been successfully undertaken in management of these lesions [28]. Aneurysmectomy is unattractive because of the lesion's proximity to major collateral vessels and venous structures. In fact arterial reconstruction following aneurysmal exclusion or excision has rarely been reported [42].

REFERENCES

1. Bedford PD, Lodge B: Aneurysm of the splenic artery. Gut 1:312, 1960
2. Boijsen E, Efsing HO: Aneurysm of the splenic artery. Acta Radiol [Diagn] (Stockh) 8:29, 1969
3. Bradley RL: Gastric hemorrhage due to ruptured aneurysm. Am J Surg 108:431, 1964
4. Brintnall BB, Laidlaw WW and Papp JP: Hemobilia: pancreatic pseudocyst hemorrhage demonstrated by endoscopy and arteriography. Digest Dis 19:186, 1974
5. Castleman B, Scully RE, McNeely BU: Case records of the Massachusetts General Hospital. N Engl J Med 289:682, 1973
6. Clark F and Murray SM: Steatorrhoea due to dissecting aneurysm of the superior mesenteric artery. Br Med J 2:965, 1962
7. DeBakey ME, Cooley DA: Successful resection of mycotic aneurysm of superior mesenteric artery: case report and review of the literature. Am Surg 19:202, 1953
8. Duke LJ, Lamberth WC Jr, Wright CB: Inferior mesenteric artery aneurysm: Case report and discussion. Surgery 85:385, 1979

9. Eckhauser FE, Stanley JC Zelenock GB, et al: Gastroduodenal and pancreaticoduodenal artery aneurysms: a complication of pancreatitis causing massive gastrointestinal hemorrhage. Surgery (in press)
10. Goldblatt M, Goldin AR, Shaff MI: Percutaneous embolization for the management of hepatic artery aneurysms. Gastroenterology 73:1142, 1977
11. Guida PM, Moore SW: Aneurysm of the hepatic artery. Report of five cases with a brief review of the previously reported cases. Surgery 60:299, 1966
12. Haimovici H, Sprayregen S, Eckstein P, et al: Celiac artery aneurysmectomy: case report with review of the literature. Surgery 79:592, 1976
13. Harris RD, Anderson JE, Coel MN: Aneurysms of the small pancreatic arteries: a cause of upper abdominal pain and intestinal bleeding. Radiology 115:17, 1975
14. Hubens A, DeSchepper A: Hepatic artery aneurysm: a pitfall in biliary surgery. Br J Surg 66:259, 1979
15. Inglis FG, McKee NH: Unusual cause of upper gastrointestinal bleeding. Rupture of splenic artery aneurysm into stomach with survival. Canad J Surg 15:276, 1972
16. Janne P, Bremen J, Bremer A: Aneurysm of the gastroduodenal artery as a cause of hemobilia. Am J Surg 133:633, 1977
17. Kraft RO, Fry WJ: Aneurysms of the celiac artery. Surg Gynecol Obstet 117:563, 1963
18. Kreel L: The recognition and incidence of splenic artery aneurysms. A historical review. Australas Radiol 16:126, 1972
19. Laipply TC: Syphilitic aneurysm of the celiac artery. Am J Med Sci 206:453, 1943
20. Lesna M, Tweedle DEF: Submucosal jejunal aneurysm. Beitr Pathol 154:190, 1975
21. Lina JR, Jaques P, Mandell V: Aneurysm rupture secondary to transcatheter embolization. Am J Roentgenol 132:553, 1979
22. MacFarlane JR, Thorbjarnason B: Rupture of splenic artery aneurysm during pregnancy. Am J Obstet Gynecol 95:1025, 1966
23. Mandelbaum I, Kaiser GD, Lempke RE: Gastric intraumural aneurysm as a cause for massive gastrointestinal hemorrhage. Ann Surg 155:199, 1962
24. Manzullo V, Bevilacqua G, DiCarlo V, et al: Su un caso di aneurisma del tronco celiaco rotto in duodeno. Minerva Chir 33:839, 1978
25. Milliard M: Fatal rupture of gastric aneurysm. Arch Pathol 59:363, 1955
26. Moore SE, Guida PM, Schumacher HW: Splenic artery aneurysm. Bull Soc Int Chir 29:210, 1970
27. Nordentoft EL, Larsen EH: Rupture of a jejunal intramural aneurysm causing intestinal bleeding. Acta Chir Scand 133:256, 1967
28. Olcott C, Ehrenfeld WK: Endoaneurysmorrhaphy for visceral artery aneurysms. Am J Surg 133:636, 1977
29. Owens JC, Coffey RJ: Aneurysm of the splenic artery including a report of six additional cases. Int Abstr Surg 97:313, 1953
30. Prasad JK, Chatterjee KS, Johnston DWB: Unusual case of massive gastrointestinal bleeding-pseudoaneurysm of the head of the pancreas. Canad J Surg 18:490, 1975

31. Probst P, Castañeda-Zuñiga WR, Gomes AS, et al: Nonsurgical treatment of splenic-artery aneurysms. Radiology 128:619, 1978
32. Ranniger K, Menguy R, Kittle CF, et al: Angiographic diagnosis of an intrahepatic aneurysm as a cause of unexplained bleeding. Radiology 90:507, 1968
33. Reuter SR, Fry WJ, Bookstein JJ: Mesenteric artery branch aneurysms. Arch Surg 97:497, 1968
34. Scheinin TM, Vanttinen E: Aneurysms of the splenic artery in portal hypertension. Ann Clin Res 1:165, 1969
35. Spanos PK, Kloppedal EA, Murray CA: Aneurysms of the gastroduodenal and pancreaticoduodenal arteries. Am J Surg 127:345, 1974
36. Stanley JC: Splanchnic artery aneurysms. In Rutherford RB (ed.) Vascular Surgery. Philadelpia, Saunders, 1977, p 673
37. Stanley JC, Frey CF, Miller TA, et al: Major arterial hemorrhage. A complication of pancreatic pseudocysts and chronic pancreatitis. Arch Surg 111:435, 1976
38. Stanley JC, Fry WJ: Pathogenesis and clinical significance of splenic artery aneurysms. Surgery 76:898, 1974
39. Stanley JC, Thompson NW, Fry WJ: Splanchnic artery aneurysms. Arch Surg 101:689, 1970
40. Thomford MR, Yurko JE, Smith EJ: Aneurysm of gastric arteries as a cause of intraperitoneal hemorrhage. Review of literature. Ann Surg 168:294, 1968
41. Verta MJ Jr, Dean RH, Yao JST, et al: Pancreaticoduodenal artery aneurysms. Ann Surg 186:111, 1977
42. Violago FC, Downs AR: Ruptured atherosclerotic aneurysm of the superior mesenteric artery with celiac axis occlusion. Ann Surg 174:207, 1971
43. Weaver DH, Fleming RJ, Barnes WA: Aneurysm of the hepatic artery: the value of arteriography in surgical management. Surgery 64:891, 1968
44. West JE, Bernhardt H, Bowers RF: Aneurysms of the pancreaticoduodenal artery. Am J Surg 115:835, 1968
45. Wolstenholme JT: Major gastrointestinal hemorrhage associated with pancreatic pseudocyst. Am J Surg 127:377, 1974

Henry D. Appelman, M.D.

Morphologic Features of Right Colonic Vascular Ectasias in Elderly Patients

ABSTRACT

A common cause of episodic, usually low-grade colonic bleeding in elderly patients has been identified as a collection of ectatic thin-walled mucosal vessels invariably associated with severely dilated, tortuous submucosal veins. Recent studies suggest that these ectasias are secondary to chronic obstruction of the submucosal veins by tension in the muscularis propria. Gross detection of these lesions in the resected specimens is best accomplished when some type of material such as silicone rubber, barium, or dye, is injected into the arteries. The microscopic features are those of mucosal vascular tangles with submucosal varices.

The abnormal intramural vasculature in the right colon which, usually in elderly patients, is a cause of chronic recurrent bleeding, has been called by a number of names. These include arteriovenous malformation [1, 9, 17, 20], including the Type I AVM of Moore, et al [13], hemangioma [15], angiodysplasia [2, 11], vascular dysplasia [6], and most recently, and probably most correctly, vascular ectasia [4, 12, 16].

GROSS IDENTIFICATION

For years, the identification of these bleeding lesions was elusive. First, the lesions are flat and small, usually less than 5 mm in diameter [5, 12]. Figure 1 is an example of one of the very few grossly visible lesions of this type that we have seen, an irregularly shaped, flat congested focus, about 5 mm across.

Henry D. Appelman, M.D.: Professor of Pathology, Department of Pathology, University of Michigan Medical Center, Ann Arbor, Michigan.

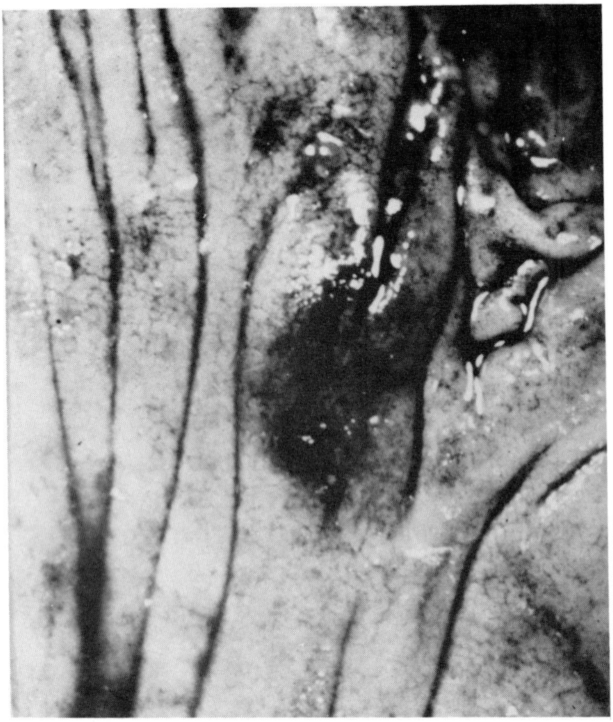

Fig. 1. In the center right, an irregular hemorrhagic or congested 5 mm focus is present above the ileocecal valve in the proximal-most ascending colon.

Obviously, lesions such as this will not be detected by barium enema examinations. Second, the patients often are not actively bleeding when operated upon, so that specific bleeding points, such as in Fig. 1, are infrequently evident [3]. Thus, the surgeon is commonly faced with the problem of resecting a lesion that is neither visible nor palpable [1, 2, 5, 13]. As a result, for many years, the cause of bleeding in these elderly patients was unexplained.

The development of selective abdominal angiographic technics finally allowed these lesions to be visualized [2, 11, 17]. A group of abnormal findings fulfill the radiographic diagnosis of vascular ectasia or angiodysplasia. These include a cluster or tuft of small vessels seen during the arterial phase, dilatation and slow emptying of tortuous intramural veins, and early filling of the extramural veins [2, 4, 11]. Such findings are now used to direct the limits of surgical resection by pinpointing the location of the distorted vasculature [1, 9, 13]. Although abnormal vessels are angiographically demonstrable, the finding of active bleeding sites, as defined by extravasation of contrast material into the colonic lumen, is uncommon.

Recently, a number of reports have lauded the diagnostic merits of colonoscopy in detecting these ectatic right colonic foci, occasionally even in the absence of diagnostic angiographic findings [14, 15, 20]. It is clear that vascular ectasias or dysplasias, once virtually defying diagnosis, are now demonstrable by either, or both, of two fairly readily available techniques, angiography and colonoscopy.

In spite of the level of angiographic diagnostic sophistication, the pathologist examining the resected specimen remained frustrated because, most of the time, there was still no grossly visible lesion [6]. Attempting to identify a vascular lesion by random sampling was usually unrewarding; serial blocking and sectioning of the resected specimen was too expensive and time consuming to be practical. The introduction of specimen angiography using a colloidal barium sulfate solution greatly facilitated gross dissection of the resected colon by identifying the location of the abnormal vessels in the specimen. The pathologist could now concentrate on the area in question, serially block and section it, and generally find the angiographically demonstrated abnormality.

In one study, injection of methylene blue dye at the time of specimen angiography seemed to be quite successful in defining bleeding sites [20]. The dye apparently turns the ectatic foci into grossly visible blue areas in the mucosa.

Hagihara et al emphasized that by careful inspection of the excised specimen in the operating room with stretching and compression of a small segment of mucosa at a time, and marking of any suspected lesions with a suture, microscopic bleeding points may be more readily found by the pathologist [9]. We have tried this in 3 patients with mixed results.

HISTOLOGIC CHARACTERISTICS

It is apparent that the use of angiographic and endoscopic techniques have improved the capabilities of detection of these right colonic bleeding lesions. It is equally apparent that, for the pathologist, there are strikingly few guidelines currently available which define these lesions histologically. In fact, there are no specific diagnostic criteria.

The few published histologic descriptions and photomicrographs share two features [2, 4, 7-10, 12, 16, 17, 20]. First, the submucosal veins are dilated. Second, these communicate with dilated thin-walled vessels in the mucosa often characterized as "distorted." Presumably this distortion is the result of both the dilatation and peculiarities of shape and, perhaps, direction or orientation. Only infrequently are the submucosal veins noted to be thick-walled or sclerotic [4, 12].

We have examined right colonic specimens with angiographically demonstrated vascular ectasias from 9 patients with the typical bleeding history. In 6 of these, specimen angiography was performed using a dilute barium sulfate suspension after which the arteries were clamped and the specimens fixed in formalin. After fixation, the specimens were oriented so as to correspond as closely as possible to the angiogram. The specific vascular lesions were found in the angiograms and the corresponding areas in the gross specimens were carefully excised and serially blocked. The barium solution effectively distended the arteries and the abnormal mucosal vessels.

On microscopic examination of these specimens, there were several changes which were noted to occur singly or in various combinations (Table 1). Presumed sites of bleeding were identified in only 4 patients. One was a large submucosal hemorrhage which had ulcerated the mucosa. The second was a cluster of ectatic mucosal and submucosal vessels, two of the latter containing organizing thrombi (Fig. 2). The third was a single dilated thrombosed mucosal vessel (Fig. 3), and the fourth was a focus of old hemorrhage in the mucosa overlying a scar containing a cluster of sclerotic vessels. It is likely that this low yield of definable bleeding sites was related to the fact that most of these patients were not actively bleeding at the time of the colectomy.

In 5 cases, mucosal ectasias were found. These are dilated, tortuous, clustered intramucosal vessels of capillary or venular type (Figs. 2 and 4). In general, these were lined only by endothelium (Fig. 3). Some of these vessels were separated from the lumen by a thin membrane of endothelium and colonic epithelium with, presumably, their associated basement membranes (Fig. 5). These ectatic mucosal vessels communicated with the submucosal venous plexus

Table 1
Histologic Features in Resected Right Colons of 9 Patients With Angiographic Evidence of Vascular Ectasias

	Age/Sex	Bleeding Points*	Mucosal Ectasia*	Submucosal Ectasia*	Submucosal Sclerosis*	Barium in Veins
Injected	58/F	+	+	+	+	+
with	72/F	+	+	+	0	+
barium	53/M	+	+	0	0	+
	80/F	0	+	+	+	+
	66/M	0	+	0	+	+
	68/F	0	0	+	+	0
Not	81/M	+	0	+	0	N/A
injected	61/M	0	0	0	+	N/A
	64/F	0	0	+	0	N/A

Legend: + indicates a change was found; 0 indicates it was not found. NA; not applicable.
*See text for definitions of these terms.

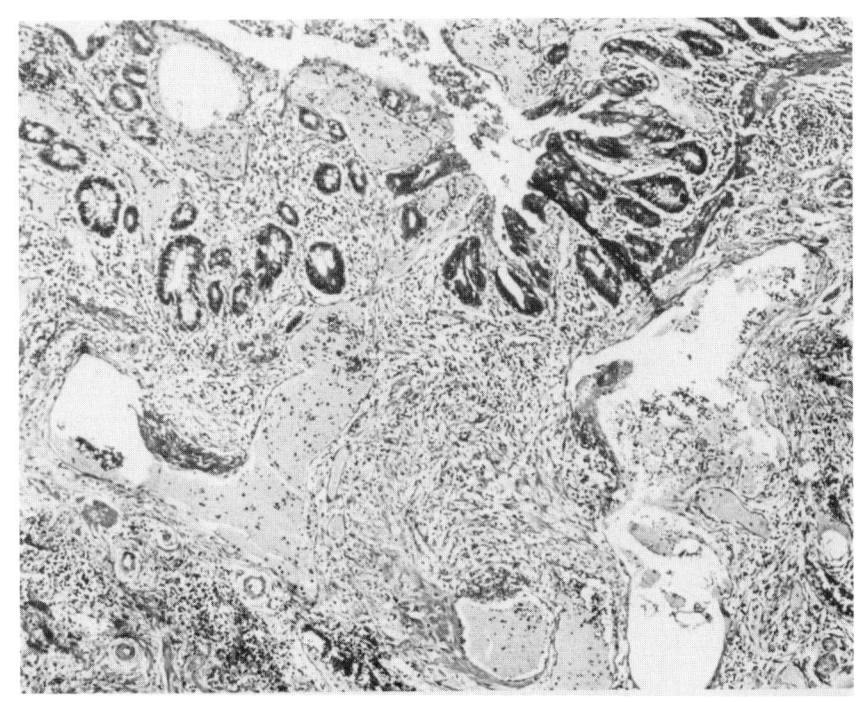

Fig. 2A. Ectatic vessels in submucosa, two of which contain mural thrombi. Ectatic vessels are also present in the mucosa. H & E. × 50.

through dilated veins which perforated the muscularis mucosae (Fig. 6). Occasionally the muscularis mucosae seemed to constrict these perforating vessels. These changes have been described and illustrated in a number of reports [2, 4, 9, 12, 20]. Dilatation (ectasia) of submucosal veins was striking (Fig. 6). This is possibly the most difficult histologic parameter to evaluate because of the large number of veins of various diameters which can be found in the submucosa. Arbitrarily, we have defined submucosal venous dilatation, or ectasia, as a vein whose diameter covers half or more of the average thickness of the submucosal layer.

Finally, in 5 patients, peculiar sclerotic changes in some of the dilated submucosal veins were noted. These involved loss of the smooth muscle from the vein wall, replacement by a mixture of collagen and mucopolysaccharide of variable thickness and exaggeration of the surrounding elastic fibers. For purposes of illustration of this sclerotic change, Figs. 7 and 8 from the most florid example have been chosen. In general, however, the venous sclerosis, when present, tended to be found in thin-walled veins, and in some veins, only part of the wall had undergone this alteration. These changes in the large submucosal

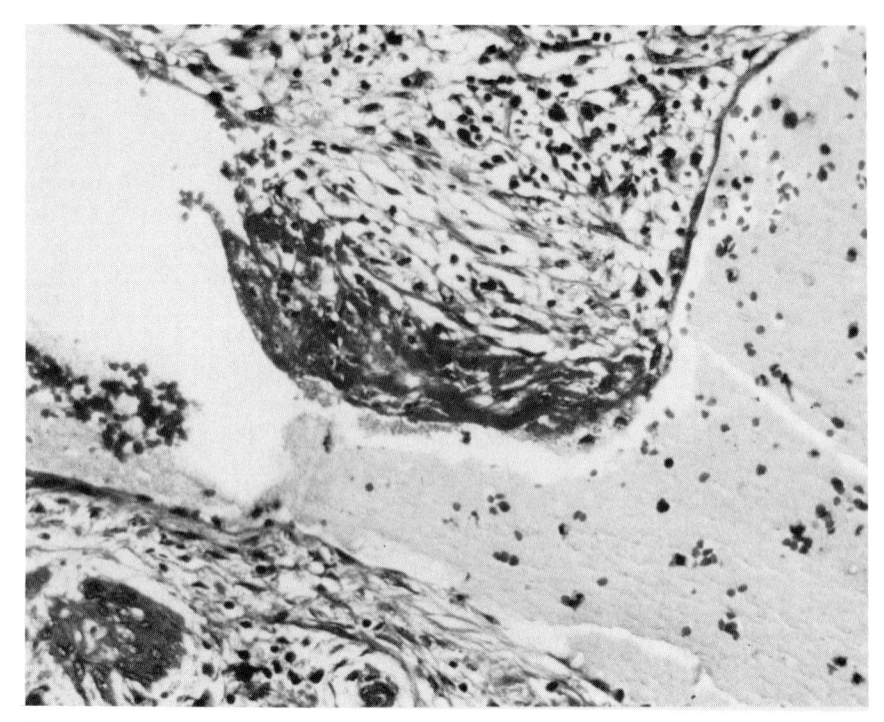

Fig. 2B. Higher power view of the thrombus in the ectasia on the left in A. The thrombus is the dense aggregate of dark fibrillar material in the center. The vessel also contains barium sulfate (gray granular material on the right) from the specimen angiography. This material also fills and distends most of the vessels in 2A. H & E. × 208.

veins were best detected using complex connective tissue stains such as the Movat Pentachrome (Fig. 8). This phlebosclerosis is similar to that found in veins subjected to significantly increased intraluminal pressures, such as might result from arteriovenous communications or from chronic obstruction.

The histologic data are summarized in Table 1. It is obvious that the likelihood of finding the mucosal vascular ectasias, the bleeding points, or the submucosal venous sclerosis, is improved dramatically by specimen angiography which distends the ectatic vessels, allowing easier detection.

It is interesting that in five of the six injected specimens, the colloidal barium solution, injected into the ileocolic, or right colic artery, under moderate pressure, was found not only in the arteries and the ectatic mucosal vessels, but passed into the submucosal veins as well.

In several studies, right colectomy specimens have been injected with a silicone rubber compound which is allowed to harden [2, 4, 7, 12]. The

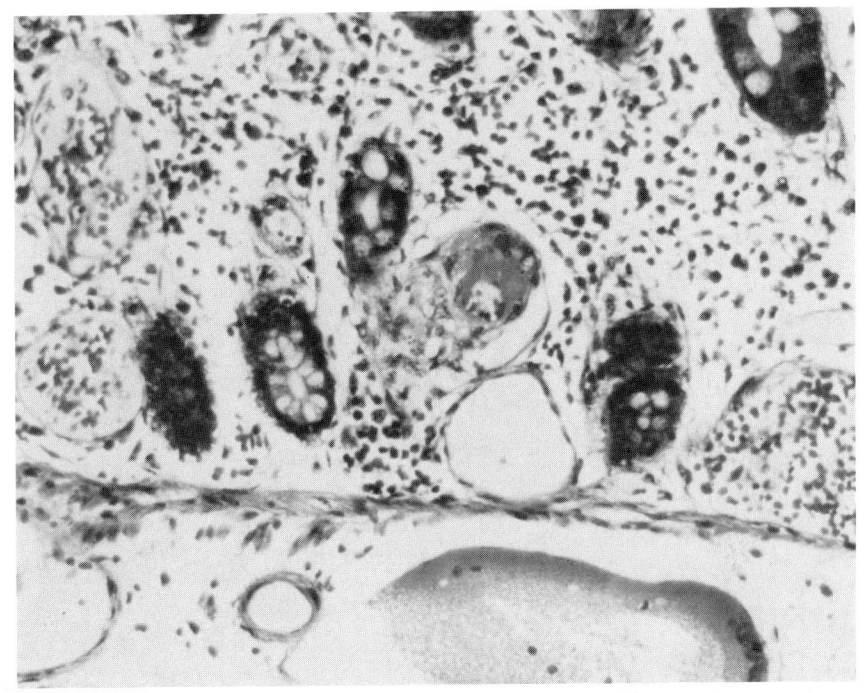

Fig. 3. In the colonic mucosa are two dilated capillary-like vessels overlying a huge superficial submucosal vein which contains barium. The uppermost mucosal vessel contains a small organizing thrombus. H & E. × 208.

specimen is fixed in formalin and cleared in methyl salicylate to produce a transparent preparation, the mucosal surface of which can be viewed with a dissecting microscope. Using this technique, the angiographically defined abnormal vasculature also appears as a cluster of dilated superficial mucosal vessels often communicating with dilated submucosal veins. These vascular aberrations are often multiple and may become confluent. Such lesions were identified by Boley et al in all 20 specimens resected from patients with angiographically demonstrated ectasias [3]. Specific bleeding sites still were infrequently identified, and, if fortuitously found, as in the barium injected specimens, appeared usually as a small thrombus in one of the dilated superficial mucosal or even submucosal vessels [4]. It seems that when these ectatic mucosal vessels rupture, they do so at small discrete sites which spontaneously close by the formation of thrombi. The small size of the bleeding points correlates with the frequent low grade blood loss that is one of the clinical manifestations. The tendency to thrombosis relates well to the intermittent character of the bleeding in many of the patients.

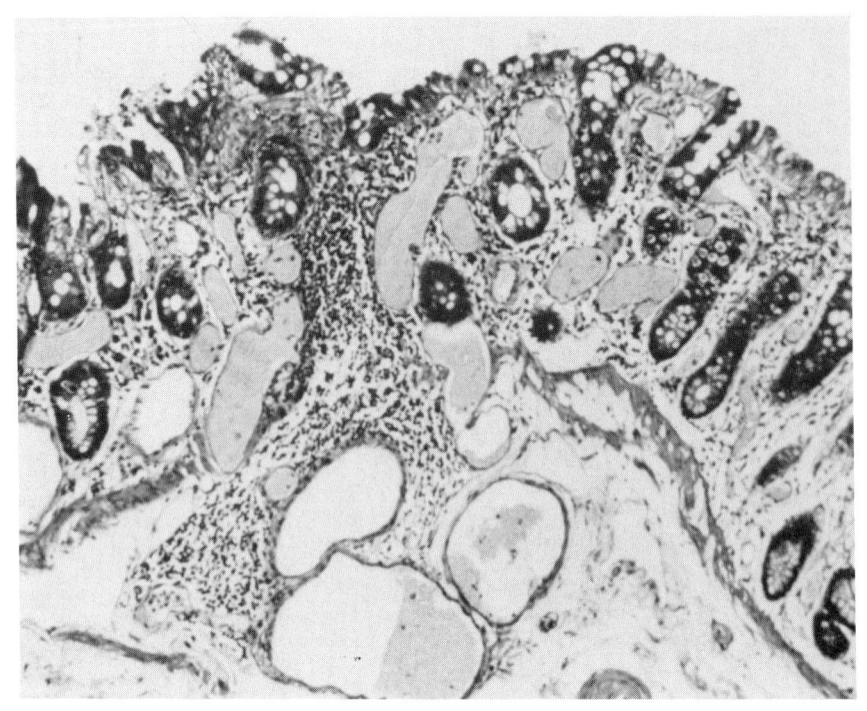

Fig. 4. Typical tangle or cluster of dilated thin-walled mucosal and submucosal vessels of capillary and venular type, most of which are filled with barium sulfate from the specimen angiography. H & E. × 83.

In some studies, atheroemboli in small arteries adjacent to the ectatic foci were noted [4, 7]. We did not find these in our cases. However, patients in the age range for colonic vascular ectasias are also in the age range for significant atherosclerosis, so that the finding of atheroemboli in these patients might not be necessarily related to the ectasias.

Based upon the studies of Boley and his co-workers, Baum and Galdibini and their colleagues, and our own efforts, it is obvious that if these lesions are to be found in resected specimens with any degree of regularity, some injection technique must be employed [4, 7, 13]. The silicone-rubber technique seems to lead to the highest, most predictable yield, yet it has been described by one of its users as "prohibitively time consuming and expensive for routine use in most laboratories" [12]. Injection of the barium sulfate solution has been relatively satisfactory in our hands, yet it probably has the same limitations as angiography, namely the inability to detect very small lesions [4], and it requires careful radiologic correlation in cutting and sampling the specimens.

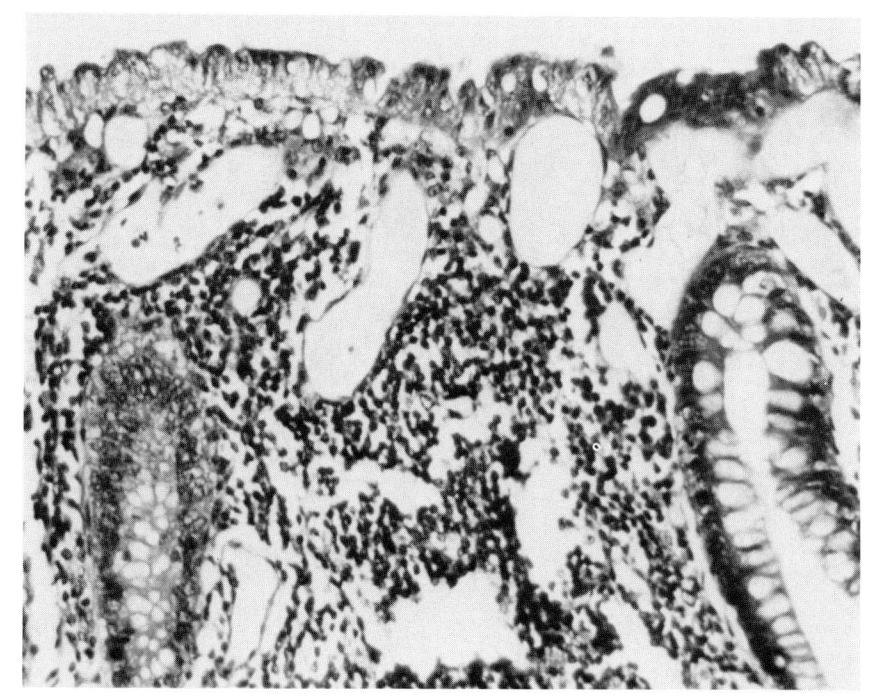

Fig. 5. Dilated mucosal vessels are separated from the lumen by a layer of endothelium, the colonic surface epithelium and, probably, the intervening basement membranes. Presumably, foci such as this are most likely to bleed. H & E. × 208.

The addition of a dye like methylene blue may provide some benefit because it induces a color change in areas of clustered vessels such as the mucosal ectasias. It is obvious, therefore, that improved gross detection techniques on the resected specimens need to be developed; techniques which are inexpensive and easily used in most pathology laboratories.

In terms of specific histologic diagnostic criteria, the following are proposed: the vascular ectasias are best identified as clusters of dilated, superficial, thin-walled mucosal vessels. These are likely to exist in combination with dilated submucosal veins. Submucosal venous dilatation alone may be difficult to define because of the different sized veins which traverse the submucosa, including some which are quite large. If partial or complete sclerosis is present in the submucosal vein walls, this aids in the diagnosis. The definition of a bleeding site from such a lesion requires the presence of the ectasia, as defined above, *plus* either an ulcer, a significant mucosal hemorrhage, or a recent thrombus in one of the superficial vessels.

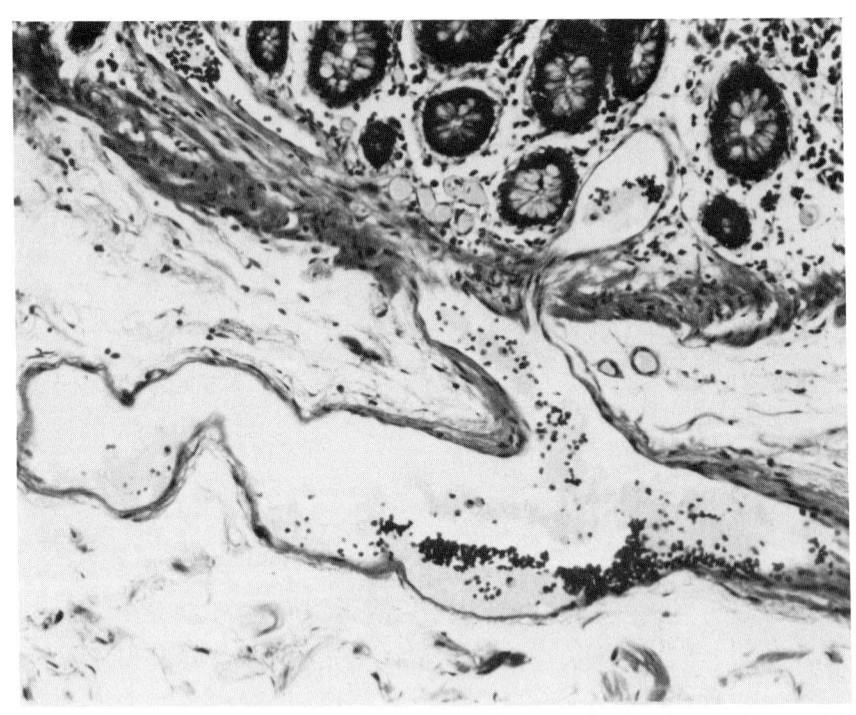

Fig. 6. Huge, irregularly-shaped, branching submucosal vein communicates with a dilated mucosal vessel through the muscularis mucosae which seems to form a constriction. H & E. × 132.

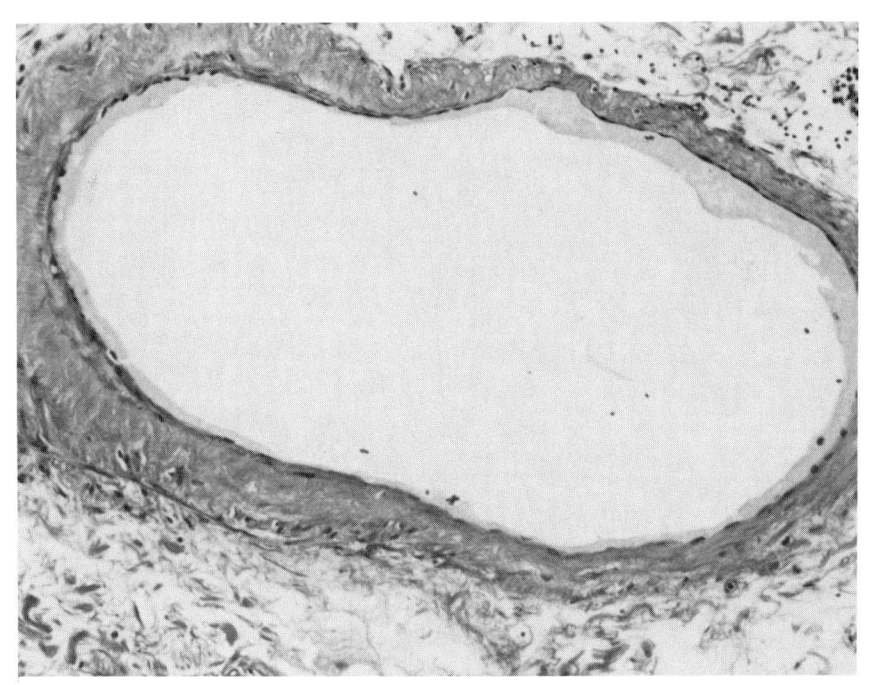

Fig. 7. This is one of the extremely dilated sclerotic submucosal veins whose wall has been altered with loss of smooth muscle and replacement by collagen and mucopolysaccharide. H & E. × 132.

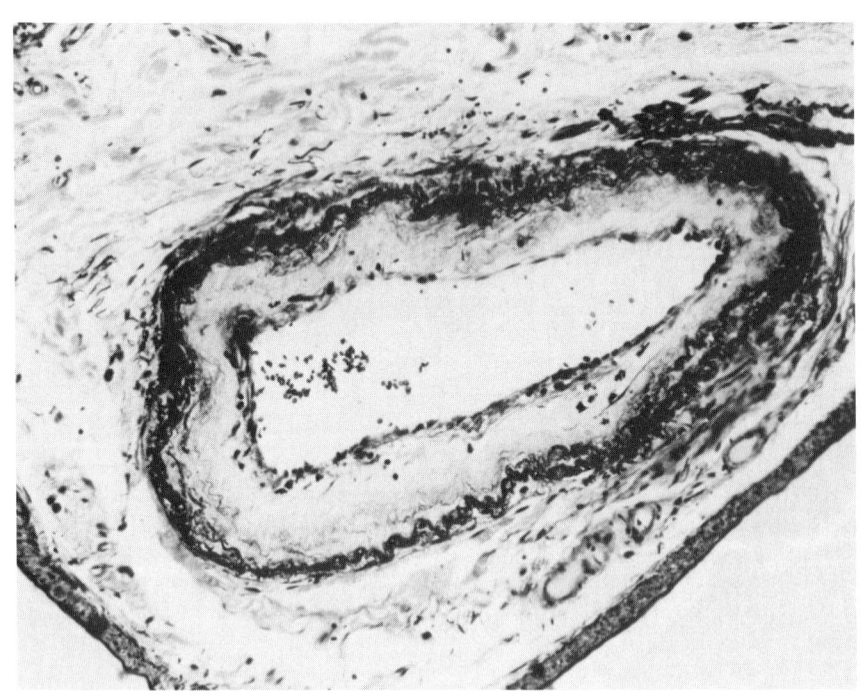

Fig. 8. Vein similar to that in Fig. 7, stained so as to demonstrate the sclerotic appearance of the wall due to replacement of muscle by collagen and mucopolysaccharide. Note the irregularly thick surrounding layer of dark elastic fibers. Movat pentachrome. × 132.

MORPHOGENESIS

It was recognized that a variety of potentially bleeding vascular lesions of the bowel existed [13]. Some were felt to be congenital, especially those occurring in patients with Osler-Weber-Rendu disease [13, 14, 18]. However, the right colonic ectasias appeared to be different [4, 13]. They occurred mainly in elderly patients, usually those over 55, and they were not associated with detectable vascular abnormalities anywhere else in the gastrointestinal tract [4, 13].

Boley and his co-workers, in an elegant study using the silicone-rubber injection technic, proposed a theory to explain the presence and development of these right colonic vascular lesions in the elderly [4]. They found that as individuals grow older, peculiar ectasias or dilatations of submucosal and mucosal vessels occur in the right side of the colon. The submucosal ectasias appear to be the most prominent feature and often are found in the absence of the mucosal ectasias. Microscopically the mucosal vessels are thin-walled, of capillary or perhaps venular type. On rare occasions, bleeding points or small ulcers may be found overlying the ectasias.

These investigators postulated that the initial alteration is a dilatation of submucosal veins, probably secondary to chronic obstruction at the point where the submucosal veins penetrate the muscularis propria. This obstruction is most likely the result of tension in the contracting muscularis propria which is presumably highest in the dilated right colon as opposed to the narrower left side. The venous ectasias occur with advancing age because the obstruction to the veins must occur over a considerable span of time before the dilatations occur.

Once the submucosal veins become dilated, secondary dilatations occur in the mucosal venules and capillaries. Our finding of histologic constrictions of vessels as they penetrate the muscularis mucosae suggests that this layer may act as a secondary point of obstruction for the mucosal veins, adding to their dilatation. Subsequent loss of the precapillary sphincter mechanism allows arterial blood to pass directly through the dilated capillary system into the veins, and this is the last evolutionary event [4]. Certainly, the ease with which both the barium sulfate suspension and the silicone-rubber material enter the dilated submucosal veins once they are injected into the arterial system suggests that arterial-venous anastomoses are already present (Fig. 9). The frequent finding of sclerotic dilated submucosal vessels, in our patient group, supports the existence of high intraluminal pressure in the venous system, possibly a manifestation of either arterial pressure transmitted to the veins via the mucosal shunts or the chronic obstruction to submucosal venous outflow, possibly at the muscularis propria.

Compelling as this explanation is, at present, it is not clear that this is the final answer. In some series the authors report lesions, presumably of this type,

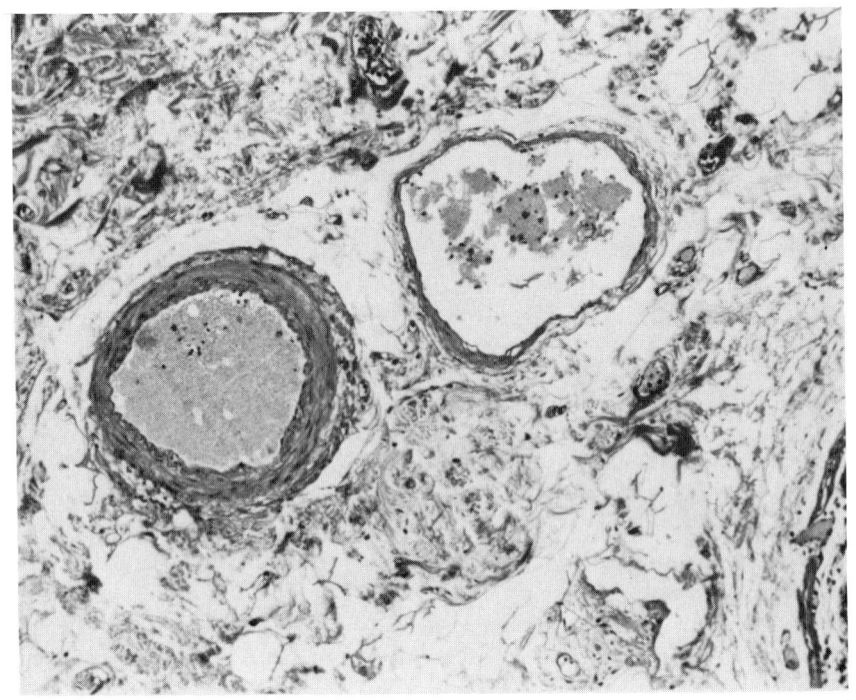

Fig. 9. In the lumens of both the submucosal artery (left) and the vein (right) barium sulfate is present, suggesting the existence of an arteriovenous shunt. H & E. × 83.

in distal small intestine and left colon [11, 16]. It remains to be seen, however, if these are identical to the right colonic lesions. In our series, and in others, at least by histologic parameters, it appears that the right colonic vascular ectasias are unique, and are thus quite different from vascular malformatiions which occur elsewhere [3, 13]. It must be recognized that right colonic mucosal and submucosal ectasias are common in elderly people. Boley et al found them in 8 of 15 right colons resected for carcinomas, all in patients over 60 years of age, none of whom were bleeding from these vessels [4]. Thus, to find them in the right colon of elderly people who are bleeding is not at all surprising, whether they are the cause of the bleeding or not [8]. Nevertheless, it is quite likely, for several reasons, that they really are the cause of bleeding in many cases. First, infrequently, they can be identified at the base of, or in, the margin of a bleeding site, usually by thromboses within them or small ulcers over them [4, 9, 10]. Second, they are present in cases with otherwise unexplained right colonic bleeding almost 100% of the time [4]. Finally, removal of the angiographically localized abnormal vasculature by right hemicolectomy generally results in cessation of the bleeding with only infrequent recurrences [19]. In fact, in those cases in which rebleeding occurs, it is likely to be due to an unrelated abnormality such as diverticulosis [17].

REFERENCES

1. Alfidi RJ, Esselstyn CD, Tarar R, et al: Recognition and angiosurgical detection of arteriovenous malformations of the bowel. Ann Surg 174:573, 1971
2. Baum S, Athanasoulis CA, Waltman AC, et al: Angio-dysplasia of the right colon: a cause of gastrointestinal bleeding. Am J Roentgenol 129:789, 1977
3. Boley SJ, DiBiase A, Brandt LJ, et al: Lower intestinal bleeding in the elderly. Am J Surg 137:57, 1979
4. Boley SJ, Sammartano R, Adams A, et al: On the nature and etiology of vascular ectasias of the colon. Gastroenterology 72:650, 1977
5. Boley SJ, Sammartano R, Brandt LJ, et al: Vascular ectasias of the colon. Surg Gynecol Obstet 149:353, 1979
6. Broor SL, Parker HW, Ganeshappa KP, et al: Vascular dysplasia of the right colon. An important cause of unexplained gastrointestinal bleeding. Digest Dis 23:89, 1978
7. Case records of the Massachusetts General Hospital (Case 36-1974). N Engl J Med 291:569, 1974
8. Fowler DL, Fortin D, Wood WG, et al: Intestinal vascular malformations. Surgery 86:377, 1979
9. Hagihara PF, Chuang VP, Griffen WO: Arteriovenous malformations of the colon. Am J Surg 133:681, 1977
10. Matsumoto M, Ishiguro M, Kato M, et al: Chronic intestinal bleeding due to arteriovenous malformation of the colon. Acta Path Jpn 28:313, 1978
11. Miller KD Jr, Tutton RH, Bell KA, et al: Angiodysplasia of the colon. Diagnost Radiol 132:309, 1979
12. Mitsudo SM, Boley SJ, Brandt LJ, et al: Vascular ectasias of the right colon in the elderly; a distinct pathologic entity. Human Pathol 10:585, 1979
13. Moore JD, Thompson NW, Appelman HD, et al: Arteriovenous malformations of the gastrointestinal tract. Arch Surg 111:381, 1976
14. Richardson JD, Max MH, Flint LM Jr, et al: Bleeding vascular malformations of the intestine. Surgery 84:430, 1978
15. Rogers BHG, Adler F: Hemangiomas of the cecum. Colonoscopic diagnosis and therapy. Gastroenterology 71:1079, 1976
16. Stewart WB, Gathright JB Jr, Ray JE: Vascular ectasias of the colon. Surg Gynecol Obstet 148:670, 1979
17. Talman EA, Dixon DS, Gutierrez FE: Role of arteriography in rectal hemorrhage due to arteriovenous malformations and diverticulosis. Ann Surg 190:203, 1979
18. Weaver GA, Alpern HD, Davis JS et al: Gastrointestinal angiodysplasia associated with aortic valve disease: part of a spectrum of angiodysplasia of the gut. Gastroenterology 77:1, 1979

19. Welch CE, Athanasoulis CA, Galdabini JJ: Hemorrhage from the large bowel with special reference to angiodysplasia and diverticular disease. World J Surg 2:73, 1978
20. Wolff WI, Grossman MB, Shinya H: Angiodysplasia of the colon: diagnosis and treatment. Gastroenterology 72:329, 1977

Norman W. Thompson, M.D., F.A.C.S.

Vascular Ectasias and Colonic Diverticula: Common Causes of Lower Gastrointestinal Hemorrhage in the Aged

ABSTRACT

Vascular ectasias and diverticular disease of the colon have been found to be the most common causes of obscure massive hemorrhage in the elderly population. The appropriate treatment of patients bleeding from vascular ectasias or diverticular disease of the colon requires a plan of management that rules out other causes of gastrointestinal hemorrhage, differentiates these two diseases, and localizes the source of bleeding. Selective visceral angiography is the single most important diagnostic study in the evaluation of patients with lower gastrointestinal hemorrhage and is the only study capable of identifying vascular ectasias with consistency. Because characteristic angiographic findings of vascular ectasias have been clarified, active bleeding from the colon is not necessary in order to make the diagnosis. The surgical treatment of venous ectasias is right colectomy and ileotransverse colostomy. Selective angiography is particularly valuable in localizing the source of bleeding in diverticulosis when a patient is actively bleeding. In most patients, transcatheter vasopressin therapy is successful in controlling the bleeding until the patient is adequately prepared for operation. Segmental colon resection has become the preferred surgical therapy for diverticular hemorrhage when preoperative localization of the bleeding point has been achieved.

Hemorrhage from the lower gastrointestinal tract, particularly when acute and massive, has been one of the most difficult diagnostic and therapeutic

---

Norman W. Thompson, M.D., F.A.C.S.: Henry King Ransom Professor of Surgery, Department of Surgery, University of Michigan Medical Center, Ann Arbor, Michigan.

problems confronting the surgeon. Frequently the source of bleeding is not detected by conventional barium roentgenographic studies or by endoscopy. Furthermore, even when a potential source of bleeding is identified, the actual bleeding site may remain occult. An exploratory laparotomy attempting to localize the source of lower gastrointestinal hemorrhage is most likely to be unsuccessful. The importance of reliable preoperative localizing studies has been emphasized in recent decades.

Accurate diagnosis of the source of lower gastrointestinal hemorrhage is the deciding factor in selecting appropriate therapeutic measures. During the past two decades, selective visceral angiography has become the single most important diagnostic technique used to localize the source of otherwise obscure gastrointestinal hemorrhage. It is now clear that angiography may be the only diagnostic study by which bleeding lesions can be identified. It is of particular value in patients with chronic iron-deficiency anemia and melena who are otherwise asymptomatic. From information obtained during the past decade in evaluating patients with obscure lower gastrointestinal hemorrhage, it has become apparent that vascular ectasias of the right colon and diverticulosis are the two most frequent causes in adults.

CLINICAL FEATURES

Both vascular ectasias and diverticulosis associated with bleeding are most likely to occur in patients 60 years of age or older [2-4, 9, 16-19]. Bleeding from either of these sources has been rare in patients under 50 years of age. The average age of the last 10 patients treated at The University of Michigan Medical Center with bleeding ectasias was 67 years, and all patients with massive diverticular bleeding were 65 years of age or older. In a large series of patients with these 2 diseases, Welch found the median age of those bleeding from vascular ectasias and those with diverticular bleeding to be 75 years [28]. Compounding the difficulty in establishing an accurate diagnosis is the fact that both of these lesions are relatively common in completely asymptomatic individuals in this age group. More than 50% of the population over 60 years of age have been shown to have diverticulosis [9, 16, 28]. Recently Boley has found vascular ectasias of the right colon in nearly 25% of individuals over 60 years of age [2-4]. It is not surprising then, that a significant number of patients who are bleeding or have bled, will be found to have both of these lesions. There appears to be no sex predilection for diverticular disease or vascular ectasias. Although the last 4 patients that we have treated with vascular ectasias were women, the overall incidence of this disease has been equally divided between the sexes. Welch found that 65% of his patients with bleeding ectasias were women [28].

Associated heart disease has been a common finding, noted in more than 50% of patients with vascular ectasias [4, 6, 11, 13, 20, 25, 28, 29]. The most common lesion noted has been aortic stenosis, occurring in nearly 25% of reported cases [7]. Although we have found aortic stenosis in only 1 of 17 patients, the majority of our patients have had significant coronary artery disease. Angina, accentuated by anemia, has been a common complaint. Several patients with hemoglobin levels as low as 5 gm% developed protracted angina but did not suffer myocardial infarctions. Although in most series of patients with diverticular hemorrhage, heart disease has not been specifically noted, hypertension and generalized atherosclerosis have been common findings in our patients. Diabetes mellitus has not been reported as being frequent in patients with vascular ectasias but has been present in the majority of our patients. During the past year, all 5 patients with bleeding vascular ectasias treated at this center, were found to be diabetics of long duration. The association of significant cardiac or vascular disease has been considered as a possible predisposing factor in those patients with bleeding ectasias [4, 20]. Baum speculated that ectasias may be the result of chronic submucosal arteriovenous shunting as a manifestation of nonocclusive mesenteric ischemia associated with low cardiac output [27]. Colonic mucosal ischemia severe enough to cause necrosis has not been found in any of our cases or those reported by others.

An important, although not definitive, feature in distinguishing diverticular from vascular ectatic bleeding, is the rate and pattern of bleeding that occurs. Bleeding from diverticulosis usually is acute and is more likely to be severe [9, 12, 16, 17, 19, 24, 27, 28]. The source of diverticular bleeding is arterial, believed to be due to the erosion by a fecalith into an arteriole in the base of a single diverticulum [16, 17, 28]. In most patients with significant bleeding, there is no history of previous diverticulitis and the acute episode usually occurs without any preceding symptoms. Massive bleeding from diverticulosis is most likely to occur in patients with diverticula involving the entire colon. Despite the great number of diverticula present, the source of bleeding is most frequently from a single diverticulum in the right colon rather than from one in the left or sigmoid colon where the diverticula are most concentrated. Olsen recognized this characteristic of bleeding diverticulosis in 1968 when he recommended subtotal colectomy rather than segmental resection of the left or sigmoid colon [19]. The use of angiography to localize the source of diverticular bleeding has confirmed Olsen's observation. Casarella at The Columbia Presbyterian Hospital and Athanasoulis at the Massachusetts General Hospital both found that two-thirds of all patients bleeding from diverticular disease did so from either the right or transverse colon, as proven angiographically [28]. In rare cases, simultaneous bleeding from two diverticula has been noted. The stool color in patients with diverticular bleeding is usually bright red or maroon although melena may occur if the rate of bleeding is slow. Despite the usual severity of diverticular hemorrhage, approximately four-fifths of patients will stop spontaneously or can be controlled with transcatheter vasoconstrictor therapy. Approximately one-fifth of those patients whose bleeding stops spontaneously will rebleed at a future date. One half of those whose bleeding can be controlled by the use of intraarterial vasopressin will rebleed. Prior to the use of angiographic techniques to diagnose and control hemorrhage, emergency operations were necessary for diverticular bleeding in approximately 15% of patients. Fewer than 10% of all patients require operative treatment today and only rarely on an emergency basis [12, 24, 27, 28].

Bleeding from vascular ectasias is characteristically recurrent and usually stops spontaneously [1-6, 11, 13, 15, 20-23, 28, 29]. Acute massive rectal hemorrhage requiring emergency measures occurs infrequently with this disease although bright red blood per rectum is not uncommon [4, 20, 28]. Approximately one-fourth of all patients have had melena or blood loss anemia with positive stool guaiac studies. Early in our experience with this entity, patients often had a long history of intermittent hemorrhage and several had undergone one or more previous explorations to determine the source of bleeding. Several patients had received 50 or more transfusions before a definitive operation was performed [18]. It is our impression that this entity is being diagnosed at an earlier stage, after fewer episodes of bleeding, fewer hospitalizations and fewer transfusions than was common five or ten years ago. Currently we are seeing more patients with anemia, referred after all conventional roentgenographic and endoscopic studies have failed to detect a source of bleeding. A single hematologist has referred 4 patients with vascular ectasias within the past 6 months after he was consulted for the evaluation of chronic blood loss anemia. Each patient had already been extensively evaluated for a source of occult gastrointestinal bleeding, although not with selective visceral angiography. The variable rate of bleeding noted in patients with vascular ectasias of the right colon is probably related to the fact that initial episodes are likely to be from small venules [2-4]. As the lesion develops, larger veins or even arteriovenous communications may be eroded, causing a more rapid rate of hemorrhage, resulting in maroon stools or hematochesia. Exsanguinating rectal bleeding caused by ectasias is rare and is more likely due to diverticulosis. The following cases are representative of patients currently being seen with vascular ectasias of the right colon.

CASE SUMMARY NUMBER 1

An 80-year-old woman was admitted to The University Hospital on July 12, 1979, for evaluation and treatment of chronic, intermittent lower gastrointestinal hemorrhage. During the preceding nine months she had been hospitalized in her community on 6 occasions for melena and anemia. She required transfusions of three units of blood during each admission. Complete gastrointestinal roentgenography had been done twice since the onset of her melena. Colonoscopy and gastroscopy were also done. Findings were limited to a small hiatal hernia without esophagitis and diverticulosis of the sigmoid and left colon. Diabetes had been diagnosed in 1952 and had been well controlled with 40 units of insulin per day. She had no complications from hypertension which had been easily controlled for 19 years. She had avoided aspirin for arthritis since her anemia had been present.

Admission hematocrit was 22 vol%. Four units of blood were administered during the first day of hospitalization.

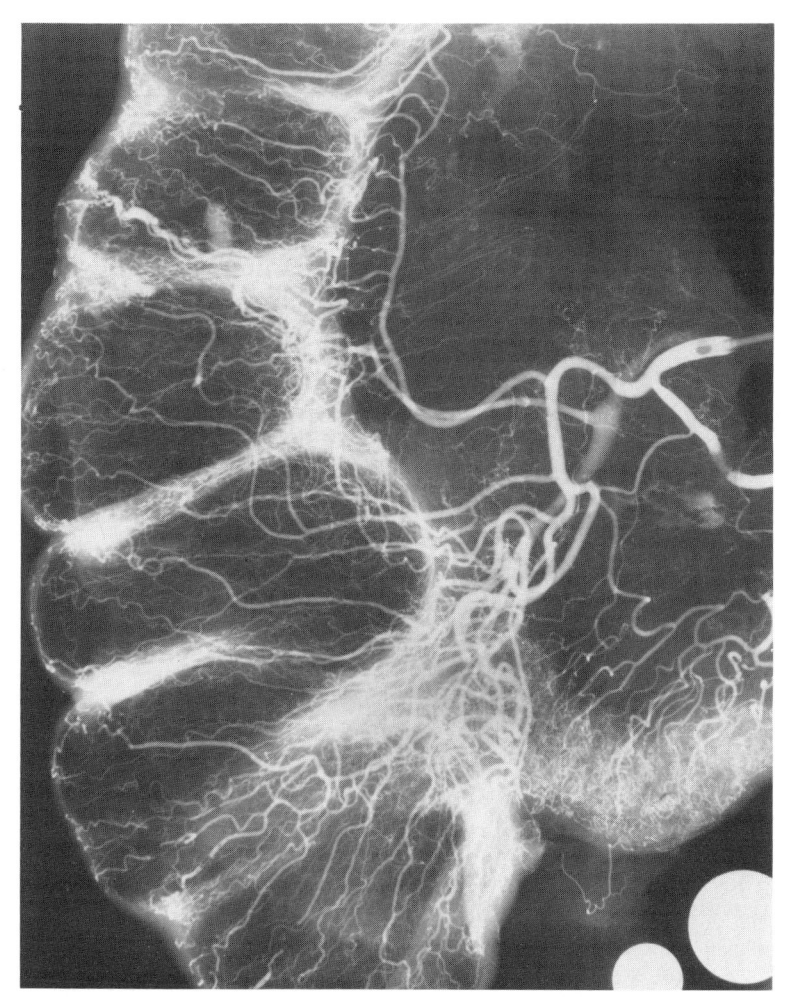

Fig. 1. Case 1. Specimen angiogram using colloidal barium. Terminal branch of right colic artery supplies several ectatic areas. Note mucosal stain in ascending colon (mid), enlarged submucosal vein, and "early filling" right colic vein.

On July 13th, selective visceral angiography was performed. The celiac and superior mesenteric artery were injected but the inferior mesenteric artery was occluded. These studies demonstrated an angiodysplastic lesion of the cecum supplied by a terminal branch of the right colic artery. The lesion was characterized by the early venous appearance of dye forming a "railroad track" pattern and a prominent draining vein running parallel to the right colic artery.

A right hemicolectomy and ileotransverse colostomy were performed on July 18, 1979. The right colon and its vessels appeared grossly normal. A specimen angiogram was obtained and the specimen opened for mucosal inspection (Fig. 1). Two mucosal "dimples," 1 mm in diameter were identified at 3 cm and 9 cm distal to the ileocecal valve. Microscopic examination of sections obtained through these locations showed dilated mucosal vessel and dilated sclerotic submucosal veins. These were considered to be venous ectasias. Her postoperative course was uneventful and she was discharged 10 days later. During a return visit in September, 1979 her hematocrit was 44 vol%. She has had no further episodes of melena.

CASE SUMMARY NUMBER 2

A 73-year-old woman was admitted to The University Hospital on July 20, 1979, with a 4 year history of anemia and intermittent rectal bleeding. For 3 years she had been treated with oral iron preparations and an occasional blood transfusion. Several complete gastrointestinal roentgenographic studies, gastroscopies and sigmoidoscopies were negative except for the presence of a small hiatal hernia and scattered sigmoid diverticula. During the past year she had increasing episodes of hematochezia and had been hospitalized on three occasions for anemia with hemoglobin levels as low as 4.2 gm%. She had received 14 units of blood during the preceding three months. Other than occasional crampy midabdominal pains and intermittent diarrhea, she had no gastrointestinal complaints. During a recent hospitalization, repeat roentgenograms and colonoscopy were normal. A selective visceral angiogram showed renal artery stenosis but no colonic lesions. Her major medical problems, in addition to bleeding included diabetes mellitus with Kimmelstiel-Wilson syndrome, mild chronic renal failure, and near blindness from macular degeneration. She also had intermittent congestive heart failure and angina. Her drug therapy included insulin, Lasix, Aldactone, Lanoxin, and Butazolidin.

She was in no distress and was not bleeding when admitted. Her blood pressure was 160/60. Initial hemoglobin was 8.5 gm% with a hematocrit of 28.5 vol%, serum creatinine was 1.6 mg%. Following initial evaluation, two units of packed red blood cells were administered. The following studies were done: barium enema and sigmoidoscopy revealing a few scattered diverticula in the sigmoid colon; upper GI series and gastroscopy revealing a small hiatal hernia without reflux. During colonoscopy two areas of bright red mucosa, 0.3 × 1 cm, opposite the ileocecal valve in the cecum were seen. A selective superior mesenteric and celiac angiogram with magnification views showed a tortuous branch of the right colic artery leading into the cecum where a mucosal stain was apparent. A dense early draining vein was also visualized. A diagnosis of cecal vascular ectasia was made. A right

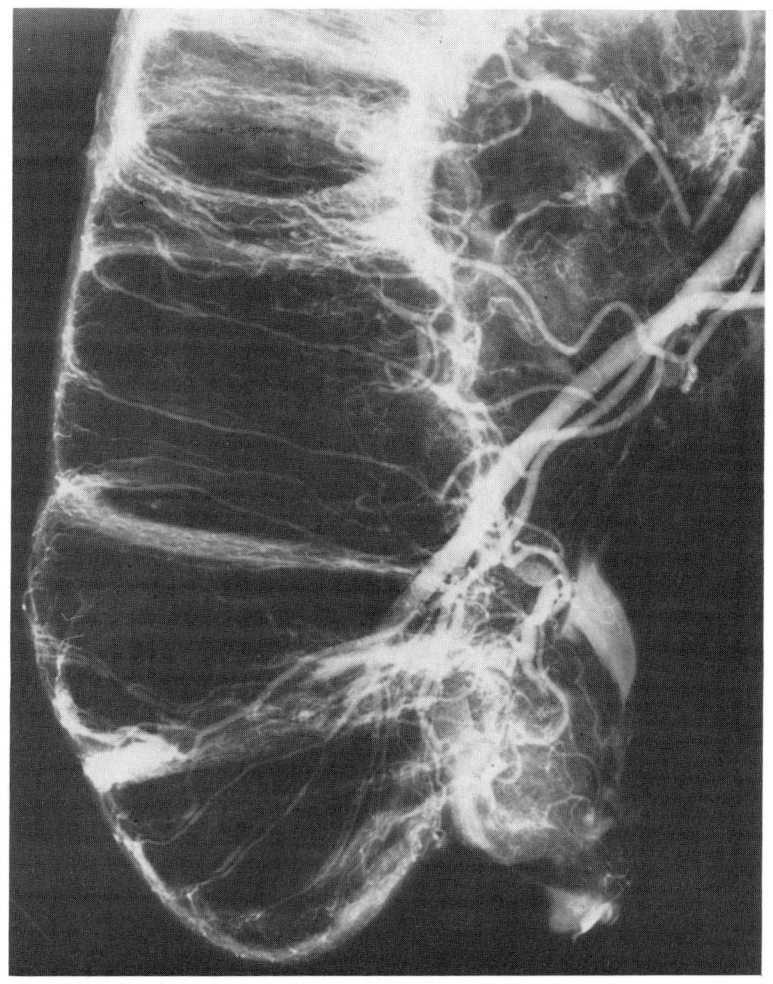

Fig. 2. Case 2. Specimen angiogram using colloidal barium demonstrates a tortuous branch of the right colic artery supplying an area of mucosal stain on the antimesenteric edge of the cecum. Note large draining vein running parallel to the right colic artery.

hemicolectomy and ileotransverse colostomy were performed. A specimen angiogram was obtained (Fig. 2). Her postoperative course was complicated by an arrhythmia which was treated with a temporary pacemaker. She was discharged on August 31, 1979 and has had no further bleeding. Her hemoglobin was 13.1 gm% and hematocrit was 40.7 vol%.

DIAGNOSIS

Selective visceral angiography has become the single most important diagnostic study in the evaluation of patients with obscure lower gastrointestinal hemorrhage [1-6, 11-15, 18, 20-22, 24-29]. Vascular ectasias of the right colon were not recognized before the use of visceral angiography [14, 18]. Diverticular hemorrhage which required emergency operation was usually treated by blind resection of either the left or the entire colon [9, 16, 17, 19].

In the patient whose bleeding has stopped and whose vital signs are stable, conventional barium roentgenograms of the colon are of value in demonstrating diverticulosis and ruling out the presence of colonic polyps, cancer or other grossly apparent lesions. There are several reports however, of bleeding diverticula and vascular ectasias, identified by colonoscopy during bleeding episodes [20, 21, 23, 28]. Although most authors have not been enthusiastic about the diagnosis of ectasias by colonoscopy, Richardson and colleagues were able to visualize the cecal lesion in 12 of 29 patients and in 7 of their last 8 patients [20]. Two of their patients were actively bleeding at the time. In 2 of our last 4 patients with suspected ectasias, tentative identification was made during colonoscopy and the findings corresponded well with lesions demonstrated angiographically.

Colonoscopy should not be considered a reliable technique in excluding the presence of vascular ectasias. Again, it is impossible to differentiate bleeding from a diverticulum and a vascular ectasia consistently without the use of selective angiography. The selective superior mesenteric angiographic characteristics of vascular ectasias are diagnostic. Although the entire mesenteric vasculature should be studied in each case, special attention should be directed to the ileocolic and right colic branches of the superior mesenteric artery. The great majority of ectasias are found in the cecum or near the ileocecal valve in the ascending colon. The most distal ectasia found in Boley's series was 23 cm from the ileocecal valve. We have found 2 ectasias in the hepatic flexure and 1 in the proximal transverse colon. The earliest and most frequent angiographic sign, as emphasized by Boley, is a densely opacified, dilated, tortuous, slowly emptying intramural vein which reflects the ectatic changes in a submucosal vein [4]. This sign has been found in 90% of patients. The second most common finding, present in about 75% of cases, is a vascular tuft in which a localized accumulation of contrast material is seen in the colonic mucosa. This finding, according to Boley, represents a more advanced lesion of the involved vessels with extension of the venous dilatation or ectasia to involve the mucosal vessels. The third sign is an early filling vein, reflecting an arteriovenous communication at the mucosal capillary level. This is considered a late sign and has been found in 60% to 70% of patients. More than 50% of patients with bleeding ectasias have had all 3 signs. The early filling vein has been present in all of our patients and usually runs parallel to the ileocolic or right colic artery which when still filled with contrast material creates the "railroad track" sign.

Extravasation of contrast material into the bowel lumen is an unusual finding in ectasias [4, 24, 27-29]. This is true because the rate of bleeding is usually too slow to demonstrate pooling within the lumen. Commonly the bleeding has stopped at the time the arteriogram has been performed. If extravasation is seen without the characteristic signs, the source of bleeding is unlikely to be an ectasia. Active bleeding is not required to make the diagnosis of vascular ectasias. Extravasation was found in only 2 of 32 patients with proven ectasias studied by Boley and in only two of 31 patients recently reported by Welch [4, 28]. We have seen extravasation of contrast material in only 1 patient with a proven vascular ectasia of the right colon. Boley has emphasized the frequent multiplicity of vascular ectasias of the right colon. In his series, he was able to identify more than one lesion in 7 of 32 patients. Only 2 patients had more than two distinct ectasias, however. We have had several patients with two distinct ectasias and would agree that local colonic excision should be avoided because of the possibility of missing an ectatic lesion that might be the source of future rebleeding.

Angiography, in the diagnosis of diverticular bleeding, is most useful when the patient is actively bleeding [17, 24, 27, 28]. In distinct contrast to bleeding vascular ectasias, the arterial bleeding from diverticula can usually be localized by the intraluminal extravasation of dye, providing the patient is bleeding at a rate of 0.5 ml per minute or more. Welch recently found that 20 of 26 patients, actively bleeding when angiographic studies were performed, had bleeding points which were demonstrable. Because many of the bleeding sites in diverticular disease are also in the right colon, the absence of the characteristic findings seen in patients with vascular ectasias is helpful in clarifying the diagnosis. When angiographic studies are done in patients suspected of having diverticular bleeding, there are no characteristic findings to confirm this diagnosis.

It is of interest that the diagnosis of diverticular hemorrhage has decreased during the past 20 years in which angiography has been used more extensively in evaluating lower gastrointestinal bleeding. Even so, the diagnosis of diverticular hemorrhage is still often made without adequate evidence. The presence of diverticulosis, demonstrated by barium enema, with no other apparent cause of bleeding was considered insufficient evidence even before angiography became available. Quinn's criteria for the diagnosis of diverticular bleeding included the passage of bright red or maroon blood by rectum, barium enema demonstration of diverticula, absence of another colonic or rectal lesion found on barium enema or sigmoidoscopy, absence of blood in the gastric aspirate and normal blood coagulation studies. These criteria are insufficient to establish the diagnosis with certainty, since they do not exclude the diagnosis of ectasia.

MANAGEMENT OF SUSPECTED LOWER GASTROINTESTINAL HEMORRHAGE

When patients present with either melena or hematochezia, the initial diagnostic studies are directed at determining whether the source of bleeding is from the upper or the lower gastrointestinal tract. A nasogastric tube is inserted into the stomach and suction is applied. If the aspirate is negative for blood, an upper gastrointestinal source of bleeding is unlikely. Sigmoidoscopy should demonstrate an obvious rectal or anal source of hemorrhage such as internal hemorrhoids or a rectal carcinoma. Coagulation studies should be performed early in the evaluation, particularly if bleeding is massive. If bleeding has stopped or is quite slow, colonoscopy may be considered. It is unlikely to be useful if the patient is bleeding rapidly enough to require urgent transfusions. If colonoscopy is unavailable or has failed to demonstrate a likely source of bleeding, a barium roentgenographic examination of the colon is indicated in the stable patient who is no longer bleeding. If the barium study is considered normal, the patient is scheduled for selective visceral angiography. When angiograms demonstrate a vascular ectasia(s) of the right colon or cecum, the patient is prepared for an elective right colectomy even if no further bleeding occurs.

If the patient is actively bleeding, angiographic studies of the superior mesenteric, celiac and inferior mesenteric arteries should be done on an emergency basis *before* a barium enema has been performed. If extravasation of contrast material is noted within the colonic lumen, in the absence of the characteristic signs of a vascular ectasia, the diagnosis of diverticular bleeding is presumed and vasopressin may be administered through the catheter. Rarely, this may be unsuccessful and an emergency operation required to control massive bleeding. If extravasation is found in the right colon and the signs of vascular ectasia are present, vasoconstricting drugs may also be administered intraarterially. In both cases bleeding is usually controlled. Because ectasias are likely to rebleed, a definitive operation should be performed when the patient has been adequately prepared and is in stable condition.

In patients with diverticular bleeding, the decision to resect the segment of colon in which the bleeding site has been identified can be individualized on the basis of history, rebleeding after discontinuance of vasopressin and the general condition of the patient. Because diverticular bleeding is less likely to recur, a conservative approach, when bleeding is controlled, is often recommended. When angiograms reveal no extravasation or evidence of an ectasia and bleeding persists, little benefit can be expected from the use of intraarterial vasoconstricting drugs. In this infrequent but frustrating situation, an emergent subtotal colectomy must be considered. Transcatheter infusion of vasopressin directly into the arterial branch supplying the bleeding point is very successful in controlling hemorrhage on a short term basis (24 to 72 hours). It is estimated that cessation of bleeding occurs in more than 90% of patients with colonic lesions shortly after starting the intraarterial infusion of 0.2 U/min of vasopressin. Usually this dose is tapered during a two or three day period and then discontinued. Should rebleeding occur, an urgent operation is usually recommended. An alternative to operation for those patients whose bleeding cannot be controlled initially or who rebleed after vasoconstriction therapy is transcatheter embolization. Various agents ranging from autologous clot to glass beads have been developed for this purpose and used rather extensively in the control of upper gastrointestinal hemorrhage. Recently Sniderman reported the successful use of absorbable gelatin sponge as a distal embolus in a poor risk patient whose bleeding vascular ectasia could not be controlled with vasopressin alone [24]. He emphasized that the risk of bowel infarction has not been adequately investigated experimentally. Similar attempts should be reserved for patients who are failures of vasopressin therapy and considered extremely poor risks for a surgical procedure.

SURGICAL TREATMENT

When the diagnosis of vascular ectasia of the colon has been established by angiographic study, the surgical treatment is right colectomy and ileotransverse colostomy. Failure to demonstrate the specific lesion grossly at operation in no way alters the indication to proceed with a right colectomy. We have been unable to identify vascular ectasias intraoperatively with but one exception. In addition to very careful inspection of the colon and its mesentery, we have also attempted to localize the lesions by the intraoperative use of the Doppler ultrasound as advocated by Cooperman and colleagues but have been unsuccessful in doing so [8]. We have had limited experience in the use of sterile methylene blue injected into the superior mesenteric artery as advocated by Fogler [11]. He reported its use in the localization of an arteriovenous malformation of the small intestine. Rapid clearing of the dye was noted in the region of the arteriovenous malformation as compared to the surrounding, normal, small intestine. Another method for intraoperative localization is the measurement of the oxygen level in a mesenteric vein, draining the suspected area of the ectasia (A-V malformation) [10]. Because it is highly unlikely that vascular ectasias can be identified intraoperatively, the importance of preoperative angiographic documentation cannot be overemphasized. It is our impression that these intraoperative techniques may be of value in patients with larger, congenital arteriovenous malformations of the intestines, in contrast to the acquired vascular ectasias of the colon under discussion. Furthermore, because the vascular ectatic changes may be multiple within the right colon, local excision, even if specific identification of one lesion is made, is no longer recommended. Despite the fact that the first patient that we identified with a vascular ectasia (A-V malformation, Type I) of the right colon was treated by local excision of the colon wall and has not rebled in 13 years, most patients are unlikely to be so fortunate. One of our patients treated by cecectomy and partial ascending colectomy rebled for the first time, five years later. He was recently reoperated upon at which time the hepatic flexure and right transverse colon were resected. Because approximately 10% of patients have been reported to rebleed eventually after partial right colectomy, most authors currently advocate excision of the entire right colon [4, 20, 28].

As emphasized by Appelman in this book, we feel that specimen angiography is essential in identifying the specific areas of the colon to be sectioned for pathological confirmation of the diagnosis. In addition to localization by specimen angiography, several ectasias have been identified by gross inspection of the mucosa after the specimen was opened. In these cases, punctate mucosal ulcerations or localized submucosal hemorrhages were identified and marked for pathological sectioning. These areas corresponded well with the localization by specimen angiography and were confirmed by histopathologic sections.

The surgical treatment of diverticular hemorrhage is also currently determined in most patients by angiographic localization of the bleeding point. With this information, the surgeon may then resect only that segment of colon in which bleeding has occurred. In more than two-thirds of patients, a right colectomy will be indicated. Whether subtotal colectomy, as advocated in the past, should be done in all patients who have bled massively from diverticulosis, remains controversial. Virtually all patients who bleed from diverticula in the right colon also have extensive diverticular disease involving the left colon as well. The same considerations must be made when the left or sigmoid colon contains the bleeding diverticulum. Those patients also usually have universal diverticulosis. From evidence accumulated during the past decade it would appear that rebleeding after segmental resection is infrequent, providing that the resected segment contains the offending diverticulum [28]. Because of the higher initial mortality and increased morbidity in elderly patients associated with subtotal colectomy, we currently favor the more conservative operation when the bleeding site has been identified. Subtotal colectomy is reserved for patients with continued bleeding presumed to be caused by diverticular disease even when a specific bleeding site has not been identified angiographically.

REFERENCES

1. Athanasoulis CA, Galdabini JJ, Waltman AC, et al: Angiodysplasia of the colon; a cause of rectal bleeding. Cardiovasc Radiol 1:3, 1978

2. Boley SJ, DiBiase A, Brandt LJ, et al: Lower intestinal bleeding in the elderly. Am J Surg 137:57, 1979
3. Boley SJ, Sammartano R, Adams WA, et al: On the nature and etiology of vascular ectasias of the colon. Gastroenterology 72:650, 1977
4. Boley SJ, Sammartano R, Brandt LJ, et al: Vascular ectasia of the colon. Surg Gynecol Obstet 149:353, 1979
5. Broor SL, Parker HW, Ganeshappa KP, et al: Vascular dysplasia of the right colon. An important cause of unexplained gastrointestinal bleeding. Am J Dig Dis 23:89, 1978
6. Cavett CM, Jelby JH, Hamilton JL, et al: Arteriovenous malformations in chronic gastrointestinal bleeding. Ann Surg 185:116, 1977
7. Cody MC, O'Donovan PB, Hughes RW: Idiopathic gastrointestinal bleeding and aortic stenosis. Am J Dig Dis 19:393, 1974
8. Cooperman M, Martin EW, Evans WE, et al: Use of doppler ultrasound in intraoperative localization of intestinal arteriovenous malformation. Ann Surg 100:24, 1979
9. Drapanas T, Pennington G, Kappelman M, et al: Emergency subtotal colectomy. Preferred approach to management of massively bleeding diverticular disease. Ann Surg 177:519, 1973
10. Evans WE, O'Dorisio TM, Milnar W, et al: Intraoperative localization of intestinal arteriovenous malformations. Arch Surg 113:410, 1978
11. Fowler DL, Fortin D, Wood GW, et al: Intestinal vascular malformations. Surgery 86:377, 1979
12. Giacchino JL, Geis WP, Pickleman JR, et al: Changing perspectives in massive lower intestinal hemorrhage. Surgery 86:368, 1979
13. Hagihara P, Chuang V, Griffen W: Arteriovenous malformations of colon. Am J Surg 133:681, 1977
14. Margulis AR, Heinbecker P, Bernard HR: Operative mesenteric arteriography in the search for the site of bleeding in unexplained gastrointestinal hemorrhage. Surgery 48:534, 1960
15. Marx EW, Gray RK, Duncan AM, et al: Angiodysplasia as a source of intestinal bleeding. Am J Surg 134:125, 1977
16. Meyers MA, Alonso DR, Gray GF, et al: Pathogenesis of bleeding colonic diverticulosis. Gastroenterology 71:577, 1976
17. McGuire HH, Haynes BW Jr: Massive hemorrhage from diverticulosis of the colon: guidelines for therapy based on bleeding patterns observed in fifty cases. Ann Surg 175:847, 1972
18. Moore JD, Thompson NW, Appelman HD, et al: Arteriovenous malformations of the gastrointestinal tract. Arch Surg 111:381, 1976
19. Olsen WR: Hemorrhage from diverticular disease of the colon. Am J Surg 115:247, 1968
20. Richardson JD, Max MH, Flint LM, et al: Bleeding vascular malformations of the intestine. Surgery 84:430, 1978
21. Rogers G, Adler F: Hemangiomas of the cecum: colonoscopic diagnosis and treatment. Gastroenterology 71:1079, 1976
22. Singh A, Shenoy S, Kaur A, et al: Arteriovenous malformations of the cecum: report of six cases. Dis Colon Rectum 20:334, 1977

23. Skibba RM, Hartog WA, Mantz FA, et al: Angiodysplasia of the cecum: colonoscopic diagnosis. Gastrointest Endosc 22:177, 1976
24. Sniderman KW, Sos TA, Casarella WA: Transcatheter alternatives to vasopressin infusion in colonic hemorrhage. Contemp Surg 15:11, 1979
25. Stewart WB, Gaithright JB, Ray JE: Vascular ectasias of the colon. Surg Gynecol Obstet 148:670, 1979
26. Sutherland DER, Chan F, Foucas E, et al: The bleeding cecal ulcer in transplant patients. Surgery 86:386, 1979
27. Talman EA, Dixon DS, Gutierrez FE: Role of arteriography in rectal hemorrhage due to arteriovenous malformations and diverticulosis. Ann Surg 190:203, 1979
28. Welch CE, Athanasoulis CA, Galdabini JJ: Hemorrhage from the large bowel with special reference to angiodysplasia and diverticular disease. World J Surg 2:73, 1978
29. Wolff WI, Grossman MB, Shinya H: Angiodysplasia of the colon: diagnosis and treatment. Gastroenterology 72:329, 1977

Gerald B. Zelenock, M.D.
Errol E. Erlandson, M.D.

Intestinal Ischemia: A Paradoxical Cause of Gastrointestinal Hemorrhage

ABSTRACT

Intestinal ischemic syndromes are infrequent causes of gastrointestinal hemorrhage. Bleeding signifies an unstable clinical situation and is a sign of advanced ischemia. Individualized treatment regimens take into account such diverse intestinal ischemic syndromes as mesenteric arterial embolization, mesenteric arterial thrombosis, low-flow nonocclusive ischemia, mesenteric venous thrombosis, isolated colon ischemia, and vasculitis. The goal of therapy is to correct the acute ischemic insult with restoration of flow through embolectomy, arterial reconstruction or infusion of vasoactive or thrombolytic drugs. Intestinal resection is reserved for nonviable gut. Contemporary clinical problems include lack of a specific diagnostic test for intestinal ischemia, operative difficulty in differentiating marginally viable from necrotic bowel, and the role of vasoactive and thrombolytic drug therapy. Optimal survival depends upon early diagnosis and treatment.

Gastrointestinal hemorrhage is a late and ominous manifestation of advanced intestinal ischemia. Recognition is often delayed because clinicians are unfamiliar with the infrequently encountered intestinal ischemic syndromes [4-6, 8, 45, 56, 68, 70]. Clinical presentation overlaps considerably with more common causes of gastrointestinal bleeding, further delaying diagnosis. In addition there is the seeming contradiction of an ischemic insult producing a bleeding lesion. This concept has been widely accepted for the stress gastritis syndromes but has not been applied to intestinal ischemia in general.

Gerald B. Zelenock, M.D.: Instructor in Surgery, Division of Peripheral Vascular Surgery, Department of Surgery, University of Michigan Medical Center; Errol E. Erlandson, M.D.: Assistant Professor of Surgery, Division of Peripheral Vascular Surgery, Department of Surgery, University of Michigan Medical Center, Ann Arbor, Michigan.

Ischemic lesions producing gastrointestinal hemorrhage are always acute processes. They may, however, occur superimposed upon chronic arteriosclerotic disease of the gut, diffuse vasculitis, or chronic cardiovascular disease. Hemorrhage implies intestinal infarction. If injury is confined to the mucosal layer of the intestinal tract, mural integrity is maintained and ultimately healing may occur. With injuries of greater magnitude, irreparable injury exists and hopes of reversing the ischemic injury are compromised by the need to resect necrotic gut. Regardless of the precipitating ischemic insult the clinical course is usually unstable. Prompt and accurate diagnosis must be followed by appropriate therapy to increase patient survival.

PHYSIOLOGIC AND ANATOMIC FACTORS IN INTESTINAL ISCHEMIA

The intestinal microcirculation has been the subject of many studies. One, two and three compartment models, a counter-current exchanger and more recently a counter-current multiplier have been proposed to explain various aspects of intestinal function and visceral blood flow [23, 43, 48]. Using these models the clinically recognized vulnerability of the villus tip to hypoxic and ischemic injury becomes understandable. Disproportionate superficial ischemia leads to early loss of mucosal integrity, submucosal hemorrhage and mucosal sloughing (Fig. 1).

A precise understanding of the regulatory mechanisms controlling splanchnic blood flow is lacking. The splanchnic circulation receives 20%-25% of the cardiac output at rest and theoretically could accommodate a flow of 5 to 6 liters per minute if all vascular beds were simultaneously dilated [23]. The sympathetic nervous system, circulating vasoactive substances, and local metabolites interact to determine not only total splanchnic blood flow but also, by affecting pre- and postcapillary sphincters, the distribution of flow in different wall compartments [23, 43, 48]. Alterations of these control mechanisms in various pathological states are the subject of intense investigation at present. An excellent review by Lanciault and Jacobson considers the visceral microcirculation in detail and relates anatomic and physiological models to clinical syndromes; a succinct explanation of the limitations of the various investigative techniques and 415 references accompany this work [43].

The gross anatomy of the splanchnic circulation has been well studied; yet considerable confusion still persists regarding normal anatomic variations and functional collateral pathways. Recognition of the marginal artery of Drummond, the arc of Riolan, the arc of Buhler and the peripancreatic anastomoses are important in assessing the functional importance of an ischemic lesion and estimating the adequacy of compensatory collaterals [12, 20, 24, 76, 77].

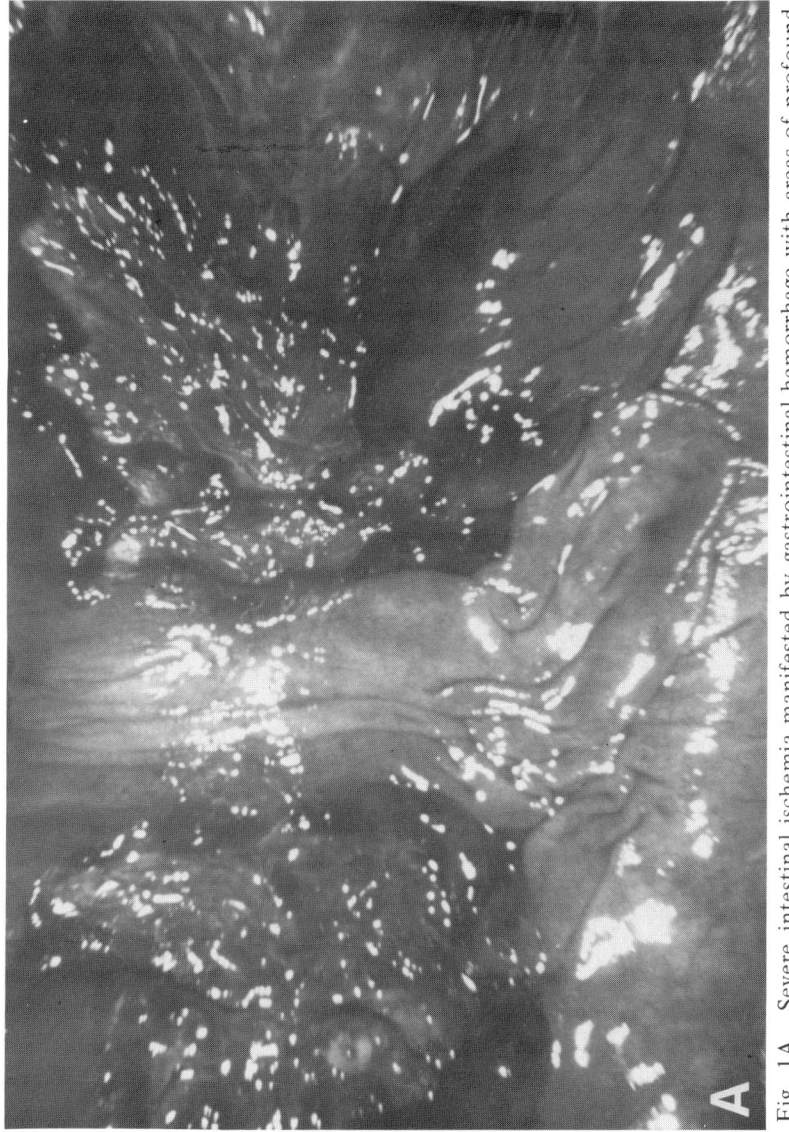

Fig. 1A. Severe intestinal ischemia manifested by gastrointestinal hemorrhage with areas of profound ischemia, submucosal hemorrhage and sloughing adjacent to relatively normal mucosa.

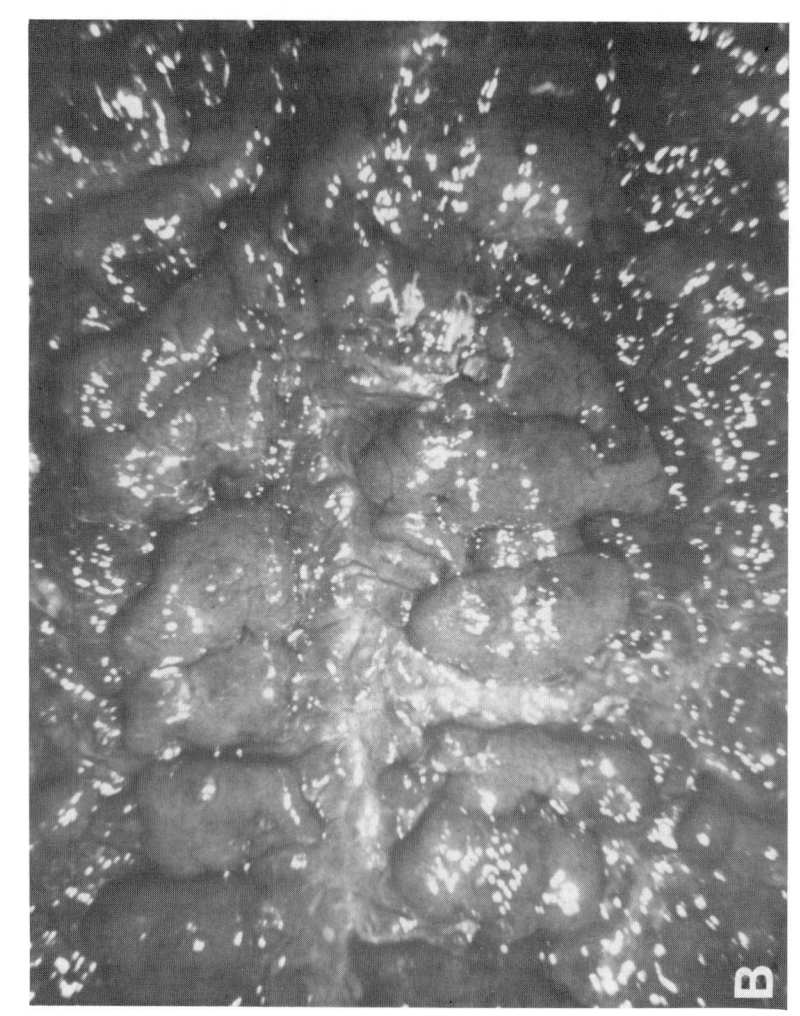

Fig. 1B. More advanced ischemic process with exposed submucosal tissue surrounding islands of necrotic mucosa.

CLINICAL SYNDROMES

Intestinal ischemic syndromes vary in etiology and clinical presentation. Recognition and classification of distinct syndromes allows selection of appropriate therapy based upon precise diagnosis, and a knowledge of the underlying pathological processes. In every instance gastrointestinal hemorrhage is a late sign of severe intestinal ischemia. In this regard, bleeding serves to emphasize the gravity of the disease state.

Superior Mesenteric Arterial Embolization

Embolization of the proximal trunk or segmental branches of the superior mesenteric artery characteristically occurs in patients with preexisting cardiac disease. The majority of such emboli are cardiac in origin and secondary to atrial fibrillation or myocardial infarction. On occasion other rhythm disturbances or anatomic cardiac lesions may give rise to this entity. Rarely the embolus arises from the proximal aorta, an atrial myxoma or a paradoxical source within the venous circulation.

Clinical manifestations are dramatic. Sudden, severe mid-abdominal pain followed by prompt evacuation of the gastrointestinal tract usually occurs. Overt gastrointestinal hemorrhage is uncommon at this point, but if actively sought, minor or occult bleeding is seen in 25%-50% of cases [1, 9]. Many patients have experienced a previous peripheral arterial embolization and virtually all have established cardiac disease [1, 9, 11, 40, 42, 57, 59, 60, 71, 75, 80]. Although 10%-33% of patients with mesenteric emboli have had previous peripheral emboli [1, 9, 40, 59] the contrary is not the case. Accordingly, most authors do not advocate routine visceral angiography in patients sustaining peripheral emboli. Even with a high index of suspicion and close clinical monitoring, mesenteric embolization may be relatively silent, being recognized late only after major complications have developed. Positive physical findings are nonspecific and often confined to the underlying cardiac disorder. Early in the course, abdominal findings invariably seem disproportionately mild for the degree of pain. As time passes and transmural infarction occurs, distention, diffuse tenderness or frank peritoneal signs evolve. Gross bleeding per rectum may be apparent at this point.

Diagnosis depends upon recognition of the typical clinical presentation and early use of visceral angiography (Fig. 2). No other diagnostic studies are sufficiently sensitive to confirm the impression of mesenteric embolus. Certain biochemical or radiological exams may exclude more common causes of gastrointestinal bleeding, but may also cause delays in diagnosis.

Early attempts at embolectomy were undertaken by Klass in 1950, and Stewart in 1951 [40, 75]. Shaw's 1957 report of the first successful superior mesenteric artery embolectomy provided the emphasis to heighten clinical recognition of this syndrome [71]. These early case reports outlined the

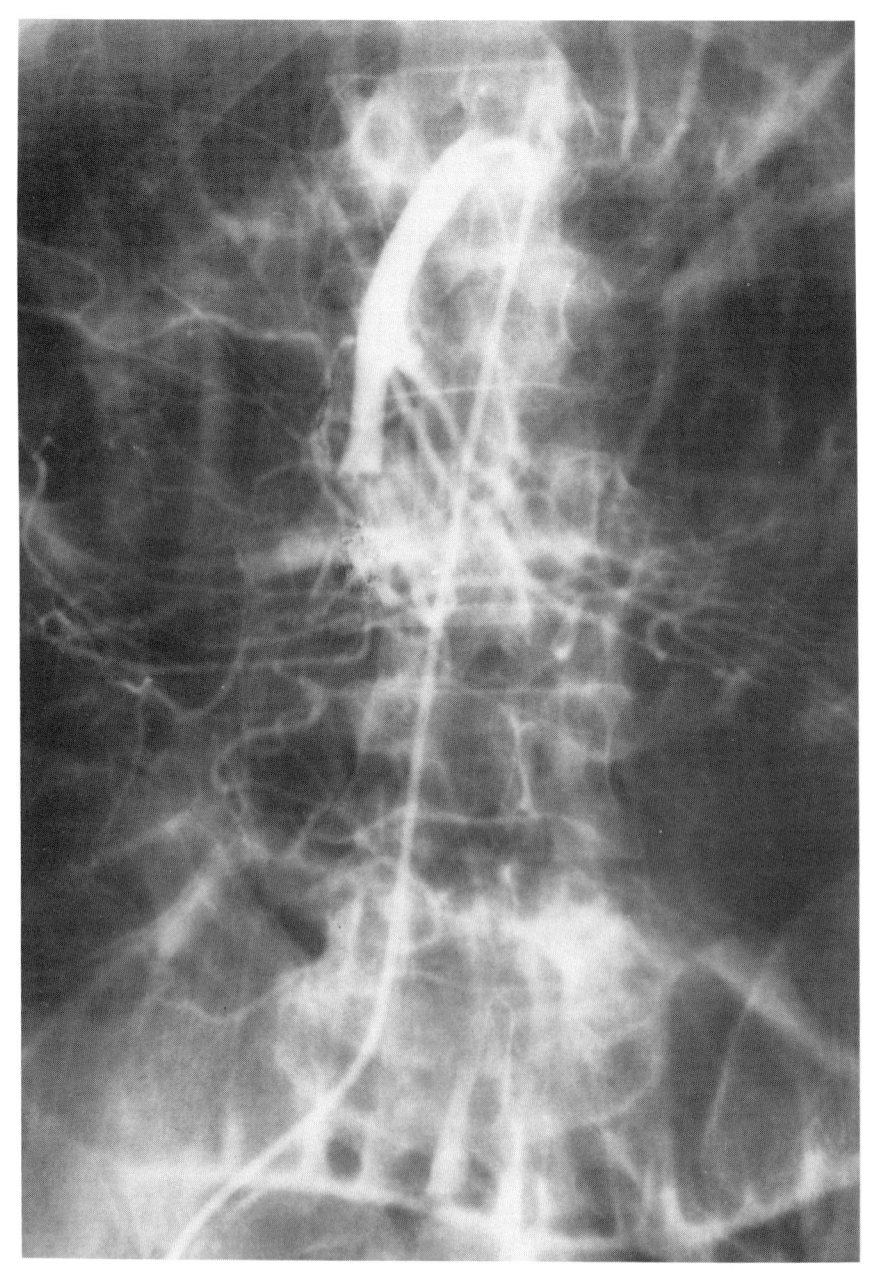

Fig. 2. Selective superior mesenteric arteriogram demonstrating an embolus lodged distal to the origins of the inferior pancreaticoduodenal artery, the middle colic artery, and the first several jejunal arcades.

therapeutic guidelines for appropriate management. They remain applicable to this day. Thromboembolectomy should be promptly performed following appropriate resuscitation. The latter should include restoration of circulating volume and prophylactic antibiotics. Anticoagulation is indicated even in a patient with minor gastrointestinal bleeding to prevent thrombosis of the more peripheral mesenteric vasculature. The superior mesenteric artery may be approached above or below the transverse mesocolon by following the middle colic artery to its origin. After proximal and distal control is obtained, a linear arteriotomy extending from the inferior pancreaticoduodenal artery to the first jejunal branches is made. Gentle passage of Fogarty embolectomy catheters is performed under direct vision, coupled with a "milking" of the mesenteric vessels to remove distal thrombus. Arteriotomies are closed primarily or with a vein patch. The exact role for selective angiographic infusion of vasoactive drugs or thrombolytic agents, as either primary therapy or as a surgical adjuvant, remains ill-defined. These techniques have some established potential and considerable theoretical appeal.

Distinguishing marginally viable but potentially salvageable gut from that which is irreparably injured remains of paramount importance. Bowel color, peristaltic activity, the presence or absence of palpable pulses and response to warming are imprecise means of assessing viability, and may occasionally be misleading. Many attempts to more accurately identify nonviable bowel are cumbersome or require sophisticated equipment and technical abilities. Scanning procedures, determination of electrical impedance in the bowel wall, and fluorescein angiography have yet to gain widespread acceptance [28, 53, 74]. A simple, accurate and effective means of determining intestinal viability using Doppler techniques has been reported by Hobson and Wright and confirmed by Cooperman and co-workers [15, 33]. It has the advantage of being widely available and simple in application. The decision for a second look procedure to assess the status of marginally viable bowel should be made at the time of original exploration. Following successful embolectomy and reestablishment of flow, gastrointestinal bleeding may be anticipated as areas of ischemic infarction are converted to hemorrhagic infarcts. Recent series have reported typical postrevascularization bleeding in up to 100% of survivors [59].

Recent reports continue to document the lethal nature of mesenteric arterial embolic insults [1, 3, 5, 8, 9, 40, 42, 58, 60, 71, 73, 75, 78, 80]. Survival ranges from 25%-44% even with a very aggressive approach to diagnosis and therapy (Table 1).

Superior Mesenteric Arterial Thrombosis

Although mesenteric artery thrombosis can occur with trauma and in patients having polycythemia, thrombocytosis, antiovulant medications, and altered aspirin sensitivity, the overwhelming majority of patients experiencing this event do so against the background of generalized atherosclerotic disease [4,

Table 1
Acute Intestinal Ischemia – Gastrointestinal Hemorrhage

Institution	Patient Population	Mortality	Comment
Albert Einstein – Montefiore Hospital (1977)	35 Embolus (46%) Thrombosis (9%) Nonocclusive (43%) Other (3%)	54% 56% 33% 40%	
Baylor University (1973)	38 Embolus (7%) Thrombosis (24%) Nonocclusive (53%) Other (16%)	89%	"Most" had gastrointestinal bleeding
Cleveland Clinic (1978)	10 Embolus (70%) Thrombosis (20%) Nonocclusive (10%)	70% 57% 100% 100%	Frequent gastrointestinal bleeding (usually occult)
Emory University (1970)	42 Embolus (36%) Thrombosis (64%)	81% 87% 78%	Occult bleeding
Hadassah University (1978)	40 Embolus (42%) Thrombosis (58%)	78% 71% 83%	Bleeding stools
Johns Hopkins Hospital (1974)	33	85%	Frequent guaiac positive secretions or bloody stools
Massachusetts General Hospital (1967)	136 Embolus (21%) Thrombosis (16%) Nonocclusive (49%) Other (13%)	92% 76% 95% 100%	Occult bleeding or chemically positive gastrointestinal secretions frequent
Massachusetts General Hospital (1978)	103 Embolus (55%) Thrombosis (45%)	85% 77% 96%	Gastrointestinal hemorrhage in 25% Post revascularization hemorrhage in all cases
Northwestern University (1975)	48 Embolus (69%) Thrombosis (31%)	83% 76% 100%	No gross bleeding noted

5, 8, 9, 16, 34, 44, 46, 49, 54, 55]. It is surprising that such events are relatively uncommon given the widespread and universal arteriosclerotic disease of the splanchnic vasculature which has been documented in both angiographic and autopsy studies [17, 18, 20, 41, 65]. The critical arteriosclerotic lesion in these cases seems to have a predilection for the more proximal portions of the main trunks (Fig. 3).

Gastrointestinal hemorrhage of even an occult nature is uncommon when these lesions are in a remediable preinfarction state [1, 5, 16]. Astute clinicians should be able to detect typical clinical manifestations of this disease prior to overt clinical catastrophes. Dunphy (1936) and Mikkelson (1957) have emphasized that half of these patients with intestinal infarction due to superior mesenteric arterial thrombosis have premonitory symptoms in the form of chronic intestinal angina [54]. The task is to recognize the characteristic picture of postprandial abdominal pain and weight loss and to be vigorous in pursuit of diagnosis. Gross hemorrhage implies a major complication, often with transmural infarction. In these circumstances the need to resect necrotic gut compromises attempts to reestablish intestinal blood flow.

Lateral aortography with selective visceral angiography is essential for diagnosis at all stages of the disease process. Despite early attempts to demonstrate flow limited absorptive defects, useful test criteria have not been forthcoming. Similarly, attempts to quantitate decreased splanchnic blood flow have not gained widespread acceptance [31].

In 1958 Shaw described the first successful superior mesenteric artery thromboendarterectomy and Derrick and co-workers performed celiac and superior mesenteric artery bypass using autologous iliac artery [18, 72]. At present bypass techniques using autologous saphenous vein or prosthetic materials are preferred by most authorities [1, 5, 16, 54, 59].

If mesenteric revascularization is performed prior to intestinal infarction operative mortality is an acceptable 5%-12%. However, once mesenteric thrombosis and visceral infarction has occurred, overall prognosis remains dismal with only occasional survivors reported (Table 1).

Low Flow Nonocclusive Ischemia

Nonocclusive ischemia is considered by many authors to be the most common cause of visceral infarction [4, 5, 8, 10, 31, 58, 63, 78]. This entity became widely recognized in the 1960's as ability to support critically ill patients improved. In adult populations, this lesion has certain similarities to necrotizing enterocolitis seen in critically ill neonates. The precise relationship between these 2 syndromes occurring at the extremes of age remains to be further defined. In elderly patient populations the central pathogenetic mechanism is intense vasospasm — often exacerbated by hypoperfusion, elevated catecholamines and angiotensin, or use of pressors and cardiac glycosides [4, 5, 8-10, 47, 63, 78]. The exact mechanisms initiating this intense vasospasm are

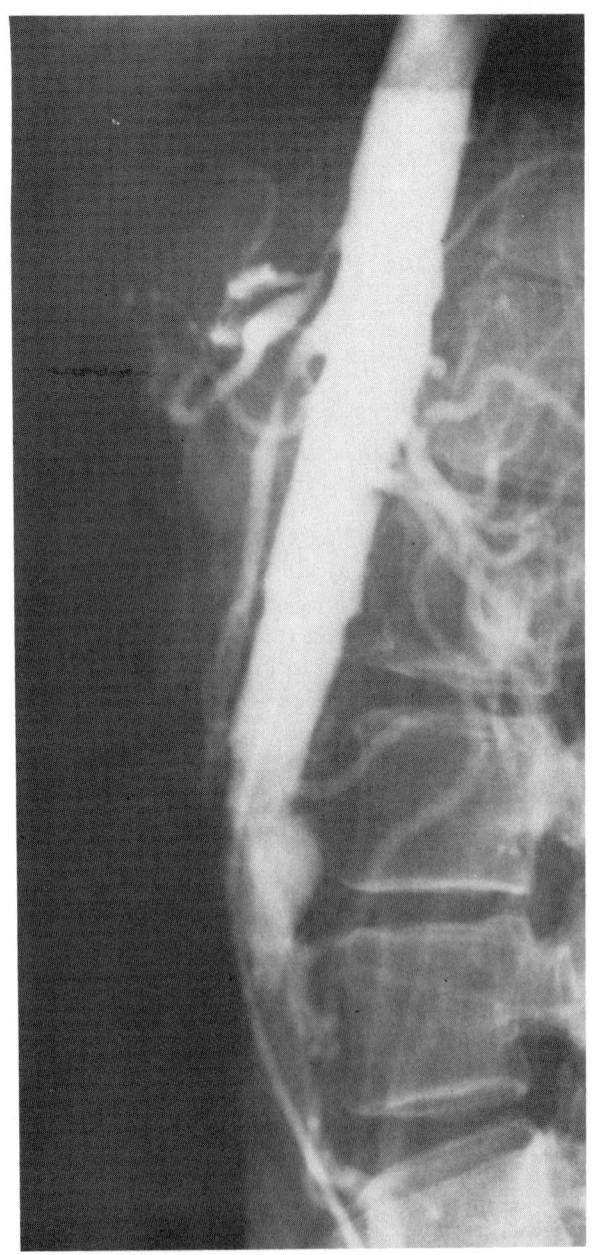

Fig. 3. High grade stenosis of the celiac and superior mesenteric arteries. These proximal arteriosclerotic lesions predispose to arterial thrombosis.

poorly understood, but persistent vasoconstriction can be demonstrated in a variety of clinical and experimental settings.

The typical patient is elderly, with atherosclerotic heart disease and congestive heart failure or a recent myocardial infarction. Frequently the patient is critically ill, in an intensive care unit and may be septic, in shock, and receiving digitalis or pressors. A recognizable precipitating event in this setting may, or may not, be present and the paucity of physical findings makes diagnosis difficult until transmural infarction occurs. Fully 75% of the documented cases of nonocclusive ischemia will have guaiac positive gastrointestinal secretions or overt gastrointestinal hemorrhage at some point during their course [63, 78]. Early symptoms and signs are protean and include abdominal pain, anorexia, nausea, vomiting, diarrhea, abdominal distention and unexplained deterioration of vital signs. Distention, peritoneal signs and frank bleeding are late manifestations of ischemic infarction and imply mucosal necrosis and sloughing.

Diagnosis, and to some extent therapy, hinge upon angiography. Whereas mesenteric embolus and thrombosis are surgical emergencies and demand urgent operative correction, nonocclusive ischemia does not involve an organic lesion as a major deficit and early operation may be ill-advised. Angiographic diagnosis often relates to exclusion of embolic and thrombotic phenomena and recognition of mesenteric vasospasm suggestive of nonocclusive ischemia. Angiographic signs of vasospasm are subtle and include: a greater degree of aortic reflux with selective injections; slow flow with decreased filling of peripheral vessels; narrowing at the origin of major arterial branches; abnormal vessel tapering; localized beading; segmental arterial narrowing; and impaired filling of intramural vessels.

Therapy is predicated upon optimizing the patient's cardiovascular status. Transfusion, colloid and crystalloid replacement, correction of underlying shock, sepsis and congestive heart failure, close monitoring in an intensive care unit with Swan-Ganz catheterization and discontinuance of drugs known to decrease splanchnic perfusion are all important in this regard. Numerous vasoactive drugs including papaverine, tolazaline, glucagon and isoproterenol may be administered peripherally or through selective superior mesenteric artery catheters. Each has its advocates but none has produced regular clinical successes. Histamine, gastrin, cholecystokinin and E type prostaglandins are similarly known to increase splanchnic blood flow [36, 63]. Their role in therapy remains ill-defined. Surgical therapy is limited to intestinal resection should transmural infarction occur. Mortality rates of 60%-70% are common, and range toward 90% with extensive intestinal infarction.

Isolated ischemia of the colon, a localized low flow state, was described in detail by Boley in 1963 [7]. Patients were typically elderly and presented with left-sided abdominal pain and gross or occult blood in the stools occasionally accompanied by watery diarrhea. In contrast to the other ischemic lesions producing gastrointestinal hemorrhage, recovery is the rule and diagnosis is more dependent upon barium contrast studies than angiography. Sequential barium enema changes of thumbprinting, ulceration and healing or scarring with stricture, follow over periods of weeks to months. Recovery is to be anticipated and clinical series report survivals in excess of 70%-80% in most instances with vigorous supportive therapy [7, 13, 19, 25, 27, 37-39, 50, 79].

Mesenteric Venous Thrombosis

Visceral infarction due to mesenteric venous thrombosis occurs without obvious cause or may occur with a variety of underlying factors. Most common are severe dehydration, intraabdominal sepsis, portal hypertension, pancreatitis, operative manipulation, hypercoagulable states, antiovulant medications, selective injection of vasoactive drugs, low flow states associated with aortic insufficiency or congestive heart failure, polycythemia and anti-thrombin III deficiency [14, 35, 51, 61, 62, 64, 66].

Clinical presentation is typically delayed. The patient's abdominal pain is frequently mild and present for 5 to 6 days prior to recognition. Lower gastrointestinal tract bleeding is a late finding and usually mild to moderate in severity. Rapid development of ascites is common and serosanguineous peritoneal fluid is an almost invariable finding at operation.

Plain films are not diagnostic. Multiple air fluid levels frequently suggest small bowel obstruction and this is often the preoperative diagnosis. Abdominal scintiangiographic techniques using technetium sulfur colloid have been reported by Smith and Selby to be of specific diagnostic utility [74]. Angiography may produce several clues to the diagnosis. Failure to opacify the superior mesenteric vein and portal vein, prolonged opacification of the bowel wall, and slow arterial phase contrast washout suggest venous obstruction.

Present treatment is limited to resection of the necrotic gut. Primary anastomosis of remaining compromised bowel is contraindicated. Anticoagulation is an important surgical adjuvant and should be instituted with systemic administration of heparin. Patients with antithrombin III deficiency may be "heparin resistant" and thus require massive heparin doses or alternate means of anticoagulation [61]. The role of arteriographic or retrograde portal infusions of thrombolytic agents remains to be defined. Prognosis is determined by the magnitude of the resection. Matthews and White reported 22 cases with 13 deaths and this greater than 60% mortality is duplicated in most clinical reports [51].

Vasculitis and Intestinal Ischemia

Segmental intestinal infarction secondary to vasculitis invariably presents as an acute abdomen or with occult gastrointestinal hemorrhage. Many underlying etiologies produce similar clinical pictures (Table 2) [22, 26, 32, 57]. Diagnosis

Table 2
Small Vessel Disease, Vasculitis, and Intestinal Ischemia

Collagen vascular and inflammatory vasculopathy
  Polyarteritis
  Dermatomyositis
  Rheumatoid arthritis
  Sjogren's syndrome
  Henoch-Schonlein purpura
  Essential mixed cryoglobulinemia
  Wegener's granulomatosis
  Giant cell arteritis
  Hepatitis B associated antigens
  Inflammatory bowel disease
  Typhoid

Local vasculopathy
  Cholesterol embolization
  Radiation
  Enteric coated potassium salts

Systemic vasculopathy
  Diabetes mellitus
  Polycythemia vera
  Kohlmeier-Degos syndrome
  Cogan's syndrome

Reactive vasculopathy
  Estrogen-progesterone compounds
  Pheochromocytoma
  Carcinoid syndrome
  Ergotism
  Buerger's disease
  Associated with renal vascular hypertension or accelerated
    phase of malignant hypertension

---

is usually made after multiple clinical laboratory studies and standard contrast studies. Therapy is, in general, supportive with management of the underlying disorder. Resection is reserved for obviously nonviable gut and occasionally recognizable late strictures.

Iatrogenic Colon Ischemia

Ischemia usually involving the left colon is a clinically recognized complication of aortic surgery (1%-2%) and colon resection [21, 29]. Sacrifice of the inferior mesenteric artery makes viability dependent upon the adequacy of preexisting collateral vessels. Pre- and intraoperative assessments of the functional status of these collaterals may be difficult. Hagihara, Ernst and Griffen have reported an incidence of endoscopically evident ischemic colitis following aortic surgery of 7% for elective procedures and up to 60% with treatment of ruptured aneurysms. They proposed criteria for a more precise estimation of colonic viability based on inferior mesenteric artery back pressure. Hobson and Wright suggest intraoperative Doppler assessment as an accurate guide to intestinal viability [33]. The validity of both methods needs further clinical documentation.

Passage of bloody, diarrheal stool following aortic surgery necessitates urgent sigmoidoscopic or colonoscopic evaluation. In many of these cases the anal sphincter is somewhat lax and guaiac positive fecal material is usually present. If ischemia is present, the rectum presents an edematous, blue submucosal hemorrhage or mucosal sloughing and ulceration with a yellow-green, shaggy pseudomembrane. These patients must be returned promptly to the operating room for attempted revascularization of the left colon. Obviously nonviable colon is exteriorized or resected.

REFERENCES

1. Bergan JJ, Dean RH, Conn J, et al: Revascularization in treatment of mesenteric infarction. Ann Surg 182:430, 1975
2. Bergan JJ, Haid SP, Conn J: Systemic effects of intestinal revascularization. Am J Surg 117:235, 1969
3. Bergan JJ, Hoehn J: Superior mesenteric artery embolectomy. JAMA 188:935, 1964
4. Bergan JJ, Yao JST: Acute intestinal ischemia. In Rutherford RB: Vascular Surgery, Philadelphia, Saunders, 1977, p 825
5. Boley SJ, Brandt LJ, Veith FJ: Ischemic disorders of the intestines. Curr Prob Surg 15:1-86, 1978
6. Boley SJ, DiBiase A, Brandt LJ, et al: Lower intestinal bleeding in the elderly. Am J Surg 137:57, 1979
7. Boley SJ, Schwartz S, Cash J, et al: Reversible vascular occlusion of the colon. Surg Gynecol Obstet 116:53, 1963
8. Boley SJ, Schwartz SS, Williams LF (eds): Vascular Disorders of the Intestine. New York, Appleton-Century-Crofts, 1971
9. Boley SJ, Sprayregan S, Siegelman SS, et al: Initial results from an aggressive roentgenotogical and surgical approach to acute mesenteric ischemia. Surgery 82:848, 1977
10. Bynum TE, Jacobson ED: Non-occlusive intestinal ischemia. Arch Intern Med 139:281, 1979
11. Carnevale NJ, Delaney HM: Cholesterol embolization to the cecum with bowel infarction. Arch Surg 106:94, 1973

12. Chiene J: Complete obliteration of the coeliac and mesenteric arteries at their origin. Br Med J 2:201, 1868
13. Coghill CL, Makkar J, Campana HA, Park YS: Ischemic colitis. Am Surg 43:137, 1977
14. Collins GJ, Zuck TF, Zajtchuk R, et al: Hypercoagulability in mesenteric venous occlusion: Report of two cases. Am J Surg 132:390, 1976
15. Cooperman M, Pace WG, Martin EW Jr, et al: Determination of viability of ischemic intestine by doppler ultrasound. Surgery 83:705, 1978
16. Crawford ES, Morris GC, Myhre HO, et al: Celiac axis, superior mesenteric artery and inferior mesenteric artery occlusion. Surgical considerations. Surgery 82:856, 1977
17. Demos NJ, Bahuth JJ, Urnes PD: Comparative study of arteriosclerosis in the inferior and superior mesenteric arteries. Ann Surg 155:599, 1962
18. Derrick JR, Pollard HS, Moore RM: The pattern of arteriosclerotic narrowing of the celiac and superior mesenteric arteries. Ann Surg 149:684, 1959
19. Detry R, Devroede G, Madarnas P, et al: Ischemic colitis associated with hypertension. Canad J Surg 22:256, 1979
20. Dick AP, Graff R, Gregg DM, et al: An arteriographic study of mesenteric arterial disease: Large vessel changes. Gut 8:206, 1967
21. Ernst CB, Hagihara PF, Daugherty ME, et al: Ischemic colitis incidence following abdominal aortic reconstruction: A prospective study. Surgery 80:417, 1976
22. Fauci AS, Haynes BF, Katz P: NIH Conference: The spectrum of vasculitis. Ann Int Med 89:660, 1978
23. Folkow B, Neil E: Gastrointestinal and liver circulations. In Folkow B, Neil E (eds): Circulation. New York, Oxford University Press, 1971, p 466
24. Fry WJ: Arterial circulation of the small and large intestine. In Strandness DE Jr (ed): Collateral Circulation in Clinical Surgery. Philadelphia, Saunders, 1969
25. Gore RM, Calenoff L, Rogers LF: Roentgenographic manifestations of ischemic colitis. JAMA 241:1171, 1979
26. Greene FL, Ariyan S, Stansel HC: Mesenteric and peripheral vascular ischemia secondary to ergotism. Surgery 81:176, 1977
27. Grimes DA, Johnson G Jr, Grice OD: The iliac steal phenomenon. Arch Surg 104:333, 1972
28. Gurll NJ, Braxton G: Potential differences as an estimate of intestinal viability. J Surg Res 18:611, 1975
29. Hagihara PF, Ernst CB, Griffen WO Jr: Incidence of ischemic colitis following abdominal aortic reconstruction. Surg Gynecol Obstet 149:571, 1979
30. Haglund U, Lundgren O: Non-occlusive acute intestinal vascular failure. Br J Surg 66:155, 1979
31. Hanson HJB, Engel HC, Ring-Larson H, et al: Splanchnic blood flow with abdominal angina before and after arterial reconstruction. Ann Surg 186:216, 1977
32. Herrington JG, Grossman LA: Surgical lesions of the small and large intestinal resulting from Buerger's disease. Ann Surg 168:1079, 1968

33. Hobson RW, Wright CB, O'Donell JA, et al: Determination of intestinal viability by doppler ultrasound. Arch Surg 114:165, 1979
34. Houle M, Kennedy A, Prior AL, et al: Small bowel ischemia and infarction in young women taking oral contraceptives and progestational agents. Br J Surg 64:533, 1977
35. Inahara T: Acute superior mesenteric venous thrombosis: treatment by thrombectomy. Ann Surg 174:956, 1971
36. Johsson K, Wallace S, Jacobson ED, et al: The use of prostaglandin E_1 for enhanced visualization of the splanchnic circulation. Radiology 125:375, 1977
37. Kaminski DL, Keltner RM, William VL: Ischemic colitis. Arch Surg 106:558, 1973
38. Karmody AM, Jordan FR, Zaman SN: Left colon gangrene after acute inferior mesenteric artery occlusion. Arch Surg 111:972, 1976
39. Kinkhabwala M, Rubinowitz JC, Dallemand S, et al: Intersplanchnic steal syndrome; another cause for reversible colon ischaemia. Br J Radiol 47:729, 1974
40. Klass AA: Embolectomy in acute mesenteric occlusion. Ann Surg 134:913, 1951
41. Kohler R, Laustela E, Harjola PT, et al: Angiographic study of arteriosclerosis in the coeliac and mesenteric circulation. Ann Chir Gynec (Finn) 57:531, 1968
42. Krausz MM, Manny J: Acute superior mesenteric arterial occlusion: A plea for early diagnosis. Surgery 83:482, 1978
43. Lanciault G, Jacobson ED: The gastrointestinal circulation. Gastroenterology 71:851, 1976
44. Laufman H, Nora PF, Mittelpunkt AI: Mesenteric blood vessels: advances in surgery and physiology. Arch Surg 88:1021, 1964
45. Law DH, Watts HD: Gastrointestinal bleeding. In Sleisenger MH and Fordtran JS (eds): Gastrointestinal Disease, 2nd ed. Philadelphia, Saunders, 1978
46. Lescher TJ, Bombeck CT: Mesenteric vascular occlusion associated with oral contraceptive use. Arch Surg 112:1231, 1977
47. Levinsky RA, Lewis RM, Bynam TE, et al: Digoxin induced intestinal vasoconstriction: The effects of proximal arterial stenosis and glucagon administration. Circulation 52:130, 1975
48. Lundgren O: Studies on blood flow distribution and counter current exchange in the small intestine. Acta Physiol Scand, Suppl 303
49. Marston A: Mesenteric arterial disease: the present position. Gut 8:203, 1967
50. Marston A, Pheils MT, Thomas L, et al: Ischaemic colitis. Gut 7:1, 1966
51. Matthews JE, White RR: Primary mesenteric venous occlusive disease. Am J Surg 122:579, 1971
52. Mattox KL, Guinn GA: Mesenteric infarction. Am J Surg 126:332, 1973
53. Meyers MB, Cherry G, Gesser J: Relationship between surface pH and pCO_2 and the vascularity and viability of the intestine. Surg Gynec Obstet 134:787, 1972

54. Mikkelsen WP: Intestinal angina: Its surgical significance. Am J Surg 94:262, 1957
55. Myers TJ, Steinberg WM, Rickles FR: Polycythemia vera and mesenteric arterial thrombosis. Arch Int Med 139:695, 1979
56. Ockner RK: Vascular disease of the bowel. In Sleisenger MH and Fordtran JS (eds): Gastrointestinal Disease, 2nd ed. Philadelphia, Saunders, 1978
57. O'Neill WM, Hammar SP, Bloomer HA: Giant cell arteritis with visceral angitis. Arch Int Med 136:1157, 1976
58. Ottinger LW, Austen WG: A study of 136 patients with mesenteric infarction. Surg Gynec Obstet 124:251, 1967
59. Ottinger LW: The surgical management of acute occlusion of the superior mesenteric artery. Ann Surg 188:721, 1978
60. Perdue GD, Smith RB III: Intestinal ischemia due to mesenteric arterial disease. Am Surg 36:152, 1970
61. Peters TG, Lewis JD, Filip DJ, et al: Antithrombin III deficiency causing postsplenectomy mesenteric venous thrombosis coincident with thrombocytopenia. Ann Surg 185:229, 1977
62. Polk HC Jr: Experimental venous occlusion. Ann Surg 163:432, 1966
63. Price WE, Rohrer GV, Jacobson ED: Mesenteric vascular diseases. Gastroenterology 57:599, 1969
64. Qureshi MA, Mansfield RD: Recurrent mesenteric venous thrombosis with recovery. Am J Surg 108:421, 1964
65. Reiner L, Jimenez FA, Rodriques FL: Atherosclerosis in the mesenteric circulation. observations and correlations with aortic and coronary atherosclerosis. Am Heart J 66:200, 1963
66. Renert WA, Button KF, Fuld SL, et al: Mesenteric venous thrombosis and small bowel infarction following infusion of vasopressin into the superior mesenteric artery. Radiology 102:299, 1972
67. Robertson GS, Lyall AD, Macrae JGC: Acid-base disturbances in mesenteric occlusion. Surg Gynecol Obstet 128:15, 1969
68. Sabiston DC (ed): Davis-Christopher Textbook of Surgery. The Biologic Basis of Modern Surgical Practice, 11th ed. Philadelphia, Saunders, 1977
69. Sachs IL, Klima T, Frankel NB: Thromboangitis obliterans of the transverse colon. JAMA 238:336, 1977
70. Schwartz SI, Storer EH: Manifestations of gastrointestinal disease. In Schwartz SI, Shires GT, Spencer FC, Storer EH (eds). Principles of Surgery, 3rd ed. New York, McGraw Hill, 1979
71. Shaw RS, Rutledge RH: Superior mesenteric artery embolectomy in the treatment of massive mesenteric infarction. N Engl J Med 257:595, 1957
72. Shaw RS, Rutledge R: Acute and chronic thrombosis of the mesenteric arteries associated with malabsorption. New Engl J Med 258:874, 1958
73. Skinner DB, Zarins CK, Moosa AR: Mesenteric vascular disease. Am J Surg 128:835, 1974
74. Smith RW, Selby JB: Scintiangiographic diagnosis of acute mesenteric venous thrombosis. Am J Radiol 132:67, 1979
75. Stewart GD, Sweetman WR, Westphal K, et al: Superior mesenteric artery embolectomy. Ann Surg 151:279, 1960

76. Turner W: On the existence of a system of anastomosing arteries between and connecting the visceral and parietal branches of the abdominal aorta. Br For Med Chir Rev 32:222, 1863
77. Verstraete M, Vandebroucke J: The clinical significance of communication between abdominal splanchnic arteries. Angiologica 7:160, 1970
78. Williams LF Jr: Vascular insufficiency of the intestines. Gastroenterology 61:757, 1971
79. Williams LF Jr, Wittenberg J: Ischemic colitis: A useful clinical diagnosis, but is it ischemic? Ann Surg 182:439, 1975
80. Zuidema GD: Surgical management of superior mesenteric arterial emboli. Arch Surg 82:267, 1961

William W. Coon, M.D.

Drug-related and Hematological Disorders Associated With Gastrointestinal Bleeding

ABSTRACT

Drug-related episodes of gastrointestinal bleeding have been linked to the administration of a number of agents, but most reports are anecdotal. Data are available to support acetylsalicylic acid (ASA) playing a role in the induction of gastric bleeding; whether certain other antiinflammatory drugs have a similar effect is not as clear. The influence of adrenal corticosteroid administration is controversial.

All drugs which significantly alter hemostasis may potentiate bleeding from a preexisting gastrointestinal lesion; although these lesions may have been unrecognized prior to the onset of hemorrhage, an extensive diagnostic evaluation will frequently result in their detection. There is no evidence that antithrombotic agents themselves are responsible for producing pathologic alterations in gastrointestinal mucosa or its accompanying vessels.

The principal hematologic disorder associated with gastrointestinal hemorrhage is thrombocytopenia which can stem from any of many causes. Less frequent but not uncommon are the many acquired derangements of blood coagulation. The recognition and management of both congenital and acquired alterations in hemostasis and other hematologic conditions responsible for gastrointestinal bleeding are briefly discussed.

DRUG-RELATED GASTROINTESTINAL BLEEDING

Acetylsalicylic Acid

Although gastrointestinal bleeding (GI) associated with drug ingestion is becoming increasingly recognized, the relative importance of drug-induced

---

William W. Coon, M.D.: Professor of Surgery, Department of Surgery, University of Michigan Medical Center, Ann Arbor, Michigan.

lesions within the spectrum of causes of gastrointestinal bleeding has not yet been established. While data are available which might possibly implicate several drugs in a causal role, most reports are anecdotal or inadequately controlled retrospective trials.

Possible mechanisms for drug-related gastrointestinal lesions are linked to mucosal or vascular injury or alterations in hemostasis: (1) initiation of or interference with healing of a gastric ulcer; (2) initiation of mucosal ulceration of the gastrointestinal tract (other than gastric ulcer) by a direct toxic effect upon mucosal cells; (3) bacterial or fungal ulceration secondary to drug-induced leukopenia or other immunodeficiency; (4) toxic vascular injury; (5) drug-induced thrombocytopenic bleeding; (6) qualitative alterations in platelet function; (7) hypocoagulability of the blood; and (8) excessive activation by drug of fibrinolytic activity.

Acetylsalicylic acid or aspirin (ASA) is the drug most frequently linked with clinically significant upper gastrointestinal bleeding. The initiation of gastric mucosal ulceration by ASA may be related to its known inhibitory effect on prostaglandin synthesis, since prostaglandins have recently been shown to have a cytoprotective effect for gastric mucosa [23]; indomethacin-induced gastric ulceration has been prevented by orally administered prostaglandins [19]. The erosive effect of aspirin appears to be mediated by a loosening of tight junctions between gastric epithelial cells with a back diffusion of acid [8]; pepsin secretion may also contribute [13]. A higher gastric acid output may potentiate the erosive effect [5], but findings in this regard have been controversial. Bile reflux from the duodenum may also have a pathogenetic role [3]. Gastric mucosal injury does not require direct contact of the drug with the gastric mucosa [9]. The volume of blood loss may be increased by the effect of ASA on prolongation of bleeding time by inhibition of platelet aggregation [21]; administration of aspirin to a patient with a preexisting bleeding lesion can significantly potentiate the blood loss [9].

When considering gastrointestinal bleeding related to ingestion of aspirin and other antiinflammatory agents, one must differentiate between small increases in fecal blood loss and major bleeding. Although an increase of a few milliliters in daily gastrointestinal blood loss occurs in the majority of subjects taking aspirin [9, 24], the incidence rate for hospital admissions for major bleeding associated with recent and heavy use of aspirin has been estimated at only 15 per 100,000 per year [18]. No method for prediction of which subjects will develop clinically significant bleeding has been found.

Gastroscopic studies have shown that aspirin produces extensive superficial gastric erosions; lesions have been less frequent after administration of indomethacin, phenylbutazone, naproxen, ibuprofen and diclofenac [10, 16]. Gastrointestinal blood loss is less with sodium salicylate, choline salicylate or suitable formulations of ASA and antacid [9, 17]. The ingestion of both ethanol and ASA appears to accentuate the erosive process [22].

The best documentation that aspirin increases the frequency of clinically significant gastrointestinal bleeding is a controlled retrospective study involving 88 patients admitted to a hospital with major GI bleeding of unknown cause [18]. A history of "heavy" ASA use (on four or more days per week) was elicited in 16% of bleeding patients but only 6.9% of matched controls. Heavy aspirin use was recorded in 23% of patients diagnosed as having gastritis and 33% of those with acute gastric ulcer. No relationship to bleeding duodenal ulcer was found. In this and other clinical studies it has not been possible to determine whether aspirin has any etiologic relationship to the development of acute gastric ulcer or whether the ingestion of ASA precipitated bleeding in a preexisting ulcer. In addition, whether the use of buffered aspirin will lower the frequency of major GI bleeding has not been determined; the amount of buffering agent present may be inadequate.

Antiinflammatory Agents

Although assumptions have been made that other antiinflammatory-analgesic agents might also induce major gastrointestinal hemorrhage and although anecdotal reports of gastrointestinal bleeding after ingestion of indomethacin [15], ibuprofen [11], phenylbutazone, etc. [1] have appeared, there is no good evidence of an increase in clinically significant bleeding episodes related to administration of these drugs.

Fortunately, the great majority of patients with apparent drug-related GI hemorrhage will respond to nonoperative management. In a recent study of endoscopically documented erosive gastritis, only 4 of 74 patients required operation for control of bleeding [14].

There is also conflicting evidence as to whether adrenocorticosteroid therapy influences the development of peptic ulcer and its complications, including gastrointestinal bleeding. Many of the earlier anecdotal reports incriminating these agents were probably linked to the fact that the diseases for which adrenal corticosteroids are administered often are associated with an increase in frequency of associated peptic ulcer. Conn and Blitzer have recently reported data showing no relationship between adrenocorticosteroid therapy and peptic ulcer [4]. However, Cantu and Prieto reported a four-fold increase in frequency of gastrointestinal bleeding in patients with intracranial operations who received high doses of corticosteroids as compared to those who had no steroid therapy; patients with prior GI complaints were excluded [2].

Other drugs have also been incriminated. Three of 600 psychiatric patients receiving high doses of reserpine developed major GI bleeding [12]. The intravenous administration of ethacrynic acid which was originally linked to bleeding in patients receiving heparin has been associated with the initiation of gastrointestinal bleeding in the absence of concomitant administration of anticoagulant [25].

Chemotherapeutic Agents

As might be expected, cancer chemotherapeutic drugs which induce gastrointestinal mucosal ulceration, particularly methotrexate, may produce GI bleeding. These agents are also linked with bleeding episodes resulting from bone marrow suppression and thrombocytopenia, or bleeding from infectious mucosal ulcers brought about by immunodeficiency, resulting either from the drug or the drug combined with the effect of the underlying disease. Similar mechanisms of bleeding are associated with many other pharmacologic agents which may produce hypoplasia or aplasia of the bone marrow by toxic or idiosyncratic mechanisms.

Anticoagulants

One of the principal complications of drugs utilized for antithrombotic therapy is bleeding. In general terms, the more effective the antithrombotic drug and the more intensive the therapy, the greater the frequency of hemorrhage. In our previously reported experience with 3862 courses of heparin and oral anticoagulant treatment in hospitalized patients [6], 6.8% of courses were associated with bleeding complications, and in 2% bleeding was major, requiring blood transfusion or termination of therapy. Twenty-two percent of these hemorrhagic complications were gastrointestinal in origin, and two-thirds of these were major. Most minor episodes of GI bleeding were related to hemorrhoids or bleeding from erosions produced by a nasogastric tube.

In 28 of 45 major episodes an underlying lesion responsible for the bleeding could be identified. In nine patients a peptic ulcer was first recognized as a result of anticoagulant-induced hemorrhage; in 7 the bleeding was manifested only by melena without hematemesis, hypotension or a major decrease in hematocrit. In contrast to these 9 patients with unrecognized peptic ulcer, only 4 of a total of 140 patients with a known history of ulcer developed bleeding during anticoagulant treatment. Nine more patients with a previously diagnosed peptic ulcer bled from sources other than their ulcer. Two patients bled from previously unrecognized operable tumors of the right colon. These observations point to the importance of a thorough diagnostic investigation of patients developing gastrointestinal bleeding during anticoagulant therapy.

What appears to be "spontaneous" bleeding into the wall of the intestine may occur during anticoagulant therapy. Intramural bleeding may produce acute abdominal pain, tenderness and signs of partial or complete bowel obstruction. The typical radiographic findings of thickened mucosal folds, bowel rigidity and luminal narrowing in conjunction with the history of anticoagulant ingestion should lead to the correct diagnosis. Occasionally, mucosal erosion will be followed by gross evidence of gastrointestinal bleeding. Conservative therapy with reversal of anticoagulant effect will usually result in gradual resolution of the hematoma.

The pathogenesis of anticoagulant-induced GI bleeding is unknown. Although toxic lesions of the vascular wall have been produced by administration of massive doses of oral anticoagulants to experimental animals, no histólogic changes in vessels have been found in humans with this complication. Most patients developing gastrointestinal bleeding without a subsequently demonstrable underlying lesion have received excessive doses of anticoagulant or have developed inordinately prolonged clotting tests as a result of other drug interactions with the anticoagulant [7]. The most frequent drug interaction recognized in recent years has been the concomitant ingestion by the patient of antiplatelet agents, particularly aspirin or one of the more than 400 proprietary preparations containing aspirin.

Other antithrombotic drugs which are used less frequently and may occasionally be associated with the development of GI bleeding include streptokinase, urokinase, ancrod and dextran.

HEMATOLOGICAL DISORDERS AND GASTROINTESTINAL BLEEDING

Diagnosis

Although recognized by every experienced clinician assessing a patient with gastrointestinal bleeding, many of us may at times neglect to assess fully the myriad hematological causes of gastrointestinal bleeding. While hematological abnormalities are primarily responsible for only a small segment of gastrointestinal bleeding disorders, they may play a secondary role in a much larger proportion of patients. Early detection of defects in hemostasis may be of major importance in the rapid and effective management of this problem. Diagnosis is dependent upon a thorough history and physical examination and appropriate interpretation of laboratory studies.

Defects in hemostasis may result from abnormalities in vascular integrity, clotting factor activity or in the number or function of platelets. The presumption that hemostatic abnormality may be present can usually be made by the time the history and physical examination have been completed. The value of a thorough family history of abnormal bleeding is of obvious importance for the detection of hereditary and familial disorders. Personal history should include data concerning episodes of spontaneous bleeding and their location and age of onset and abnormal bleeding during prior dental procedures or operations. Bleeding at an early age after minor trauma, particularly hemarthrosis, is indicative of a severe clotting factor deficiency, usually one of the hemophilias.

A careful drug history is important because some patients neglect to tell the physician they are receiving anticoagulants, and many will not mention ingestion of aspirin or one of the proprietary preparations containing salicylates. A physical examination with findings suggesting the presence of splenomegaly, chronic hepatic or renal disease, obstructive jaundice, collagen vascular disease, severe malnutrition, sepsis, major burns, or massive blood loss points to the immediate need for more extensive laboratory investigations of hemostatic function. The usual screening procedures (Table 1) which will detect most hemostatic abnormalities include bleeding time, platelet count, prothrombin time and partial thromboplastin time. In selected circumstances, a Rumpel-Leede test, blood smear for platelet morphology and abnormal cells, platelet aggregation studies, a quantitative assessment of fibrinogen level, thrombin time, or tests for fibrinolysis or fibrin split products may be indicated. Abnormalities in one or more of these procedures may then lead to more definitive tests for a specific hemostatic defect.

Table 1
Screening Procedures for Bleeding Disorders

Procedure	Factors Measured	Clinical Disorders
Rumpel-Leede test	Capillary fragility; platelet activity	Hereditary vascular disorders; drug toxicity; thrombocytopenia
Bleeding time	Platelet function	Hereditary vascular disorders; von Willebrand's disease; thrombocytopenia; thrombasthenia; aspirin ingestion
Platelet count	Platelets	Thrombocytopenia
Clot retraction	Platelet enzyme activity	Thrombocytopenia; thrombasthenia
Partial thromboplastin time	Factors I, II, V, VIII, IX, X, XI, XII; Fletcher and Fitzgerald	Hereditary plasma factor deficiencies; liver disease; heparin effect
Prothrombin time	Factors I, II, V, VII, X	Vitamin K deficiency; Coumadin, heparin, or propylthiouracil effect; hereditary plasma factor deficiencies
Thrombin time	Fibrin degradation products	Intravascular coagulation; heparin effect; primary and secondary fibrinolysis
Fibrinogen	Fibrinogen	Intravascular coagulation; fibrinolysis
Euglobulin lysis	Plasmin activity	Fibrinolysis

If specific abnormalities are detected, it is important to assess which deviations from normality may be of significance in contributing to perpetuation of bleeding (Table 2).

Spectrum of Hematological Disorders

No attempt will be made in this review to enumerate all of the hemostatic (Table 3) and hematological abnormalities which might result in gastrointestinal bleeding. The following brief comments are meant to point out the spectrum of diseases which may enter into the differential diagnosis. Some general guidelines for approach to management of the more common disorders are listed in Table 4.

Congenital abnormalities in vascular or platelet function or both are comparatively rare. Gastrointestinal bleeding related to a congenital abnormality in vascular connective tissue may be an important clinical presentation in patients with pseudoxanthoma elasticum and Ehlers-Danlos syndrome [25]. Hereditary telangiectasia (Osler-Weber-Rendu disease), a vascular defect with occasional associated abnormalities in platelet function, is responsible for episodic, slow, but often persistent gastrointestinal blood loss; a careful mirror or endoscopic examination of the pharynx and esophagoscopy may detect lesions missed on routine physical examination. More common is von Willebrand's disease, a combined deficiency of factor VIII coagulant and von Willebrand's factor (which is essential for normal platelet function).

Drugs which alter platelet function can appreciably accentuate the magnitude of hemorrhage if administered to patients with von Willebrand's disease. In

Table 2
Relationship of Laboratory Abnormality to Risk of Bleeding

Test	Normal	Lesion Present; Bleeding Possible	Risk of "Spontaneous" Bleeding
Bleeding time (min)	< 6	> 10	> 15
Platelet count (per μl^3)	200,000	50,000	10,000
Prothrombin time (sec)	12	> 16	35
Partial thromboplastin time (sec)	30	45	60
Thrombin time (sec)	8	16	60
Fibrinogen (mg%)	150	< 100	30
Euglobulin lysis time (min)	90	< 60	< 30

Table 3
Bleeding Disorders Which May Be Associated With Gastrointestinal Bleeding

---

Hereditary and familial
  Hereditary telangiectasia
  Hemophilia A (factor VIII deficiency)
  Hemophilia B. (factor IX deficiency)
  von Willebrand's disease
  Other rare factor deficiencies (V, X, XI)
  Familial thrombocytopenias and thrombocytopathies
  Henoch-Schönlein purpura

Acquired
  Platelet factor deficiencies (quantitative or qualitative, primary or secondary)
  "Hypoprothrombinemias" (acquired "deficiencies" of factors II, VII, X, associated with severe liver disease, oral anticoagulants, propylthiouracil toxicity, etc.)
  Disseminated intravascular coagulation (consumption coagulopathy)
  Fibrinolytic bleeding
  Circulating anticoagulant (lupus erythematosis, dysproteinemias, heparin or oral anticoagulant therapy, etc.)

---

more general terms, any agent which alters normal hemostasis will aggravate bleeding if given to a patient with a congenital or acquired clotting factor deficiency. Spontaneous bleeding into the gastrointestinal tract in both classical hemophilia and von Willebrand's disease may occur in the absence of radiographically or operatively demonstrable lesions. GI bleeding in conjunction with other hereditary clotting factor deficiencies is rare.

Acquired abnormalities in platelet number or function are a frequent contributor to gastrointestinal bleeding, particularly in a secondary role of increasing the volume and duration of blood loss in a patient with a specific gastrointestinal lesion. In addition to vascular purpuras (Henoch-Schönlein, etc.), idiopathic thrombocytopenic purpura and thrombotic thrombocytopenic purpura, secondary thrombocytopenias related to immune destruction, decreased synthesis, and splenic sequestration should be considered. Patients with chronic renal disease may have both defective vascular integrity and quantitative or qualitative deficiencies in platelets. Vascular and platelet abnormalities, liver failure, renal failure or an antibody specific for factor VIII may be responsible for gastrointestinal bleeding in collagen disease, particularly systemic lupus erythematosis. Qualitative as well as quantitative platelet defects are found frequently in patients with myeloproliferative disorders and associated gastrointestinal bleeding. Primary thrombocythemia results occasionally in gastrointestinal bleeding, presumably from small hemorrhagic mucosal infarcts. A similar process has been described in patients with homocystinuria.

Table 4
Management of More Common Coagulation Abnormalities Associated With Active Bleeding

Hemophilia A	Rapid infusion of 25 U/kg of factor VIII concentrate. Continued factor VIII replacement in amounts to compensate for continued blood loss. Repeat original dose at 12 hr intervals for 3-5 days and then every 24 hr for another 3-5 days
Hemophilia B	Twenty-five U/kg prothrombin complex concentrate. Follow regimen outlined above
von Willebrand's disease	Plasma, 10 ml/kg, or cryo-factor VIII, one bag/10 kg, plus platelet concentrate one bag/10 kg. Additional doses to compensate for continued blood loss
Bleeding associated with severe liver disease	Fresh platelet-rich plasma, 2-3 units, and one or more additional units every 4-6 hours. Vitamin K_1, 10 mg slowly. Assess need for additional platelet concentrate and prothrombin complex
Bleeding associated with chronic renal disease	Platelet concentrates. Assess need for hemodialysis
Bleeding associated with collagen disease or dysproteinemias	Steroids, immunosuppressive agents, exchange transfusions
Bleeding associated with anticoagulants	Heparin: protamine sulfate, 50-100 mg intravenously; oral anticoagulants: vitamin K_1, 25-50 mg intravenously slowly; infusion of plasma or whole blood with massive bleeding
Consumption coagulopathy	Platelet concentrates, 1 bag/10 kg, plus whole blood or plasma plus erythrocyte concentrates. Cryoprecipitate (source of fibrinogen and factor VIII) and prothrombin complex concentrate may also be required

In addition to the hemostatic abnormalities linked to bleeding in patients with agnogenic myeloid metaplasia, an estimated 6%-8% of these individuals develop portal hypertension and esophageal varices; these lesions should be considered in every patient with this disorder who develops gastrointestinal bleeding.

Patients with isolated splenic vein thrombosis may also bleed from esophageal varices. Although pancreatitis is the most common cause of splenic vein thrombosis, it is essential in the operative management (splenectomy) to rule out other etiologic factors, principally lymphoma or pancreatic carcinoma.

Hemorrhagic necrosis of the GI tract, frequently multifocal and usually confined to mucosa only is common in patients with leukemia. Bleeding is frequently aggravated by an accompanying thrombocytopenia and may become refractory if ischemic necrosis is extensive.

Leukemia, idiopathic thrombocytopenic purpura, and hemophilia may also be responsible for intramural hematomas and produce a clinical picture similar to that seen in patients receiving anticoagulant therapy. These hematomas may occur spontaneously or may be initiated by minimal abdominal trauma.

Certain acquired abnormalities of blood coagulation may accentuate bleeding from a specific gastrointestinal lesion or, less frequently, may be associated with GI bleeding in which no specific source of bleeding can be demonstrated. The latter situation is more common in conjunction with hemorrhage secondary to disseminated intravascular coagulation.

Although gastrointestinal bleeding in patients with chronic liver disease is usually secondary to esophageal or gastric varices, peptic ulcer, or gastritis, an associated coagulative abnormality may have a major effect upon volume of blood loss and therapeutic efforts to control the bleeding. The spectrum of hemostatic defects may include all phases of hemostasis: vascular, platelet and multiple clotting factor deficiencies. In addition to a decrease in synthesis of vitamin-K dependent clotting factors II, VII, IX, X, decreases in fibrinogen (rare) and factors V, XI, and XIII have been described. Chronic intravascular coagulation with increases in fibrin and fibrinogen degradation products and enhanced secondary fibrinolysis is not uncommon, particularly after operations upon the liver. An adequate definition of the hemostatic defect is essential to rational therapy.

In patients with obstructive jaundice or malabsorption from other causes without severe underlying liver disease, the vitamin-K dependent clotting factor abnormality is usually relatively mild and can be satisfactorily corrected by serial administration of small amounts of vitamin K_1, or in the face of severe bleeding, by stored plasma. Recently, melena secondary to vitamin K deficiency was encountered in patients receiving parenteral hyperalimentation with inadequate vitamin replacement.

An accurate prior diagnosis of hematological disease and an appreciation of the lesions and hemostatic abnormalities which may accompany that diagnosis are the most important elements in prevention and management of associated gastrointestinal bleeding.

REFERENCES

1. Boston Collaborative Drug Surveillance Program. Hospital admissions due to adverse drug reactions. Arch Intern Med 134:219, 1974

2. Cantu RC, Prieto A: Evaluation of the increased risk of gastrointestinal bleeding following intracranial surgery in patients receiving high steroid dosages in the immediate postoperative period. Int Surg 49:325, 1968
3. Cochran KM, Mackenzie JF, Russell RI: Role of taurocholic acid in production of gastric mucosal damage after ingestion of aspirin. Br Med J 1:183, 1975
4. Conn HO, Blitzer BL: Non-association of adrenocorticosteroid therapy and peptic ulcer. N Engl J Med 294:473, 1976
5. Cooce AL: The role of acid in the pathogenesis of aspirin-induced gastrointestinal erosions and hemorrhage. Am J Dig Dis 18:225, 1973
6. Coon WW, Willis PW III: Hemorrhagic complications of anticoagulant therapy. Arch Intern Med 133:386, 1974
7. Coon WW: Anticoagulant therapy for venous thromboembolism. Postgrad Med 63:157, 1978
8. Davenport HW: Salicylate damage to the gastric mucosal barrier. N Engl J Med 276:1307, 1967
9. Grossman MI, Motsumoto VK, Lichter RJ: Fecal blood loss produced by administration of various salicylates. Gastroenterology 40:383, 1961
10. Halvorsen L, Dotevall G, Sevelius H: Comparative effects of aspirin and naproxen on gastric mucosa. Scand J Rheumatol 2 (Suppl):43, 1973
11. Holdstock DJ: Gastrointestinal bleeding: a possible association with ibuprofen. Lancet 1:541, 1972
12. Hollister LE: Hematemesis and melena complicating therapy with rauwolfia alkaloids. Arch Intern Med 99:218, 1957
13. Johnson LR: Pepsin secretion during damage by ethanol and salicylic acid. Gastroenterology 62:412, 1972
14. Lee ER, Dagradi AE: Hemorrhagic erosive gastritis. Am J Gastroenterol 63:201, 1975
15. Lee P, McCusher S, Allison A, et al: Adverse reactions in patients with rheumatic diseases. Ann Rheum Dis 32:565, 1973
16. Lehtola J, Sipponen P: A gastroscopic and histological double-blind study of the effects of diclofenac sodium and naproxen on the human gastric mucosa. Scand J Rheumatol 6:97, 1977
17. Leonards JR, Levy G: Gastrointestinal blood loss from aspirin and sodium salicylate tablets in man. Clin Pharmacol Ther 14:62, 1973
18. Levy M: Aspirin use in patients with major upper gastrointestinal bleeding and peptic ulcer disease. N Engl J Med 290:1158, 1974
19. Lippman W: Inhibition of indomethacin-induced gastric ulceration in the rat by perorally administered synthetic and natural prostaglandins. Prostaglandins 7:1, 1974
20. McKusick VA: Hereditable Disorders of Connective Tissue (ed 4). St. Louis, C.V. Mosby, 1972, p 292, p 498
21. Mielke CH Jr: Aspirin as an antiplatelet agent: template bleeding time as a monitor of therapy. Am J Clin Pathol 59:236, 1973
22. Needham CD, Kyle J, Jones PF, et al: Aspirin and alcohol in gastrointestinal hemorrhage. Gut 12:819, 1971
23. Robert A, Nezamis JE, Lancaster C, et al: Cytoprotection by prostaglandins in rats. Gastroenterology 77:433, 1979

24. Scott JT, Porter IH, Lewis SM, et al: Studies of gastrointestinal bleeding caused by corticosteroids, salicylates and other analgesics. Q J Med 30:167, 1961
25. Slone D, Jick H, Lewis GP, et al: Intravenously-given ethacrynic acid and gastrointestinal bleeding. JAMA 209:1668, 1969

Index

Abdominal organs, examination of, prior to surgery, 138
Acetylsalicylic acid (ASA; aspirin), 156, 407–409
Acidity control in treatment of bleeding ulcers, 118–123
   stress ulcers, 175–177
Acute gastric erosions, *see* Erosive gastritis
Acute gastric mucosal hemorrhages, diagnosing, 54
Acute gastric mucosal lesions, surgery for, 142–143
Adenomatous polyps in bleeding infants and children, 18
Age, surgery and
   decision to operate, 8, 9
   peptic ulcer surgery, 84–85
Air contrast barium enemas for chronic bleeding, 30, 31, 35
Air contrast gastrointestinal series for chronic bleeding, 30, 32, 35
Anal fissure in bleeding infants and children, 14, 16
Anatomy
   of gastroesophageal varices, 278–280
   and intestinal ischemias, 390–392
   and portosystemic shunts, 319–320
Aneurysms, *see* Splanchnic artery aneurysms
Angiography, *see* Diagnostic angiography; Therapeutic angiography
Antacids, acidity reduction with, 121–122

Anticoagulants, bleeding associated with, 410–411
Anticholinergic drugs, acidity reduction with, 120–121
Antiinflammatory agents, bleeding associated with, 409
Argon laser photocoagulation, 192–193
Arterial embolization
   selective
     complications of, 226
     in control of lower gastrointestinal hemorrhages, 225
     in control of upper gastrointestinal hemorrhages, 205–211
     superior mesenteric, 393–395
Arterial flow, hepatic, vasopressin action on, 266
Arterial thrombosis, superior mesenteric, 395–397
Arteriovenous malformations
   in bleeding infants, 18–19
   diagnosing lower gastrointestinal hemorrhages due to, 66–67
ASA (acetylsalicylic acid; aspirin), 156, 407–409
Associated conditions
   of chronic blood loss, 25–29
     bleeding diathesis, 26, 27
     colitis, 26, 29
     colonic cancer, 26, 27
     colonic polyps, 26, 27
     drugs, 25–26; *see also* Drug-related bleeding

419

Associated conditions *(continued)*
  gastric cancer, esophagitis, gastritis
    and asymptomatic peptic ulcer,
    26, 28
  genetic disorders, 26–27
  miscellaneous lesions, 26, 28–29
  vascular malformations, 26–28
  and decision to operate, 9–11
Asymptomatic peptic ulcers associated
  with chronic bleeding, 26, 28

Balloon catheters
  esophageal variceal bleeding treated
    with, 292
  upper gastrointestinal hemorrhages
    controlled with, 211–212
Balloon tamponade
  gastroesophageal, variceal bleeding
    controlled with, 275–293
  results of esophageal, in cirrhotic
    patients, 299
Barium enemas, air contrast, 30, 31, 35
Bipolar electrocoagulation, 198–199
Bismuth compounds, acidity control with,
    123–124
Bleeding adults, 3–12
  abstract on, 3–4
  decision to operate on, 8–11
  estimating rate of bleeding in, 7–8
  history of, 4–5
  laboratory tests for, 5–6
  monitoring, 7
  physical examination of, 5
  radiology and endoscopy for, 6–7
Bleeding diathesis
  chronic bleeding and, 26, 27
  and rebleeding after surgery, 152
Bleeding infants and children, 13–22
  abstract on, 13
  causes of rectal bleeding in, 15
  general considerations on, 13–14
  management of, 21–22
  specific conditions affecting, 14–21
    anal fissure, 14, 16
    duplications, 16
    esophageal varices, 20–21
    intussusception, 16
    lymphoid nodular hyperplasia, 18

Meckel's diverticulum, 16
miscellaneous, 18–19
peptic ulcer, 19–20
polyps, 17–18
Bleeding peptic ulcers, 81–93
  abstract on, 81–82
  diagnosing upper gastrointestinal
    hemorrhages due to, 54
  in infants and children, 19–20
  management of, 89–90, 95–112
    abstract on, 95–96
    approaches and technique, 106–109
    the hemorrhage, 105–106
    medical, *see* Medical management, of
      bleeding peptic ulcers
    nature of disease and, 96–104
    the patient, 104–105
    the ulcer, 106
    See also Electrocoagulation;
      Photocoagulation; Therapeutic
      angiography
  potential prospective studies on, 89
  rebleeding, *see* Rebleeding, peptic ulcers
    and
  and tenets of ulcer bleeding, 84–88
  See also Upper gastrointestinal bleeding
Bleeding site(s)
  importance of finding, in chronic
    bleeding, 25
  multiple, and rebleeding after surgery,
    149
  surgery with no external evidence of,
    138–139
Bowel
  inflammatory disease of, 67
  small bowel x-ray, 30, 32

Carcinomas, *see* Neoplasms
Cardiovascular hemodynamics, portal
  hypertension and, 244–248
Carcinoembryonic antigens for chronic
  bleeding, 33–34
Catastrophic hemorrhages, and decision to
  operate, 8
Celiac artery aneurysms, 346
Chronic bleeding, 23–38
  abstract on, 23–24
  conditions associated with, 25–29

bleeding diathesis, 26, 27
colitis, 26, 29
colonic cancer, 26, 27
colonic polyps, 26, 27
drugs, 25-26, *see also* Drug-related bleeding
gastric cancer, esophagitis, gastritis and asymptomatic peptic ulcer, 26, 28
genetic disorders, 26-27
miscellaneous lesions, 26, 28-29
vascular malformations, 26-28
and decision to operate, 11
diagnosis of, 29-36
approach to, 34-36
methods of, 29-34
importance of finding source of, 25
lesions not associated with, 29
presentation of, 24-25
Chronic duodenal ulcers, surgery for, 141-142
Chronic gastric ulcers, surgery for, 140-141
Cirrhotic patients
with gastrointestinal bleeding, prognosis in, 233
See also Elective portosystemic shunts; Portacaval shunts; Portal hypertension
Coagulation abnormalities, *see* Hematologic disorders
Coagulation supplementation for stress ulcers, 177-178
Colic artery aneurysms, 351-352
Colitis associated with chronic ulcers, 26, 29
Colonic cancer
associated with chronic bleeding, 26, 27
diagnosing lower gastrointestinal bleeding due to, 67
Colonic diverticula, *see* Vascular ectasias
Colonic ischemias, iatrogenic, 401-402
Colonic lavage for chronic bleeding, 33
Colonic polyps associated with chronic bleeding, 26, 27
Colonic trauma, lower gastrointestinal bleeding due to, 73
Colonic vascular ectasias, *see* Right vascular ectasias
Colonoscopy, 47-48
for chronic bleeding, 30-32, 35

Combination therapy, acidity reduction with, 123
Complications
of diagnostic endoscopy, 44-46
of gastroesophageal variceal bleeding, 287-288
of selective arterial embolization, 226
of therapeutic angiography, 225-227
of transhepatic obliteration of gastroesophageal varices, 226-227
of vasopressin infusions for variceal bleeding, 266
Continuing (recurring) bleeding, and decision to operate, 9, 10
Contraindications, endoscopy, 44-46
Coronary vein embolization for variceal bleeding, 216-223
Cronkhite-Canada syndrome, 17

Diagnosis
of bleeding esophageal varices, 297-298
of bleeding due to immunosuppression, 336-337
of chronic bleeding, 29-36
approach to, 34-36
methods of, 29-34
and decision to operate, 9
of hematologic disorders associated with gastrointestinal bleeding, 411-413
of hemobilia, 342-343
incorrect, and rebleeding after surgery, 148
of vascular ectasias, 382-384
See also specific diagnostic methods; for example: Colonoscopy; Diagnostic angiography
Diagnostic angiography, 51-78
abstract on, 51-52
for chronic bleeding, 30, 33, 35
indications for, 52
for lower gastrointestinal hemorrhages, 64-76
technique used, 52-53
for upper gastrointestinal hemorrhages, 53-64
Diagnostic endoscopy, 39-50
abstract on, 39-40
for bleeding adults, 6-7

Diagnostic endoscopy *(continued)*
  determining mortality risk in patients with bleeding peptic ulcers with, 88
  lower, 46–48
  upper, 40–46
    accuracy of, 41–42
    causes of bleeding determined with, 43–44
    for chronic bleeding, 30, 33, 35
    complications and contraindications for, 44–46
    facilities and equipment for, 40
    technique, 41
    timing of, 42–43
    usefulness of, 46
Diverticula
  chronic blood loss not associated with, 29
  diagnosing lower gastrointestinal hemorrhages due to bleeding of, 65
  jejunal, 70
  See also Colonic diverticula; Meckel's diverticulum
Drug-related bleeding, 407–411
  chronic, 25–26
  history of drug ingestion and decision to operate, 9, 10
  See also Erosive gastritis
Drugs
  for bleeding stress ulcers, 175–181
  See also specific drugs
Duodenal ulcers
  chronic, surgery for, 141–142
  diagnosing lower gastrointestinal hemorrhages due to, 67, 69
Duplication in bleeding infants and children, 16

Ectasias, *see* Vascular ectasias
Elderly, the, lower gastrointestinal bleeding in, *see* Right colonic vascular ectasias; Vascular ectasias
Elective mesocaval shunts, 321–322
Elective portacaval shunts, 295–297, 320

Elective portosystemic shunts, 295–297, 311–326
  abstract on, 311
  anatomic and technical considerations in, 319–320
  history of, 311–314
  indications for, 314–317
  physiological considerations in selection for, 317–319
  results of, 320–323
Elective splenorenal shunt of Warren, results of, 322–323
Electrocoagulation, 194–199
  bipolar, 198–199
  in control of upper gastrointestinal hemorrhages, 212
  monopolar, 194–196
  for occlusion of bleeding vessels, 107
Electrofulguration, monopolar, 196–198
Embolization
  arterial, *see* Arterial embolization
  coronary vein, variceal bleeding control with, 216–223
  for occlusion of bleeding vessels, 107
Emergency portacaval shunts for bleeding esophageal varices, 295–310
  diagnosis of, 297–298
  general therapy measures, 298
  specific medical therapy, 298–300
  surgery, 300–307
Endoscopic hemostats for bleeding stress ulcers, 181–182
Endoscopy
  diagnostic, *see* Diagnostic endoscopy
  fiberoptic, 291–293
  interoperative, for acute gastric erosions and stress ulcers, 186–187
  intraoperative, prior to surgery, 137
  therapeutic, *see* Electrocoagulation; Photocoagulation
Enemas, air contrast barium, for chronic bleeding, 30, 31, 35
Erosive gastritis (acute gastric erosions)
  pathophysiology of, 155–158
  prevention and treatment of, 167–188
    abstract on, 167–171
    in actively bleeding patients, 172–173
    with interoperative endoscopy, 186–187
    nonoperative therapy for active bleeding, 181–184

INDEX

pharmacologic intervention for stress bleeding, 175–181
prophylaxis, 173–175
surgery for, 184–186
Esophageal balloon tamponade, results of, in cirrhotic patients with bleeding esophageal varices, 299
Esophageal variceal bleeding
emergency portacaval shunts for, 295–310
diagnosis, 297–298
general therapy measures, 298
specific medical therapy, 298–300
surgery, 300–307
in infants and children, 20–21
injections for, using fiberoptic endoscope, 291–293
Esophagitis associated with chronic bleeding, 26, 28

Fiberoptic endoscopy, esophageal variceal injections using, 291–293
Flexible fiberoptic sigmoidoscopy, 46–47
Fluorescin string tests for chronic bleeding, 34

Gastric artery aneurysms, 346–348
Gastric cancer associated with chronic bleeding, 26, 28
Gastric decompression for acute gastric erosions and stress ulcers, 175
Gastric erosions, *see* Erosive gastritis
Gastric lavage for bleeding ulcers, 115–116
stress ulcers, 181
Gastric mucosal barrier concept, 157–158
Gastric mucosal hemorrhages, acute, 54
Gastric mucosal lesions, surgery for acute, 142–143
Gastric ulcers, chronic, surgery for, 140–141
Gastritis
associated with chronic bleeding, 26, 28
See also Erosive gastritis
Gastroduodenal artery aneurysms, 348–350
Gastroenteritis, infectious, in bleeding infants and children, 19

Gastroepiploic artery aneurysms, 346–348
Gastroesophageal variceal bleeding
balloon tamponade in control of, 275–293
abstract on, 275
anatomy of varices and, 278–280
complications, 287–288
historical background to, 276–278
and physiology of variceal bleeding, 280–284
results, 286–287
technique, 284–286
complications of transhepatic obliteration of gastroesophageal varices, 226–227
coronary vein embolization for, 216–223
Gastrointestinal series, air contrast, for chronic bleeding, 30, 32, 35
Generalized juvenile polyposis, 17
Genetic disorders
associated with chronic bleeding, 26–27
hereditary juvenile polyposis, 17

Hemangiomas in bleeding infants and children, 18–19
Hematologic disorders, bleeding due to, 411–416
diagnosis of, 411–413
spectrum of disorders, 413–416
Hemobilia, 339–344
diagnosis of, 342–343
etiology of, 340–342
treatment of, 343
Hemodynamics
hemodynamic categorization of portacaval shunts, 318
hemodynamic effects of intraarterial vs. intravenous vasopressin, 266–268
of portal hypertension, 235–251
abstract on, 235–236
cardiovascular hemodynamics, 244–248
historical summary on, 236–237
pathogenesis and natural history of portal hypertension, 237–240
splanchnic hemodynamics, 240–244
Hemolytic-uremic syndrome, 19
Hemostats, endoscopic, for bleeding ulcers, 181–182

Henoch-Schonlein purpura, 19
Hepatic arterial flow, vasopressin action on, 266
Hepatic artery aneurysms, 350–351
Hepatic reserve, portacaval shunts, gastrointestinal hemorrhages and, 253–260
Hereditary juvenile polyposis, 17
Hernia, chronic blood loss not associated with hiatus, 29
Hypertension
  and decision to operate, 9
  See also Portal hypertension

Iatrogenic colonic ischemias, 401–402
Iatrogenic sepsis, prevention of, in treatment of acute erosive gastritis, 173–174
Identification of right colonic vascular ectasias, 359–361
Ileal artery aneurysms, 351–352
Immunosuppressed patients, bleeding in, 329–338
  abstract on, 329–330
  diagnosis and treatment of, 336–337
  etiology of, 330–333
  incidence of, and mortality in, 333–335
Indications
  diagnostic angiography, 52
  elective portosystemic shunts, 314–317
  surgery in case of type II hemorrhages, 133–134
Infectious gastroenteritis in bleeding infants and children, 19
Inflammatory bowel disease, gastrointestinal bleeding due to, 67
Interoperative endoscopy for acute gastric erosions and stress ulcers, 186–187
Intestinal ischemias, 389–406
  abstract on, 389–390
  clinical syndromes of, 393–402
    iatrogenic colonic ischemias, 401–402
    low flow nonocclusive ischemias, 397–400
    mesenteric venous thrombosis, 400
    superior mesenteric arterial embolization, 393–395
    superior mesenteric arterial thrombosis, 395–397
    vasculitis, 400–401
  physiologic and anatomic factors in, 390–392
Intestinal variceal bleeding, lower gastrointestinal hemorrhages due to, 73, 76
Intraarterial vasopressin
  for bleeding stress ulcers, 182
  in control of lower gastrointestinal hemorrhages, 223–225
  in control of upper gastrointestinal hemorrhages, 203–205
  hemodynamic effects of intravenous vs., 266–268
  selective, 262–264
Intragastric vasoconstrictors for bleeding ulcers, 116–117
Intraoperative endoscopy prior to surgery, 137
Intravenous vasopressin for variceal bleeding
  bleeding esophageal varices, 299, 300
  effects of infusions into varices, 268
  high doses of, 262–264
  hemodynamic effects of intraarterial vs., 266–268
Intussusception in bleeding infants and children, 16
Ischemias, *see* Intestinal ischemias

Jejunal artery aneurysms, 351–352
Jejunal diverticula, lower gastrointestinal bleeding due to, 70
Juvenile polyps, 17

Laboratory tests
  for bleeding adults, 5–6
  for chronic bleeding, 30, 35
Laparotomy for chronic bleeding, 34
Laser photocoagulation, 190–194

INDEX

Lavage
  colonic, for chronic bleeding, 33
  See also Gastric lavage
Lesions
  associated with chronic bleeding, 26, 28–29
  factors influencing formation of, in stress ulcers, 159–160
  mucosal, surgery for, 142–143
  not associated with chronic bleeding, 29
  See also Erosive gastritis
Ligations, transesophageal varix, 300–302
Liver, *see* Cirrhotic patients; *and entries beginning with terms:* hepatic, transhepatic
Low flow nonocclusive ischemias, 397–400
Lower gastrointestinal hemorrhages
  angiographic diagnosis of, 64–76
  endoscopic diagnosis of, 46–48
  therapeutic angiography for, 223–225
  vascular ectasias as cause of, 375–388
    abstract on, 375–376
    case studies of, 378–382
    clinical features of, 376–378
    diagnosis of, 382–384
    management of suspected hemorrhages, 384–386
    See also Right colonic vascular ectasias
Lymphoid nodular hyperplasia, 18

Malformations, *see* Arteriovenous malformations; Vascular malformations
Mallory-Weiss tears, upper gastrointestinal hemorrhages due to, 54
Management
  of bleeding infants and children, 21–22
  of common coagulation abnormalities, 415
  of gastrointestinal bleeding due to immunosuppression, 336–337
  of peptic ulcers, 89–90, 95–112
    abstract on, 95–96
    approaches and technique, 106–109
    of hemorrhages, 105–106
    medical, *see* Medical management, of bleeding peptic ulcers

  nature of disease and, 96–104
  the patient, 104–105
  the ulcer, 106
  See also Electrocoagulation; Photocoagulation; Therapeutic angiography
  of suspected lower gastrointestinal bleeding due to vascular ectasias, 384–386
  See also specific modes of management; for example: Drugs; Surgery
Marginal ulcers, upper gastrointestinal hemorrhages due to, 54
Meckel's diverticulum
  in infants and children, 16
  lower gastrointestinal hemorrhages due to, 69–70
Meckel's scans for chronic bleeding, 34
Medical management
  of bleeding esophageal varices, 298–300
  of bleeding peptic ulcers, 87–88, 113–128
    abstract on, 113–114
    initial therapy, 114–117
    new therapies, 123–124
    with reduction of gastric acidity, 118–123
Mesenteric arterial embolization, superior, 393–395
Mesenteric arterial thrombosis, superior, 395–397
Mesenteric artery aneurysms, superior, 354–355
Mesenteric venous thrombosis, 400
Mesocaval shunts, elective, 321–322
Milk drips, acidity reduction with, 122–123
Monitoring of bleeding adults, 7
Monopolar electrocoagulation, 194–196
Monopolar electrofulguration, 196–198
Morbidity, and bleeding peptic ulcers, 87
Mortality
  in cases of gastrointestinal hemorrhage due to immunosuppression, 333–335
  in patients with bleeding peptic ulcers, 87
    determining risk of, with endoscopy, 88
  from portacaval shunts, 316
  from variceal hemorrhages in cirrhotic patients, 296

Mucosal lesions, acute gastric, surgery for, 142–143
Multiple bleeding sites, and rebleeding after surgery, 149

Nasogastric aspirate for chronic bleeding, 30, 31, 35
Nd: YAG laser photocoagulation, 193–194
Neoplasms
    upper gastrointestinal hemorrhages due to, 55–56
    See also specific neoplasms; for example: Colonic cancer; Gastric cancer
New ulcers, as cause of rebleeding after surgery, 149–150
Nodular hyperplasia, lymphoid, 18
Nonocclusive ischemias, low flow, 397–400
Nontransplant immunosuppression, 335
Nutritional support for acute gastric erosions and stress ulcers, 174–175

Occlusion
    of bleeding vessels, 107
    See also Electrocoagulation; Embolization; Photocoagulation; Vasopressin infusions

Pain, and decision to operate, 9, 10
Pancreatic artery aneurysms, 348–350
Pancreaticoduodenal artery aneurysms, 348–350
Patient history
    bleeding adults, 4–5
    for chronic bleeding, 29–30
Patient selection for portosystemic shunts, 317–319
Peptic ulcers
    asymptomatic, chronic bleeding due to, 26, 28
    See also Bleeding peptic ulcers; Duodenal ulcers; Gastric ulcers; Marginal ulcers; Stress ulcers
Perforation, and decision to operate, 8
Peutz-Jeghers syndrome, 17
Pharmacologic action of vasopressin, 264–266
Pharmacology, see Drugs
Photocoagulation, 189–194
    for occlusion of bleeding vessels, 107
    laser, 190–194
Physical examination
    of abdominal organs prior to surgery, 138
    of bleeding adults, 5
    for chronic bleeding, 29–30, 35
Polyps
    in bleeding infants and children, 17–18
    colonic, associated with chronic bleeding, 26, 27
Portacaval shunts
    elective, results of, 320
    gastrointestinal hemorrhages, hepatic reserve and, 253–260
    hemodynamic categorization of, 318
    See also Emergency portacaval shunts
Portal hypertension, hemodynamics of, 235–251
    abstract on, 235–236
    cardiovascular hemodynamics, 244–248
    historical summary on, 236–237
    pathogensis and natural history of portal hypertension, 237–240
    splanchnic hemodynamics, 240–244
Portosystemic shunts, see Elective portosystemic shunts
Preoperative factors influencing survival in portacaval shunts, 304–307
Prevention of acute gastric erosions, see Erosive gastritis, prevention and treatment of
Primary operations, inadequate, and rebleeding after surgery, 150–152
Prognosis
    for cirrhotic patients with gastrointestinal hemorrhages, 233
    in patients with portal hypertension, 246
    See also Mortality; Survival
Prophylaxis
    for acute gastric erosions and stress ulcers, 173–175

INDEX

portosystemic shunts as, 295
Prostaglandins, acidity reduction with, 123
Psychological preparation for surgery, 137
Purpura, Henoch-Schonlein, 19

Radiology
  for bleeding adults, 6–7
  See also Diagnostic angiography;
    Fluoroscopy; Therapeutic
    angiography; X-rays
Rate of bleeding
  and decision to operate, 9
  estimating, in adults, 7–8
Reactionary hemorrhages, 147–148
Rebleeding
  and decision to operate, 9, 10
  from peptic ulcers
    increased risk of, with each bleeding
      episode, 85
    severity of initial bleeding and risk of,
      85–86
  after surgery, 147–153
  surgery to prevent, 86–87
H_2-receptor antagonists, acidity reduction
  with, 119–120, 123
Recurring (continuing) bleeding, and
  decision to operate, 9, 10
Right colonic vascular ectasias in the
  elderly, 359–374
  abstract on, 359
  gross identification of, 359–361
  histologic characteristics of, 361–370
  morphogenesis of, 371–373

Scanning for chronic bleeding, 34
Secondary hemorrhages, following surgery
  for bleeding ulcers, 147–148
Selective arterial embolization
  complications of, 226
  for control of lower gastrointestinal
    hemorrhages, 225
  for control of upper gastrointestinal
    hemorrhages, 207–211
Selective intraarterial vasopressin infusions
  for variceal bleeding, 262–264

Sepsis, prevention of iatrogenic, in
  treatment of acute erosive
  gastritis, 173–174
Sigmoidoscopy
  for chronic bleeding, 30, 31, 35
  flexible fiberoptic, 46–47
Small bowel x-rays for chronic bleeding,
  30, 32
Splanchnic artery aneurysms, 345–357
  abstract on, 345
  celiac artery aneurysms, 346
  gastric or gastroepiploic artery
    aneurysms, 346–348
  gastroduodenal, pancreaticoduodenal
    and pancreatic artery aneurysms,
    348–350
  hepatic artery aneurysms, 350–351
  jejunal, ileal and colic artery aneurysms,
    351–352
  splenic artery aneurysms, 352–354
  superior mesenteric artery aneurysms,
    354–355
Splanchnic hemodynamics in portal
  hypertension, 240–244
Splenic artery aneurysms, 352–354
Splenorenal shunts of Warren, results of
  elective, 322–323
Stress ulcers
  diagnosing upper gastrointestinal
    hemorrhages due to, 54
  hypothesis on, 158–162
  pathophysiology of, 158
  prevention and treatment of, 167–188
    abstract on, 167–171
    in actively bleeding patients,
      172–173
    with interoperative endoscopy,
      186–187
    nonoperative therapy for active
      bleeding, 181–184
    pharmacologic intervention, 175–181
    prophylaxis, 173–175
    recent experimental developments in,
      162–164
    surgery for, 142–143, 184–186
String tests, fluorescin, for chronic
  bleeding, 34
Superior mesenteric arterial embolization,
  393–395
Superior mesenteric arterial thrombosis,
  395–397

Superior mesenteric artery aneurysms, 354–355
Surgery
 for acute gastric erosions, 184–186
 for bleeding peptic ulcers, 86–87
  age and, 84–85
  rebleeding, *see* Rebleeding, from peptic ulcers
  decision to operate on adults, 8–11
 for lower gastrointestinal bleeding due to vascular ectasias, 385–386
 for stress ulcers, 142–143, 184–186
 for upper gastrointestinal hemorrhages, 129–145
  abstract on, 129–131
  management of type II hemorrhages, 132–134
  plan of operation, 137–139
  specific surgical therapies, 139–143
  transoperative approach to, 133–137
  when to operate, 131–132
 See also Elective portosystemic shunts; Portacaval shunts
Survival in portacaval shunts, preoperative factors influencing, 304–307
Systemic intravenous vasopressin for bleeding esophageal varices, 299, 300

Tamponade, *see* Balloon tamponade
Technetium-labeled injections, scanning for chronic bleeding following, 34
Tests
 fluorescin string, 34
 See also Laboratory tests
Therapeutic angiography, 203–230
 abstract on, 203–204
 complications of, 225–227
 for control of lower gastrointestinal hemorrhages, 223–225
 for control of upper gastrointestinal hemorrhages, 204–223
  with balloon catheters, 211–212
  with electrocoagulation, 212
  with intraarterial vasopressin, 204–205
  with selective arterial embolization, 207–211
  variceal bleeding controlled by coronary embolization, 216–223
Therapeutic endoscopy, *see* Electrocoagulation; Photocoagulation
Thrombosis
 mesenteric venous, 400
 superior mesenteric arterial, 395–397
Transesophageal varix ligation, 300–302
Transfusions
 for bleeding stress ulcers, 182–183
 decision to operate and difficulties with, 9, 10
Transhepatic obliteration of gastroesophageal varices, complications of, 226–227
Transplant immunosuppression, incidence of, and mortality due to gastrointestinal bleeding in cases of, 334
Trauma, colonic, diagnosing lower gastrointestinal hemorrhages due to, 73
Tumors
 presence of, and decision to operate, 9, 10
 See also Neoplasms
Type II upper gastrointestinal hemorrhages, surgery for, 132–134

Upper gastrointestinal bleeding
 angiographic diagnosis of, 53–64
 endoscopic diagnosis of, 40–46
  accuracy of, 41–42
  for chronic bleeding, 30, 33, 35
  complications and contraindications, 44–46
  determination of causes of bleeding with, 43–44
  facilities and equipment for, 40
  technique, 41
  timing of, 42–43
  usefulness of, 46
 surgery for, 129–145
  abstract on, 129–131

management of type II hemorrhages,
  132–134
plan of operation, 137–139
specific surgical therapies, 139–143
transoperative approach to, 133–137
when to operate, 131–132
therapeutic angiography for, 204–223
  with balloon catheters, 211–212
  with electrocoagulation, 212
  with intraarterial vasopressin
    infusions, 204–205
  with selective arterial embolization,
    207–211
  variceal bleeding controlled by
    coronary vein embolization,
    216–223
See also Bleeding peptic ulcers
Uremic-hemolytic syndrome, 19

Variceal bleeding
  lower gastrointestinal hemorrhages due
    to intestinal, 73, 76
  vasopressin in management of, 261–273
    abstract on, 261–262
    appraised, 268–270
    hemodynamic effects of intravenous
      vs. intraarterial vasopressin,
      266–268
    high dose intravenous, 262–264
    pharmacologic action of vasopressin,
      264–266
    selective intraarterial vasopressin
      infusions for, 262–264
  See also Esophageal variceal bleeding;
    Gastroesophageal variceal
    bleeding
Varices
  chronic bleeding not associated with, 29
  ligation of transesophageal, 300–302
  transhepatic obliteration of
    gastroesophageal, 226
Vascular ectasias, 375–378
  abstract on, 375–376
  case studies of, 378–382
  clinical features of, 376–378
  diagnosis of, 382–384
  and management of suspected lower
    gastrointestinal hemorrhages,
    384–386
  See also Right colonic vascular ectasias
Vascular malformations associated with
  chronic bleeding, 26–28
Vasculitis, 400–401
Vasoconstrictors, intragastric, for bleeding
  ulcers, 116–117
Vasopressors, occlusion of bleeding
  vessels with, 107
Vasopressin infusions
  complications of, 225–226
  intraarterial
    for bleeding stress ulcers, 182
    in control of lower gastrointestinal
      hemorrhages, 223–225
    in control of upper gastrointestinal
      hemorrhages, 204–205
    hemodynamic effects of intravenous
      vs., 266–268
    selective, 262–264
  intravenous, see Intravenous vasopressin
    for variceal bleeding
  in management of variceal hemorrhages,
    261–273
    abstract on, 261–262
    appraised, 268–270
    hemodynamic effects of intravenous
      vs. intraarterial vasopressin,
      266–268
    high dose intravenous, 262–264
    pharmacologic action of vasopressin,
      264–266
    selective intraarterial infusions,
      262–264
Venous thrombosis, mesenteric, 400

X-rays, small bowel, for chronic bleeding,
  30, 32